Applied Neurosciences for the Allied Health Professions

Commissioning Editor: Rita Demetriou-Swanwick
Development Editor: Veronika Watkins/Clive Hewat
Project Manager: Sruthi Viswam
Designer/Design Direction: Miles Hitchen
Illustration Manager: Jennifer Rose

Applied Neurosciences for the Allied Health Professions

Edited by

Douglas McBean BSc(Hons), PhD
Senior Lecturer in Physiology & Neuroscience, Queen Margaret University, Edinburgh, Scotland

Frederike van Wijck BSc, MSc, PhD, MCSP, FHEA
Reader in Neurological Rehabilitation, Glasgow Caledonian University, Glasgow, Scotland

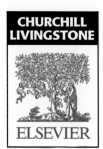

CHURCHILL
LIVINGSTONE

ELSEVIER

Edinburgh London New York Oxford Philadelphia St Louis Sydney Toronto 2013

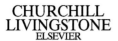

CHURCHILL
LIVINGSTONE
ELSEVIER

ISBN 978-0-7020-3028-4

British Library Cataloguing in Publication Data
A catalogue record for this book is available from the British Library

Library of Congress Cataloging in Publication Data
A catalog record for this book is available from the Library of Congress

Notices
Knowledge and best practice in this field are constantly changing. As new research and experience broaden our understanding, changes in research methods, professional practices, or medical treatment may become necessary.

Practitioners and researchers must always rely on their own experience and knowledge in evaluating and using any information, methods, compounds, or experiments described herein. In using such information or methods they should be mindful of their own safety and the safety of others, including parties for whom they have a professional responsibility.

With respect to any drug or pharmaceutical products identified, readers are advised to check the most current information provided (i) on procedures featured or (ii) by the manufacturer of each product to be administered, to verify the recommended dose or formula, the method and duration of administration, and contraindications. It is the responsibility of practitioners, relying on their own experience and knowledge of their patients, to make diagnoses, to determine dosages and the best treatment for each individual patient, and to take all appropriate safety precautions.

To the fullest extent of the law, neither the Publisher nor the authors, contributors, or editors, assume any liability for any injury and/or damage to persons or property as a matter of products liability, negligence or otherwise, or from any use or operation of any methods, products, instructions, or ideas contained in the material herein.

your source for books, journals and multimedia in the health sciences

www.elsevierhealth.com

Working together to grow
libraries in developing countries

www.elsevier.com | www.bookaid.org | www.sabre.org

ELSEVIER   BOOK AID International   Sabre Foundation

The
Publisher's
policy is to use
**paper manufactured
from sustainable forests**

Contents

Contributors

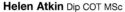

Helen Atkin Dip COT MSc
Advanced Occupational Therapy Research Fellow, School
of Health Community and Education Studies, Northumbria
University; Occupational Therapist, Walkergate Park,
Centre For Neurorehabilitation and Neuropsychiatry,
Newcastle upon Tyne, UK

Barbara J. Chandler BMedSci MBBS MD FRCP
Consultant Rehabilitation Medicine, NHS Highland,
Raigmore Hospital, Inverness, UK

Jan Gill BSc(Hons) PhD
Reader in Physiology, Queen Margaret University,
Edinburgh, UK

Helen Kelly BSc (Hons) PhD
Lecturer in Speech and Hearing Sciences, University
College Cork, Cork, Republic of Ireland

Chris Price MD
Clinical Senior Lecturer in Stroke Medicine, Newcastle
University, Newcastle upon Tyne, UK

Paulette van Vliet PhD
Professor of Stroke Rehabilitation, University of Newcastle,
Newcastle, Australia

Acknowledgement

With love and thanks to Mag, Paul, JohnJo and Frances.

Thanks also to Fred – a supportive colleague and friend along the journey.

Douglas McBean

With love to Chris, for his unfailing encouragement.

With thanks to Douglas, for his friendship, expertise and wit. Finally, our sincere thanks to all the students, patients and research participants we have had the privilege to work with over the years, for their inspiration and searching questions that have led us to writing this book.

Frederike van Wijck

Why this book?

Neurological rehabilitation is at the core of a range of allied health professions, including physiotherapy, occupational therapy, speech and language therapy, prosthetics and orthotics – to name but a few. Across the life span, people with neurological conditions require rehabilitation services; from children with cerebral palsy needing gait training following surgery, to young adults with traumatic brain injury, preparing for return to work, to older people coping with the impact of Parkinson's disease. With an aging population worldwide, it is increasingly important that rehabilitation be effective. For this to occur, it needs to be grounded in science.

Science offers the robust and systematic framework that aims to describe, explain and predict phenomena. As an allied health professional working in rehabilitation, you require science to describe and explain the phenomena you treat on a daily basis. You require science to generate hypotheses about which treatment would work best in a specific case. The scientific method is also required to establish the effectiveness of interventions, as evidence-based practice is the hallmark of the health professions.

Therapists working in neurological rehabilitation in particular need a sound understanding of neuroscience in order to provide effective, patient-centred interventions. You will require a good knowledge of the normal structure and function of the nervous system at the molecular, cellular, organ and system levels, as well as an understanding of the effects of neurological conditions on the patient as an individual. These conditions may not only impair posture, movement and activities of daily living, but also functions such as attention, perception, decision-making, planning, memory as well as communication, emotion and motivation, sleep and sexuality. During the rehabilitation process, patients often need to learn new skills or relearn skills they mastered previously. An important question is therefore how, as a therapist, you may optimise learning in neurological rehabilitation. To do so, you will require a good understanding of factors promoting and inhibiting functional recovery and learning, which include both pharmacological and behavioural interventions.

Having taught a module on applied neurosciences to undergraduate, pre-registration and postgraduate students for over a decade however, we have not been able to identify a single textbook that we think covers the required material in a comprehensive manner, and presents this at an accessible level that highlights the clinical relevance of the material. We have therefore written this book with the intention to fill this gap.

Aims of this book

The aim of this textbook is to provide undergraduate and pre-registration postgraduate students in a range of allied health professions with an accessible and comprehensive foundation in neurosciences to help them understand some of the most commonly found problems in neurological rehabilitation, and inform their clinical practice. Given the scope and depth of the field of "neurosciences", we have had to limit this text to what we felt would suffice as a foundation. As allied health professionals in neurological rehabilitation come across a wide range of complex issues, we felt it would probably be more useful to provide a general introduction to a range of topics. However, as a consequence it was not possible to do justice to more advanced or in-depth material, which can be found in numerous excellent textbooks and papers. For those who are interested in further literature, we have provided signposts to additional sources of information.

Content of this book: a bird's eye view

In people with neurological conditions (e.g. stroke, multiple sclerosis or cerebral palsy), problems may be complex and affect a range of different functions, e.g. mobility, communication and mood. Multidisciplinary team input is essential to ensure that rehabilitation meets the person's needs, and therefore this book covers a range of topics that will give you an insight into the impact of neurological conditions on a wide range of functions – and how these may be managed using both behavioural and pharmacological interventions. But first, the book will lay the foundation of basic neuroscience.

Chapters 1–8 will provide you with the required basic knowledge and understanding of the normal structure and function of the nervous system at different levels of analysis, i.e. from the organism as a whole, through to the molecular where this is appropriate. The following topics will be covered:

- Introduction to neuroscience
- Basic neuroanatomy and neurophysiology
- Lifespan changes in the nervous system (i.e. neurodevelopment and ageing)
- Introduction to pharmacology
- Introduction to the brain–behaviour relationship
- Motor control and learning.

Chapters 9–14 will then explore some of the most commonly found disorders you are likely to come across in neurological rehabilitation settings. Each of these will be described and explained, linking back to basic neurosciences described chapters 1–8. The text will refer to a range of management strategies for these disorders, covering both behavioural (e.g. physiotherapy, occupational therapy, and speech and language therapy) and pharmacotherapeutic interventions. Case studies will be used extensively to highlight the clinical relevance of the topics discussed, while self-assessment questions will be included for you to check your progress – and encourage you to consider how this material may inform your clinical practice. Topics discussed will include disorders of the following functions:

- Attention and memory (e.g. amnesias)
- Perceptuo-motor control (e.g. dyspraxia)
- Communication (e.g. aphasias)
- Executive function (e.g. executive dysfunction)
- Emotion and motivation (e.g. depression)

- Sexual function and continence
- Sleep
- Pain.

Finally, chapter 15 will synthesise key points from this book, highlighting the relevance for allied health professionals working in rehabilitation, and summarise current principles underpinning best practice. It will also look to the future by identifying gaps in evidence-based practice and suggesting ideas for future research, as well as explore what the future of rehabilitation may have in store.

How to use this book

Each chapter will open by indicating the aims for the section, in order to focus your attention on key points to be addressed. The main text comprises core material, and definitions of key concepts will be provided throughout each chapter.

A variety of supplementary information boxes point you towards additional information:

- Case Studies will highlight clinical relevance of the material.
- Research boxes will stimulate (we hope!) your interest in more advanced material and/or original research studies.

Suggestions for further reading are included at the end for the real enthusiasts!

As students are expected to vary in their background knowledge regarding this topic, we have organised the material in such a way that general neuroscience and key concepts are introduced in Chapters 1–8. Those already familiar with this material may wish to use it as a refresher, or move straight onto the more problem-orientated material in Chapters 9–14.

An introduction to neuroscience

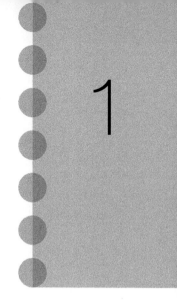

CHAPTER CONTENTS

LEARNING OUTCOMES

At the end of this chapter, you should be able to:

- identify the key players involved in the birth of 'neuroscience' and subsequent development to where we are now
- indicate the different levels of analysis that can be used to investigate neuroscience
- discuss some of the different methodologies that can be used to study the functional activity within the brain
- discuss the advantages and disadvantages of the aforementioned imaging techniques.

Welcome to applied neuroscience

As soon as people hear the term 'neuroscience' they think 'Okay ... this is going to be difficult'. This is probably, in part, due to the fact that we are all aware that there is probably more that we do not know about the brain and the nervous system than we do know. The aim of this book is to make neuroscience understandable and useful to allied health professionals working in neurological rehabilitation.

So what is neuroscience all about – and how does it inform clinical practice?

Neuroscience refers to the scientific investigation of the nervous system in all its aspects. Although the brain has fascinated us for hundreds and hundreds of years, the actual term 'neuroscience' is relatively new. In fact the Society for Neuroscience was only founded in 1970! Before we go on to the specifics, let us ask ourselves exactly what we already know about the brain. How about some apparently simple questions:

- How much does it weigh?
- What percentage of the total amount of oxygen does it use in rest?
- What is the smallest working unit – how many?
- Does it change after reaching adulthood?
- What happens when it gets damaged?

It is hoped that you will be able to find the answers to these questions and more as we work our way through this book together.

Why would allied health professionals (AHPs) need to study neuroscience? A large proportion of people requiring support from AHPs are those with injury, disease or degeneration of the nervous system (e.g. stroke, multiple sclerosis, head injury, motor neurone disease). For example, the incidence of stroke in the United Kingdom is 150 000 per year (UK Department of Health figures from 2005) and 52% of stroke survivors return home with lasting disability (Wolfe 2000). In the UK, 300 000 people live with stroke-related disability at any one time (Adamson et al., 2004).

Given nervous system pathology, the main challenge for AHPs is how to provide effective intervention, aimed at optimising function, autonomy and quality of life. It is this that requires the knowledge of each aspect of neuroscience. Problems encountered in patients may include:

- reduced control of movement *(e.g. incoordination)*
- difficulty with functional tasks *(e.g. dyspraxia)*
- altered sensation and perception *(e.g. hemianopia)*
- impaired attention and memory *(e.g. neglect)*
- impaired speech and language *(e.g. dysphasia)*
- altered motivation and emotion *(e.g. depression)*.

Let us start with a simple, everyday concept about the nervous system, but one that is central to rehabilitation – damage and recovery. We can probably all think of examples of how the nervous system is able to recover following trauma, e.g. the stroke patient with an initial loss of motor and speech function who recovers some degree of function through therapy; or the person with a brain tumour who following surgery relearns how to plan and manage his time by working with a clinical psychologist; or the child with cerebral palsy who learns to use his bicycle. So what can we learn from examples such as these? Firstly, the brain is adaptable insofar as it is able to show neuroplasticity, i.e. there is leeway or spare material and/or different ways of something being done. Think of the brain as a lump of plasticine which has been shaped into a bowl. The bowl of plasticine can be broken up, remodelled and turned into a different bowl. Two different ways of using the material, but both performing the same task.

Underneath these examples lies the assumption that our ability to move, communicate, think and plan are all governed by the brain. Although we now take this notion for granted, this was not always the case! So before we study the nervous system in more detail, we invite you to go back in history, to appreciate how our current understanding of the brain and its relationship with behaviour, thinking and emotion evolved from the work of some of the giants in the field.

The history

Now for a concise history of the study of the nervous system, starting back in the days of the Greek and Roman Empires.

Hippocrates (c. 460–377 BC), widely regarded as the 'Father of Western Medicine', was a Greek physician who instituted a shift in the thinking and practice in medicine. Before Hippocrates, religion was the accepted paradigm to describe, explain and predict events – and doctors were in fact priests, whom patients would seek in temples for religious healing through prayer and purification. Under the influence of Hippocrates, medicine moved away from religion and towards the use of nature to diagnose, explain and treat illness. Doctors were trained as physicians – students of nature – and they practised a craft instead of religious rituals. In contrast to his predecessors, who believed that the heart was the centre for the soul and control of the body, Hippocrates believed that the mind was in the brain and controlled the body, but that it was something intangible. Hippocrates was uniquely different from his contemporaries in that he believed that disease and head injuries, not demons and evil spirits, caused madness and affected coordination. Hippocrates was prolific and wrote an impressive body of work, known together as the Corpus Hippocraticum, comprising treatment manuals, speeches, notes and books. One important point to make here is that there is no evidence that Hippocrates and his physicians ever dissected a human – or in fact any organism. At the time of Hippocrates, the Greeks believed that interfering with the human body after death was tantamount to sacrilege, while many Greeks were also believers in reincarnation. So it is not entirely clear on what evidence the Hippocratic Corpus was based.

Plato (428–348 BC), a Greek philosopher, agreed with Hippocrates in believing that the mind was in the head. However, he also believed that the mind and the body were separate, and that we reach the truth not via our senses but through our thoughts, i.e. by logic and reasoning. In other words, the senses cannot be trusted.

Aristotle (384–322 BC) was both Plato's student and rival – anyone know that feeling! Aristotle was a keen dissector, who studied the anatomy of almost 50 species. In contrast to Plato, Aristotle felt that he could trust his senses. From his observations that the heart moved and was filled with blood, and that it felt warm, he deduced that this organ was vital to life – the heart was 'the acropolis of the body' (Finger 2000). In contrast, the brain looked still and bloodless, and he deduced from this that the brain must act as a cooling system for the heart! So Aristotle's model was that the heart was the seat of our emotions. He also argued that the mind and the brain were one, and that the mind was entirely physical – in other words, we can only understand the mind by studying the body.

Remember that, so far, human autopsy was not allowed in the Golden Age of Greece, due to religious beliefs. However, after Hippocrates' death, much changed in Greek society, and Alexandria in Egypt had developed itself into one of the great places for academic study, of which medicine was one.

Human dissection was led by **Herophilus of Chalcedon** and **Erasistratus**, around 300 BC. Erasistratus was also the first to notice and comment on the fact that the human brain had many more wrinkles in comparison to the animal, which he equated to a greater 'brain power'. However, this was an opinion, which was later questioned by Galen.

Galen (AD 129–199) was a Graeco-Roman physician to the gladiators and is widely regarded as the founder of experimental physiology. Like Aristotle, Galen felt that the truth is only conveyed through the senses, but unlike any of his predecessors, he took systematic observation and dissection to a new height. Thereby, he introduced a paradigm shift in medicine and transformed it into an applied science. Galen's interest in understanding how the body works may have been inspired by his father, who was an architect, and Galen diligently dissected animals in an attempt to reveal their internal structure. However, he did not perform human autopsies, as the Roman religious and legal systems did not permit this. His knowledge and understanding of human anatomy and physiology were most likely based on his observations of wounded gladiators – of which there appeared to be plenty. In contrast to Aristotle, however, Galen noted that the brain did not feel cool, and that nerves went to the brain – not the heart. He could, therefore, not accept Aristotle's model of the brain as a 'radiator'. By additionally noting that the cerebrum felt softer compared to the cerebellum, Galen postulated that the former was the seat of sensation, while the latter was the commander of muscles. Although this model would inevitably be considered rather crude and simplistic today, an element of truth remains, albeit based on a different rationale. So far, so good. However, Galen also postulated a physiological model of the brain, which was based on hydraulics. He thought that nerves were hollow, and that body fluids (the cerebrospinal fluid or CSF) moved between nerves and ventricles (the cavities within the brain). Moreover, Galen believed that the CSF was the psychic fluid (the fluid of the mind) and when he discovered the ventricles, where the CSF collects, he believed that he had found the seat of the mind. Clearly,

although Galen was a brilliant anatomist, his model of the physiology of the nervous system was deeply flawed. However, his theories would not be challenged for centuries.

It is then safe to say that we had a bit of a gap, of about 1300 years, which takes us through the Middle Ages – a time of intellectual darkness and untested beliefs in the absence of any experimentation – a time when Galen's ideas became dogma. Interest in research began to gather some pace again with the Renaissance in the 14th century.

Andreas Vesalius (1514–1564), was a rather adventurous Flemish anatomist, who took considerable risk by illegally removing cadavers from cemeteries and collecting recently deceased bodies from the gallows, in order to study their anatomy. He carefully noted his observations and compiled the beautifully crafted *De humanis corporis fabrica* (on the workings of the human body), a groundbreaking publication of 663 pages long, produced at the tender age of 28 years (Vesalius, 1543). Vesalius worked as a member of the academic faculty in Padua, where people from all over the world came to observe his anatomical lessons. Gradually, Vesalius realised that many of the statements made by Galen could not be supported by his own observations. It took him a while to realise the reasons for these discrepancies; Galen had only ever performed dissections on animals! Vesalius' contribution to medical science was, therefore, the introduction of a *human* anatomy. Finally, Vesalius also discredited Aristotle's idea that the mind, and the seat of our feelings, was in the heart – he insisted that it was in the brain. He must have been quite insistent as no one has since doubted his assertion!

As we saw above, human autopsies were generally not accepted in Vesalius' time and the University of Padua was an exception. It required another paradigm shift for society to accept the practice of opening the human body after death – which eventually came from an unexpected source.

The French philosopher, **René Descartes** (1596–1650) sought certainty in his understanding of natural phenomena. He believed that, to this purpose, one required domains of 'pure' knowledge that could not be doubted. To Descartes, these were geometry and motion. According to Descartes' world view, everything could be understood in terms of mathematics, even the human body. The clock – a recent invention at the time – served as a new metaphor for the human body. (In fact, at the time of Descartes, society was infatuated with mechanical puppets and animated fountains, which would entertain the public by simulating motion.) By seeking to describe and explain natural phenomena only in terms of mathematics, Descartes reduced the complexity of these phenomena – an example of reductionism. According to this way of thinking, as long as the body is in good working order, a person should be healthy (a view still quite apparent in some branches of Western medicine today). However, there was one fundamental problem with this model; Descartes was also deeply religious and could not accept that all there was to a human was just machinery! Furthermore, what would distinguish a human from an animal? He therefore postulated another entity: the mind. The mind was everything that the body was not, i.e. not mechanistic, immaterial, conscious, non-spatial, and – most importantly – immortal. By postulating the two mutually exclusive entities of body and mind, Cartesian dualism was introduced. (In fact, Descartes perpetuated Plato's mind–body dualism by asserting that the human body and the senses were entirely mechanical and material, but the mind was something else.) By taking on Descartes' view that the mind and the body were completely different entities, and that the mind would survive death, society came to accept the ethics of opening the body after death; it was no longer sacrilege. Thus, by setting in motion a fundamental shift in thinking, Descartes' philosophy eventually opened the doors to human dissection.

However, by postulating two different entities, Descartes had also created a new problem for himself: how do the body and the mind interact if they have nothing in common? Descartes tried to solve his problem by postulating that the seat of the non-material mind was the pineal gland. It does not take long to realise that this was an entirely unsatisfactory solution to the mind–brain problem. This book is not the place to go into this problem fully, but it is worth pointing out that it still persists in society today; we use terms such as 'psychosomatic disorders' to denote problems for which we have no physical explanation and instead postulate a non-mechanistic cause. Other terms, such as 'mental health' indicate how deeply rooted Cartesian dualism is in Western society today.

Opposition to Cartesian dualism has been offered ever since by various philosophers. **John Locke** (1632–1704) was a British philosopher who put forward the idea that the mind and the body were two aspects of the same unified phenomenon, i.e. the mind needs the body to gain experience through the senses and the body needs the mind to store and use this experience. This argument, supported by fascinating case studies from neurological rehabilitation, is brilliantly presented in Damasio's book entitled *Descartes' Error* (1994).

Although neuroanatomy had made significant advances by the 17th century, there was no generally accepted theory on how the nervous system actually worked. Some scientists proposed that nerve conduction occurred through animal spirits being transported through hollow nerves, others thought that fluids leaking onto muscle tissue sparked contraction, whilst others again thought that vibration caused the transmission of information. However, none of these theories were deemed satisfactory. Crucially, Anton van Leeuwenhoek who invented the microscope, was unable to confirm that nerves were in fact hollow – a fundamental requirement for the animal spirit theory. The proposition that the nervous system could be working on the principle of electricity began to be considered instead. Electrotherapy was gaining popularity for the treatment of all sorts of ailments, and experimentation with this electricity was widespread.

Luigi Galvani (1737–1798) is one of the names associated with what was to become the new discipline of neurophysiology. A physician and scientist, Galvani undertook much of his work at home. Unhindered by ethical considerations imposed on research today, he experimented with frogs and other animals, as well as people. Serendipitously, he discovered that muscle contractions in frog legs could be triggered by electricity.

Galvani systematically experimented with electricity and muscle contraction, culminating in his famous treatise in 1791. His assistant Aldini then developed a technique whereby brain stimulation could evoke muscle contractions (e.g. eye openings) in the heads of fresh victims of the guillotine (just imagine…). Together, these experiments gave rise to a new theory that the nervous system worked on the principle of electricity.

Up until this time, scientists thought that the outer layer of the brain (the 'bark', or cortex in Latin) was an amorphous substance without specialised functions. However, **Franz Gall** (1758–1828) had different ideas. Gall was a German physician who postulated that there was a relationship between the metrics of one's cranium – which in turn would be reflected in the measurements of one's brain – and those of one's faculties, and he was responsible for the pseudo-science of phrenology (the science of mind). Phrenology supported the idea that personality and the relative development of different parts of the brain could be read from the pattern of bumps on the skull. Gall, and his pupil Spurzheim, caused a storm with their public sessions, in which people could have their skulls measured and their personalities determined. However, they faced fierce opposition and by 1840 phrenology as a science ceased to exist. However, Gall and Spurzheim made some interesting contributions; one was that they introduced the idea of 'functional localisation' in neuroscience; the idea that different parts of the brain play a specific role in human behaviour. Their other contribution was that they used a form of measurement to substantiate their claims, i.e. cranioscopy. However, theirs was pseudo-science, with many faculties being poorly defined (e.g. 'sense of metaphysics' or 'poetic talent') – and what about the assumption that the dimensions of the cranium are reflected in the dimensions of the brain? On Descartes, who had a noteworthy skull with a rather low forehead, Spurzheim commented that 'Descartes was not so great a thinker as he was held to be'! (Finger 2000).

But a threat was on the horizon, with the French physiologist, *Pierre Flourens* (1794–1867) having been requested to put phrenology to the test. To this effect, Flourens carried out a series of ablation experiments, meaning that he destroyed parts of the brain (mainly in pigeons) and observed the resultant deficits. According to Flourens, his results indicated that no one function could be localised in a particular part of the brain (but remember this was in pigeons after all). This episode was the actual start of the whole localisation of function debate.

This debate was advanced significantly by *Paul Broca* (1824–1880); a French surgeon who was one of the first modern brain surgeons. Broca was carrying out an autopsy on a patient who had had an abscess on the brain and had lost the ability to speak. The lesion he found was localised in the 3rd frontal convolution of the left hemisphere (Finger 2000). Broca, through his careful examination of this case study, firmly established a link between a particular area of the brain and a particular ability. You can imagine he had to work hard to convince his audience; Gall had also proposed a speech area, but at a different location in the frontal lobe. The difference was that Broca had clear neurological evidence of a lesion. Broca's area is now universally recognised as the motor-speech area of the brain.

More support for the functional organisation of the cortex was found in the work of *Wilder Penfield* (1891–1976), a neurosurgeon who specialised in the treatment of epilepsy. Surgical interventions for epilepsy are usually a last resort, but if a patient's health and safety are severely compromised, surgical destruction of the brain area causing the 'electrical storms' may be indicated. Naturally, it is essential that healthy brain tissue is spared. The way the surgeon would determine which tissue was functioning normally was by... talking to the patient during the operation. As the brain itself has no pain sensors, patients only required local anaesthetic. Penfield would carefully stimulate areas of the brain and note the patient's responses. These would come in the forms of movement, sensations or experiences. By systematically noting his observations, Penfield was able to compile a detailed map of brain areas in relation to the behaviours or sensations associated with them. These maps are known as the 'homunculus' (Latin for 'little man'), of which there is a motor and sensory version – the sensory version can be seen in Figure 1.1. These maps are still widely used in textbooks today. In chapter 5, we will discuss these maps in more detail, and consider the impact of experience and learning.

By the 19th century, much progress had been made in gross neuroanatomy and in neurophysiology, but the smallest functional unit of the nervous system had not yet been identified. Technological

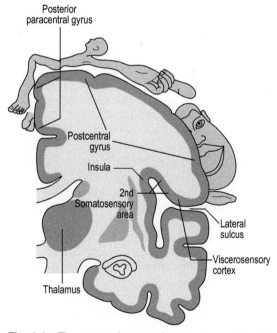

Fig. 1.1 • The sensory homunculus. From Haines, D.E. (2005) *Fundamental Neuroscience for Basic & Clinical Applications* (3rd ed), with permission

developments that facilitated this were microscopy and histological staining techniques. It was **Santiago Ramón-y-Cajal** (1852–1934) who discovered the neurone in 1891 (although this was not his term). Together with Golgi, who developed the stain that Cajal used under his microscope, they were given the Nobel Prize in 1906 for their contributions to neuroanatomy.

An enthusiastic supporter of the so-called neurone doctrine was **Charles Sherrington** (1857–1952), pathologist and neurophysiologist, who left a remarkable legacy for neuroscientists and clinicians alike. Sherrington dedicated an extraordinarily productive life to the examination of the nervous system, and was particularly interested in how individual neurones were integrated to produce complex actions. He introduced the term synapse (from the Greek synapsis, meaning 'to clasp') in 1897 – without the necessary technology to actually observe the inter-neuronal gap. Sherrington proposed the important idea that complex coordinated actions (e.g. stepping, scratching, shaking) were produced by integrated basic reflex actions – a process he called 'chaining'. Thus, using excitatory and inhibitory mechanisms at the synapses, complex behaviours could be configured from simple, automatic actions. Most of Sherrington's work took place in the laboratory, often using decerebrated animals (i.e. a cut is made through the midbrain of an anaesthetised animal). Sherrington was the first to describe the components of the now ubiquitously known knee-jerk reflex, and described the mechanism of reciprocal innervation. He also discovered the mechanism for 'proprioception' or 'kinesthesia', and mapped dermatomes. The metaphor of the brain that he used was that of a telephone exchange – a centre for the integration of higher functions – and with this theory, he entered the still unresolved domain of the mind–body problem towards the end of his career, for which he also could not provide a satisfactory answer. In 1932, he was honored with the Nobel Prize for his work, which had influenced medicine the world over. For example, in the context of rehabilitation, his ideas were fundamental to the Bobaths, who devised an approach for assessing and treating children and adults with neurological conditions that – albeit in modernised form – is still used today.

So far, this overview has looked at a selected group of giants in their fields, and considered their contributions to neuroscience. Clearly, this synopsis does not do justice to all the important discoveries in this field, and we, therefore, recommend *Minds Behind*

the Brain: A History of the Pioneers and their Discoveries (Finger 2000) if you are interested in reading more about this fascinating part of our history.

So what does history teach us? Mainly that the study of the brain has been a bumpy ride, with radical shifts in thinking, long spells of inactivity and the co-existence of opposing views. The study of the brain has been influenced strongly by both religious beliefs and technological developments. Contemporary technologies have often provided metaphors to enable scientists to think about this most complex organ in the universe (e.g. the clock, telephone exchange or, as we will see in chapter 7, the computer). One important learning point that arose at various times in the history of neuroscience is *the necessity of observation and experimentation* – without these, science becomes dogma and discoveries and progress are stifled.

Neuroscience today

The story continues, with models in neuroscience often confined to a particular level of analysis. At the molecular level, we may be interested to find out how botulinum toxin affects spasticity in children with cerebral palsy. At the cellular level, we might be interested to understand how neurones are affected in degenerative conditions such as multiple sclerosis. At the organ level – which, in the case of the nervous system would be identical to the system level – medical specialists might wish to study the effects of brain cooling on brain function after injury. At the cognitive level, psychologists might wish to study memory function in people with Alzheimer's disease – and how this changes following music therapy, for example. Similarly, the effects of neuropsychological interventions on challenging behaviour following brain injury might be examined.

In the following section, we will bring ourselves up to date with the ways in which we have enhanced our understanding of how the brain operates.

For each level of analysis indicated above, there are specific tools for the purpose of examination and outcome assessment. For example, cell recording and staining are used at the cellular level (remember Cajal, who discovered the neurone using staining techniques). At the system level, brain imaging might be used to record changes in brain structure and activity (more about this is to follow). At the cognitive level, specific neuropsychological tests to examine attention and memory, thinking and planning might be utilised. To study at the behavioural level, a range of options are available, including naturalistic observation, surveys and questionnaires, interviews and performance measurements.

Significant advances have been made in recent years in the area of brain imaging, which is used increasingly in routine clinical practice. From the section below, we would like you to understand which techniques there are, what information they obtain, why they might be used, and what their main strengths and limitations are. This field is developing fast, but you should have at least a basic knowledge and understanding of the most commonly used techniques today.

Functional imaging of the brain

As functional imaging techniques have developed over the years, they have become more and more associated with experiments trying to identify which regions of the brain are linked with specific sensory, motor and cognitive functions. When trying to identify which is the most appropriate imaging technique to use, it is important to consider the resolving power, or **resolution**. There are two aspects of the resolution that need to be considered, namely spatial and temporal, and there is a great deal of discussion as to which of these is the more important. The answer to that question is probably that which one is best is very much dependent on what is being measured:

- The *spatial resolution* is how far apart two discrete brain areas have to be before the image can show them as two separate areas. The smaller the spatial resolution value is, the better the information relating to localised brain activity will be.
- The *temporal resolution* is the timescale over which measurements can be made. If the functional change to be measured is happening over a very quick timescale then the temporal resolution of the technique being used would have to be low in order to catch the event.

Direct imaging techniques

As we have learned from the work by Galvani and others the brain is essentially an electrical device, so, ideally, we would want a technique that could directly measure the electrical activity, e.g. EEG

(electroencephalography). Some of the earliest attempts to measure such activity directly involved what could be perceived as the very simple process of attaching electrodes to the scalp. It should be noted, however, that in order for these surface electrodes to measure the electrical activity of the brain, the technique was dependent on the electrical activity passing, or 'leaking' through the meningeal layers, the bone of the skull and the skin of the scalp. One drawback to this technique is the fact that the bone of the skull acts as an electrical insulator, so the only way for the current to 'leak' from the tissue itself to the surface is via the sutures and small holes in the bone. The first recorded EEG was carried out by the German neuropsychiatrist, Hans Berger in 1924. With his two electrode set-up (two silver wires inserted into the scalp at the front and back of the head) he was able to record α-rhythms (8–13 Hz). Berger was also the first person to note that the EEG could be altered or distorted by various diseases, including epilepsy (see Fig. 1.2). EEG technology has advanced over the years to such an extent that the simple two electrode set-up of Berger has been replaced by a geodesic sensor net which can contain up to 256 separate electrodes, evenly spaced out over the surface of the skull. Net systems such as this allow high-resolution EEG recording, however, the cost of such a system can be in the region of tens of thousands of pounds. The cost is important given the obvious limitations of the technique, i.e. measurements restricted to brain surface and the currents are 'leaking' through the skull.

Indirect techniques

Indirect techniques include positron emission tomography (PET) and functional magnetic resonance imaging (fMRI), both of which rely on the ability to detect changes in local brain metabolism, i.e. which substances does the brain require to sustain it? These metabolic changes include:

- changes in blood flow to an area
- changes in O_2 content of the blood
- changes in brain cell glucose metabolism.

Positron emission tomography

The basic concepts underlying PET were first discussed in the 1950s, however the major developments with the technology have taken place since the 1970s. PET was one of the first true functional

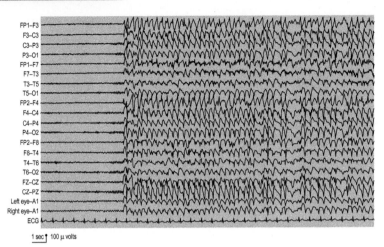

Fig. 1.2 • Rapid generalised epileptiform spikes and slow waves following a few seconds of a normal EEG. Recorded on a 30-year-old woman who walked in for follow-up of her epilepsy. She was confused but ambulatory and able to speak. From Drislane, F.W. (2000) with permission of Academic Press

imaging techniques. There is still a great deal of on-going debate regarding the exact nature of the link between the local metabolic change being detected by PET and the actual neuronal activity in the area. The rationale for there being a link is the fact that there will be an increase in metabolic activity in those areas of the brain that are more functionally active, i.e. those with increased neuronal activity. However, one should still not ignore the fact that PET does not directly monitor brain function.

PET works using one of a number of radioactive tracers labelled with ^{13}N, ^{15}O, and ^{18}F, which can be either injected or inhaled – the route being dependent on the parent molecule, e.g. radiolabelled water ($H_2{}^{15}O$) is commonly used in studies based on blood flow and would be injected. The techniques used for administration of the compounds result in them being present in the brain within about 60 seconds or so. As these molecules radioactively decay, they emit positrons. The emission of the positrons is followed by the subsequent emission of gamma (γ)-rays and it is this process that underlies the construction of the PET image.

We shall now consider what could be seen as a typical PET procedure. The radiolabelled water ($H_2{}^{15}O$) would be injected and, after a few minutes to allow for the tracer to reach the brain, a baseline image would be recorded. After the baseline had been established, the patient (or participant) would then be subjected to some form of procedure or stimulation. The PET scanner would then be used to record a post-stimulus image. The computer then simply subtracts the baseline reading from the stimulated image – the result being that those areas activated by the stimulus are 'highlighted' on the image. The

PET scanner therefore works on the simple premise that the areas which are more active will be exposed to, and as a result take up more of, the tracer. These more active areas will then experience more positron decay, hence the increase in the recorded image.

Before deciding which imaging technique is the most appropriate one to use, it is important to identify the advantages and disadvantages associated with the technique. Although the dose used is relatively low and safe, one cannot ignore the fact that PET does involve the administration of a radioisotope and, due to the fact that the measured signal can be quite low, a number of repeat scans may be required. One way to avoid the repeat administration of radioisotope to an individual is to carry out the procedure on a number of different people, however, that will remove the possibility of looking at brain activation on an individual basis. As stated above, one must also consider the resolution of the technique and this can be where PET falls down in some ways. As it has a temporal resolution of about 40 seconds, and this is affected by the half-life of the isotope being used, it can take a few minutes to obtain both the resting and stimulated images. If you think that an action potential only lasts for a few milliseconds, you can see that this level of temporal resolution does not allow for rapid detection. Coupled with this poor level of temporal resolution, PET has what is considered to be a moderate level of spatial resolution of around 5 mm. A level of spatial resolution of this magnitude is what is responsible for the – currently – rather 'blurred' images seen with PET. Another factor to consider when assessing the practicality of PET is the fact that a supply of radioisotopes is required and that a number of the isotopes are short-lived, e.g. $H_2{}^{15}O$ has a half-life of only 2 minutes. With a half-life as short as this, a local cyclotron is required to produce the radioisotope, and this must be accompanied by suitable facilities to handle the isotope.

Functional magnetic resonance imaging

A major advantage of fMRI, compared to PET, is that it does not require the administration of ionising radiation. The procedure does, however, require the person to be placed in a very strong magnetic field of 1.5 to 3 T (tesla) which is almost 50 000 to 100 000 times stronger than the Earth's magnetic field at the equator (3.1×10^{-5} T). A magnetic field of this intensity is necessary in order to affect the nuclei of the hydrogen atoms in the body. Despite being in such a strong magnetic field the patient is not aware of the 'pull' on their hydrogen atoms!

When you start to think of the molecules that make up the human body it becomes easy to appreciate that hydrogen atoms are widespread (water, fat, protein) and, from our perspective, are abundant in the brain. It is the abundance of hydrogen, coupled with the fact that it contains protons with a property known as nuclear spin, that make it play an important part in fMRI. It is the proton which is found in the nucleus of the hydrogen atom that exhibits the property of 'nuclear spin', i.e. the proton is a charged sphere spinning on its own axis, generating its own little magnetic field. One way to think of the proton is that it is like a little bar magnet. All of these little 'bar magnets' in our body are randomly orientated; however, when the patient is placed into the large magnetic field of the MRI scanner they align either against the field or along the field – the 'equilibrium situation'. This equilibrium situation can be disturbed by the application of electromagnetic radiation (radiofrequency region 40–100 MHz) so that there is a change between the two states. The exact frequency depends on the size of the magnetic field. The disturbance caused by applying the radiofrequency radiation can be monitored. A signal with an intensity linked to the number of proton nuclei that are disturbed can be calculated at a suitable frequency. The scanner can be set up so that different parts of the brain are subjected to different magnetic fields, with each part of the brain responding to a different frequency. As a result, signals from different parts of the brain will be discernible from each other.

As you will already be aware, O_2 is transported round the bloodstream in the form of oxyhaemoglobin (oxy-Hb). When oxy-Hb gives up its O_2, the resulting deoxy-Hb is carried on in the red cells. The oxy- and deoxy- forms of haemoglobin have different magnetic properties, with deoxy-Hb being paramagnetic and oxy-Hb being diamagnetic. Diamagnetic molecules will create their own little magnetic field when exposed to an external magnetic field which is contradictory to the field, and this will create a repulsive effect. Paramagnetic molecules, on the other hand, are magnetic in the presence of an external magnetic field, with a strength directly proportionate to the field applied. When an area of the brain becomes more active there should be an increase in flow to the area, with an increase in oxy-Hb (and a resultant decrease in deoxy-Hb). This change in the ratio of paramagnetic to diamagnetic molecules will produce less distortion in the overall magnetic field – the tissue appears brighter. This is known as the **B**lood **O**xygenation **L**evel-**D**ependent Contrast, or BOLD contrast.

Unlike PET scans, where multiple subjects may need to be used, one advantage of MRI is that single subjects can be used. This is a result of the better detection levels of fMRI. A second advantage that fMRI has over PET is that multiple scans can be carried out on a patient, if required, as no radioactive tracer administration is necessary. As fast scan rates can be achieved, fMRI is considered to have a better temporal resolution than PET. MRI scanners can scan every 3 seconds with a spatial resolution of 2–3 mm (possibly even 1 mm in certain circumstances). Further advantages are the fact that it is non-invasive and the cost is relatively low. It is for these reasons that fMRI is the most popular of these functional imaging techniques.

In summary, the neuroscientist has a range of different tools in his 'toolkit'. Neuroimaging techniques, which have developed rapidly over the last few decades, can be divided into those that convey the structure, and those that convey the activity of the brain. In some cases, technologies can be combined to convey both. Neuroimaging has made a tremendous contribution to our understanding of the impact of injury and illness, ageing and degeneration on the brain, the relation between the brain, behaviour and emotion, as well as the response of the brain to behavioural and pharmacological interventions. However, it is important to understand the limitations of these techniques, most commonly spatial and temporal resolution, although these keep improving all the time. Additionally, most devices require the person to be absolutely motionless, as motion artefacts (even swallowing in some cases) can confound the results.

For some populations (e.g. young children, people in pain, or those who experience anxiety or confusion), neuroimaging may not be feasible for those reasons.

Now that we have given a brief overview of key discoveries in the history of brain research, coupled with some basic information on modern investigative neuroimaging techniques, we can move forward to our study of the wider field. Before we get into the 'meat' of neuroscience, let us begin with a look at the 'bones' of some fundamental neuroanatomy and neurophysiology in Chapter 2.

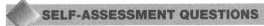

SELF-ASSESSMENT QUESTIONS

1. Highlight the key methodological differences between fMRI and PET.
2. Indicate the main advantages and disadvantages of fMRI and PET.
3. Is there any rationale for considering that one of these techniques (fMRI and PET) is safer than the other?

Further reading

BNA, 2003. Neuroscience: Science of the Brain – An introduction for young students. The British Neuroscience Association, UK.

Gross, C.G., 2009. A Hole in the Head: More tales in the history of neuroscience. MIT Press, USA.

Mulert, C., Lemieux, L., 2009. EEG – fMRI: Physiological basis, technique, and applications. Springer, New York.

Paulsen, J.S., 2009. Functional imaging in Huntingdon's disease. Exp. Neurol. 216, 272–277.

Piccini, P., Whone, A., 2004. Functional brain imaging in the differential diagnosis of Parkinson's disease. Lancet Neurol. 3, 284–290.

Posner, M.I., Raichle, M.E., 1994. Images of Mind. Scientific American Library, New York.

Sacks, O., 1985. The Man Who Mistook his Wife for a Hat and other clinical tales. Picador, London.

References

Adamson, J., Beswick, A., Ebrahim, S., 2004. Is stroke the most common cause of disability? J. Stroke Cerebrovasc. Dis. 13 (4), 171–177.

Damasio, A., 1994. Descartes' Error. Emotion, reason and the human brain. Penguin Books, New York.

Drislane, F.W., 2000. Presentation, evaluation, and treatment of nonconvulsive status epilepticus.

Epilepsy Behav. 1: 301–314. Academic Press.

Finger, S., 2000. Minds Behind the Brain: A history of the pioneers and their discoveries. Oxford University Press, New York.

Haines, D.E., 2005. Fundamental Neuroscience for Basic and Clinical Applications, third ed. Churchill Livingstone, UK.

Vesalius, A., 1543. Andreae Vesalii Bruxellensis, scholae medicorum Patauinae professoris, de Humani corporis fabrica Libri septem. (Andreas Vesalius of Brussels, professor at the school of medicine at Padua, on the fabric of the Human body in seven Books).

Wolfe, C.D., 2000. The impact of stroke. Br. Med. Bull. 56 (2), 275–286.

Basic neuroanatomy and neurophysiology

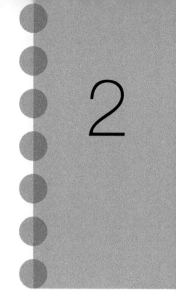

LEARNING OUTCOMES

At the end of this chapter you should be able to:

- identify the major subdivisions of the brain and the key brain areas contained within them
- identify the names and key functions of the 12 cranial nerves
- describe the structure of both the neurone and the synapse
- describe the events taking place during an action potential, with particular emphasis on the movement of sodium and potassium ions.

Introduction

When trying to navigate around the complexities of the human nervous system, it is always a much less daunting prospect if you have a good map.

Before we go on and look at the workings of the nervous system in the rest of the book, it is important that we find our bearings. The simplest way to subdivide the human nervous system is into central and peripheral sections. This, and subsequent divisions, can be seen in Figure 2.1.

As we advance through this book we shall deal with various areas of the brain and it is important that you have a clear understanding of at least the simplest level of brain anatomy. The three primary brain regions (forebrain, midbrain and hindbrain) can be further sub-divided as shown in Table 2.1.

In order to fully appreciate the orientation of the brain it is often useful to imagine a sagittal section through the brain from front to back. This results in a view of the inner and cortical surfaces, as seen in Figure 2.2.

The forebrain

The **telencephalon** comprises the majority of the two cerebral hemispheres that make up the cerebrum. The top, visible surface of the cerebral hemispheres is the cerebral cortex which sits on top of the sub-cortical structures of the limbic system and the basal ganglia. The name cortex derives from the Latin word for the bark of a tree. The **cerebral cortex** is about 3 mm thick, covers the two hemispheres of the brain and has a ridged surface comprised of grooves (sulci) and peaks (gyri). The larger grooves that can be seen on the cortical surface are the fissures. This groove/peak structure significantly increases the surface area of the cortex, taking it up to approximately $0.25\,\text{m}^2$ $(2500\,\text{cm}^2)$. The cortex can be further

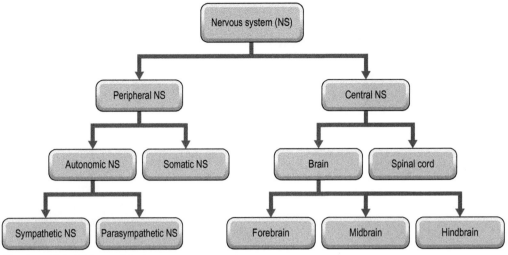

Fig. 2.1 • Subdivisions of the human nervous system

Table 2.1 Anatomical subdivisions of the brain		
Forebrain	Telencephalon	Cerebral cortex Basal ganglia Limbic system
	Diencephalon	Thalamus Hypothalamus
Midbrain	Mesencephalon	Tectum Tegmentum
Hindbrain	Metencephalon	Cerebellum Pons
	Myelencephalon	Medulla

subdivided into four lobes: frontal, occipital, parietal and temporal (Fig. 2.3) and the location of cortical structures are often identified in relation to the various lobes.

Limbic system

In 1937 the American neuroanatomist, James Papez, proposed the concept of a group of interconnected brain structures which linked up to form a circuit controlling both motivation and emotion. However, it was over 10 years before Paul McLean coined the term 'limbic', from the Latin word *limbus* meaning border or edge. The most notable structures of the limbic system are the hippocampus and the amygdala, which are involved in memory function and fear, respectively.

Basal ganglia

The basal ganglia are a collection of subcortical nuclei consisting of the caudate nucleus, the putamen, the nucleus accumbens, the substantia nigra and the globus pallidus. The primary function of these interconnected nuclei is an involvement in the control of movement. A better understanding of the role played by the basal ganglia can be achieved when there is a degeneration of specific neurones in the midbrain that project to the caudate and the putamen (i.e. the nigrostriatal dopaminergic pathway). This form of degeneration results in Parkinson's disease (PD), the symptoms of which include limb rigidity, poor balance, muscle weakness, tremor and a difficulty in initiating movements. Chapter 6 will explain the function of the basal ganglia in more depth.

Diencephalon

The diencephalon is the second major division of the forebrain and contains the hypothalamus and thalamus. The **thalamus**, which gets its name from the Greek word *thalamos* (or inner chamber), consists of two lobes divided into a number of nuclei, including the lateral geniculate nucleus (LGN) and the medial geniculate nucleus (MGN). The LGN is part of the visual pathway and processes neuronal impulses coming from the retina at the back of the eye and forwards it on in the direction of the visual cortex. The MGN, however, is involved in the processing

Fig. 2.2 • Sagittal section of the brain. From
Drake et al., (2004) with permission

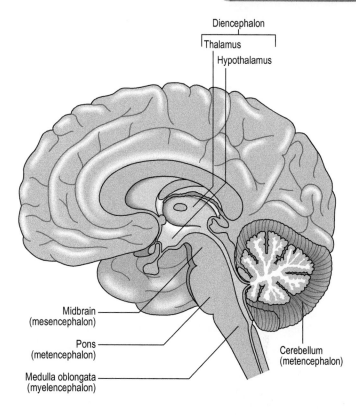

Diencephalon

Thalamus

Hypothalamus

Midbrain
(mesencephalon)

Pons
(metencephalon)

Medulla oblongata
(myelencephalon)

Cerebellum
(metencephalon)

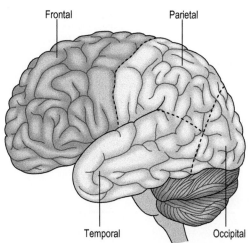

Frontal

Parietal

Temporal

Occipital

Fig. 2.3 • External appearance of the brain, showing the
lobes. From Kindlen (2003) with permission from Elsevier

of information from the cerebellum and passing it on
to the primary motor cortex.

The **hypothalamus**, which sits just under the
thalamus, although relatively small, is no less important. Its major function is to control the autonomic
nervous system and the endocrine (hormone) system,
which it does via the HPA (hypothalamus–pituitary–
adrenal) axis. As a result of this link, the hypothalamus is able to organise behaviours relating
to the survival of the species, i.e. fighting, feeding,
fleeing and mating.

The midbrain (mesencephalon)

The major structures of the **tectum** appear as four
bumps on the brain stem (the corpora quadragemina
or four bodies). The two **superior colliculi** are
involved in the processing of visual information, with
the two **inferior colliculi** involved in auditory processing. In some ways it makes good sense to have
brain areas processing auditory and visual information located so close together, when you think of
how often we use auditory and visual information
in conjunction with each other. The **tegmentum**
sits beneath the tectum and consists of a portion of
the reticular formation, several nuclei controlling
eye movements, the red nucleus, the substantia nigra
and the ventral tegmental area.

The **reticular formation** (RF), from the Latin *reticulum*, diminutive *rete*, meaning net, is a complex

13

network of over 90 nuclei receiving sensory information via various pathways and projecting on to the cerebral cortex, thalamus and spinal cord. As a result of this complex afferent processing role the RF is able to play a key role in sleep, arousal, attention, muscle tone and movement, as well as a variety of vital reflexes.

A cluster of axons originating in the **red nucleus** form one of the two major fibre tracts that process motor information received from the cerebral cortex and cerebellum and forward it on to the spinal cord. The **substantia nigra** is the starting point for the aforementioned nigrostrial neurones that project to the caudate and the putamen of the basal ganglia (see earlier mention of PD in this chapter).

Hindbrain

The hindbrain is split into two major parts: the metencephalon and myelencephalon. The **metencephalon** contains the pons and the cerebellum. The **cerebellum** (or 'little brain') is involved in the control of coordinated movements. This key role for the cerebellum becomes much more apparent when it is damaged, with the resultant impairment of walking, standing and coordinated movements, including speech. The cerebellum receives a large amount of sensory information from the visual, auditory, vestibular and somatosensory pathways, along with input about individual muscle movements being directed by the brain. Simply put, the cerebellum integrates and modifies motor outflow. The **pons** (or 'bridge') contains yet another portion of the reticular formation, including more nuclei involved in sleep and arousal. It also contains a large nucleus relaying information from the cerebral cortex to the cerebellum.

The myelencephalon contains one very important structure, the medulla oblongata ('oblong marrow') containing the nuclei involved in the control of vital functions, i.e. the regulation of the cardiovascular system, respiration and skeletal muscle tone.

Cranial nerves

The cranial nerves are nerves that emerge directly from the brain, rather than from a segment of the spinal cord. The cranial nerves are involved in a number of different processes (see Table 2.2). The fibres in the cranial nerves are either afferent (i.e. carrying information to the brain) or efferent (i.e. carrying

Table 2.2 The cranial nerves

Number	Name	Function(s)
I	Olfactory	Smell
II	Optic	Vision
III	Oculomotor	Eye movement Control of pupil size through PNS
IV	Trochlear	Eye movement
V	Trigeminal	Touch to the face Pain Jaw muscle movement
VI	Abducens	Eye movement
VII	Facial	Taste Facial muscle control
VIII	Auditory	Hearing Balance
IX	Glossopharyngeal	Taste Control of muscles of throat and larynx
X	Vagus	Internal organs (via parasympathetic NS) Control of pain associated with the viscera
XI	Spinal accessory	Neck and throat muscles
XII	Hypoglossal	Tongue movement

information from the brain). It is possible for the same cranial nerve to contain both afferent and efferent fibres (e.g. cranial nerve V, the trigeminal).

The neurone

We will revisit many of the brain areas mentioned above during the course of this book to gain a deeper understanding of the various roles that they play. Having laid down a few landmarks to help us navigate our way through the complex heterogeneous organ that is the brain, we now need to turn our attention to how the various parts communicate with each other. In order to fully appreciate the intricate workings of the nervous system (both central and peripheral) we have to go right back to basics and discuss the structure and function of the basic unit, i.e. the neurone. Neurones (or nerve cells) contain the exact same cellular organelles as the other cell types in the body. What makes them different from the other cells, however, is the projection that is the axon (Fig. 2.4).

Neurones can be considered to be the wiring system of the body, allowing complex information to pass quickly over relatively long distances. The electrical signals are supplemented by the release of chemical neurotransmitters at the gaps (synapses) between the neurones in a pathway. There are a number of different neurotransmitters found in the body and we shall discuss the role played by quite a few as we make our way through the chapters of this book. Some examples that we shall discuss include acetylcholine, serotonin and dopamine. Neurotransmitters can be classified as either excitatory (stimulating the next neurone in a pathway to fire) or inhibitory (preventing the next neurone from firing). The ability to 'switch on' or 'switch off' neuronal firing gives a much greater level of control over the functions of the nervous system.

The synapse

The meeting point of two separate neurones in a pathway, where the signal is passed from the terminal of the first neurone on to the cell body of the second neurone, is known as the synapse. Rather than having the electrical signal jumping the gap between the two neurones, the terminal of the first (or presynaptic) neurone releases a neurotransmitter which acts on specific receptors on the cell body of the second (or postsynaptic) neurone. This conversion from electrical to chemical to electrical allows the signal to pass quickly and efficiently along the neuronal pathway. The synaptic connections start to form in the very early stages of foetal development and continue to form postnatally (see Chapter 3). Our ability to learn and develop new skills as we grow – even well into old age – is a direct consequence of synaptic development. A sound understanding of the workings of the synapse is crucial for understanding the effects of different types of drugs, which will be introduced in Chapter 4.

Human nervous system

Our nervous system contains approximately 10 billion neurones and 100–500 billion neuroglia. The neuroglia are the non-neuronal cells of the

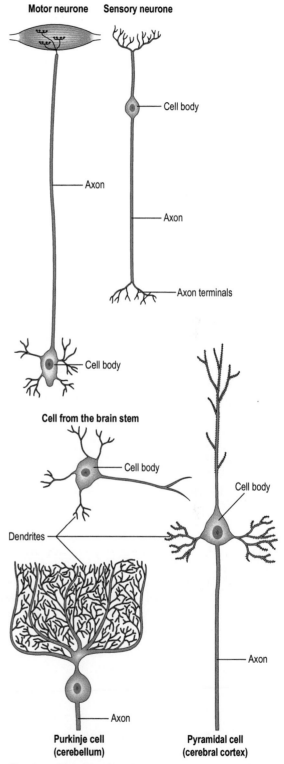

Fig. 2.4 • Examples of different types of neurones. From Kindlen (2003) with permission from Elsevier

nervous system and they are present to support the structure and the function of the neurones. There are four main types of neuroglia in the central nervous system (astrocytes, oligodendrocytes, ependymal cells and microglia) each with a distinct role in the system. The astrocytes regulate extracellular K^+ levels, aid with the formation of the blood–brain barrier and monitor neurotransmitter levels. The oligodendrocytes are the myelin-producing cells of the CNS. The ependymal cells line the ventricles of the brain and are responsible for the production of the cerebrospinal fluid (CSF). Finally, the microglia are the immune defence cells of the CNS.

Most neurones consist of three main parts (see Fig. 2.4): the cell body, the dendrites and the axon. The outer membrane of the **cell body** is the part of the neurone which is responsive to the neurotransmitter stimulus of the pre-synaptic neurone. It is the dendrites (the branch-like projections on the cell body; from the Greek word *Dendron* meaning 'tree') which receive the stimuli from the adjacent neurones. The dendrites also have the ability to respond to stimuli from the environment or the sensory organs. Neurones are connected to other neurones, forming neural networks which are often dedicated to specific functions. More about neural networks and the impact of injury and disease, as well as the effects of interventions, will be discussed later in the book.

In order for a signal to be processed along a neuronal pathway it is important that stimulus received by the cell body reaches the terminal, thereby allowing further release of a transmitter to act on the next neurones. It is the **axon** which carries the signal from cell body to neuronal terminal. In order to maintain fast transmission of the electrical signal down the axon, it important that the axon is well insulated, and this is achieved by coating the axon with **myelin**. The myelin is produced by the glial cells, namely **Schwann cells** in the periphery and **oligodendrocytes** centrally. To aid optimal transmission of the signal it is important that there are regular, small breaks or gaps in the myelination, known as nodes of Ranvier. These nodes promote the process of saltatory conduction.

The nerve impulse

In order for the nerve impulse to be generated and propagated there has to be a voltage difference across the neuronal membrane. This difference is known as the **membrane potential**. If you were to place a microelectrode inside the cell and a second one outside the cell when these were connected to a voltmeter, it would record a difference in the range of 5–100 mV. The net charge inside the cell is negative with respect to the outside of the cell, and it varies with the state the cell is in:

- Resting (resting potential)
- Active, excited state (action potential) where charge is reversed, and the inside is positive with respect to the outside.

When the neurone is at rest, the balance of ions is such that it creates a resting membrane potential of -70 mV, i.e. the inside of the cell is negative with respect to the outside. This potential comes about due to the uneven distribution of various anions and cations across the cell membrane, including Na^+, K^+, Ca^{2+}, Cl^- and HCO_3^-. The most important ions from the perspective of the nerve impulse are Na^+ and K^+ and the concentrations of these can be seen in Table 2.3.

Table 2.3 shows that there are 14 times more Na^+ ions outside cell than inside, and 37 times more K^+ ions inside cell than outside. This uneven distribution is brought about by the action of the membrane-situated Na^+/K^+ pump, moving two K^+ ions into the cell and three Na^+ ions out of the cell. The uneven distribution leads to concentration gradients across the membrane, which can be utilised to create the nerve impulse, or *action potential*.

Action potential

During an action potential the membrane potential changes from -70 mV (the resting membrane potential) to approximately $+30$ mV and back to -70 mV. This is brought about by the opening of Na^+ channels and the inflow of positive charge (Na^+), followed by the closure of the Na^+ channel, the opening of the K^+ channel and the resultant outflow of positive charge (K^+) (see Fig. 2.5, Box 2.1).

Table 2.3 Intra- and extracellular ionic concentrations at rest		
Anions	**Intracellular (mmol/l)**	**Extracellular (mmol/l)**
Na^+	10	140
K^+	150	4

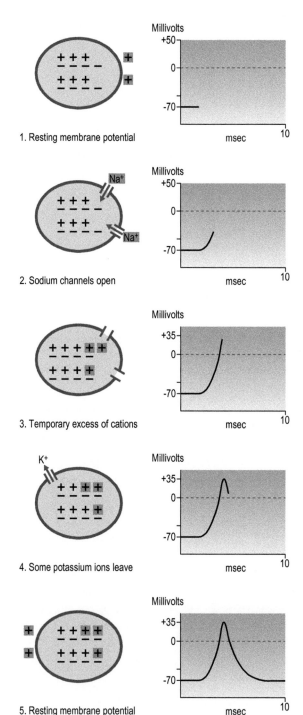

1. Resting membrane potential

2. Sodium channels open

3. Temporary excess of cations

4. Some potassium ions leave

5. Resting membrane potential

Fig. 2.5 • The action potential; ion channel opening and ionic movements. From Kindlen (2003) with permission from Elsevier

Local anaesthetics

Let us take you for a moment to the waiting room of your favourite dentist. As you wait nervously for your appointment time to come around do you ever wonder exactly how the magic pain-removing injection that you sometimes get actually works? The term local anaesthetic is very familiar to us and what we shall do in this section is link the mechanism of action of these agents to the nerve physiology covered thus far.

The concept of local anaesthesia use was brought to prominence by Dr W.S. Halsted in 1884, who utilised the anaesthetic properties of cocaine during various surgical procedures. Local anaesthetics are used to produce a reversible loss of sensation in a specific part of the body. They act by reducing the rate, and extent, of depolarisation of the cell membrane of those neurones that come into contact with the agent. This reduction comes about through the blockade of the sodium (Na^+) channels in the membrane by the local anaesthetic molecules. If the Na^+ channels are blocked then no Na^+ influx can occur, the threshold potential cannot be reached and the action potential cannot fire. Although they are referred to as local anaesthetics, the action of these agents is not restricted to the pain fibres, which explains the numbness and loss of movement that can be experienced.

Local anaesthetics are classified, according to their chemical structure, as either esters (e.g. novocaine, procaine, benzocaine) or amides (e.g. lidocaine, mepivacaine). Local anaesthetics are not only used for dental work and can, in fact, be administered in a variety of ways:

Topical	applied directly to surface
Infiltration	applied directly into the tissue
Nerve block	injected into, or near to, the nerve plexuses
Field block	injected to anaesthetise regions distal to the site of injection
Spinal	injected into the cerebrospinal fluid
Epidural	injected into the epidural space

Transmission of signals between neurones

When the action potential has travelled to the end of the axon, its arrival promotes the release of a chemical neurotransmitter. These neurotransmitters diffuse across the synapse and then excite or inhibit the next neurone. At an *excitatory* synapse the neurotransmitter depolarises the post-synaptic membrane (i.e. makes it more positive), the membrane potential moves closer to threshold, and, therefore, the post-synaptic neurone is more likely to fire. Conversely, at an *inhibitory* synapse the neurotransmitter hyperpolarises the post-synaptic membrane (i.e. makes it more negative), the membrane potential moves away from threshold), and the post-synaptic neurone is prevented from firing.

The neuromuscular junction

Although we have been talking about the brain and the associated afferent and efferent neuronal connections, there is one 'special' synapse that we should mention before we move on. In later chapters we shall discuss the motor systems within the body so it is, therefore, of the utmost importance that you understand the functioning of the skeletal neuromuscular junction. The skeletal neuromuscular junction is the specific type of synapse that is found between the terminal efferent neurone in a motor pathway and the designated muscle fibres (see Fig. 2.6). The junction is critical in the control of the musculoskeletal system.

When the action potential reaches the end of the efferent motor fibre, the neurotransmitter **acetylcholine** (ACh) is released. The ACh diffuses across the synapse and binds to nicotinic cholinergic receptors, resulting in the generation of an end-plate potential on the muscle fibre. As a result, the muscle fibre is brought to threshold and the spread of excitation produces a muscle action potential. The muscle action potential promotes the entry of calcium, the interaction of the troponin-tropomyosin complex and the contraction of the muscle. The

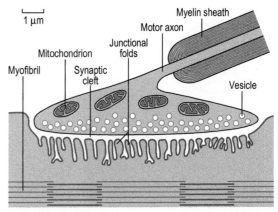

Fig. 2.6 • The neuromuscular junction. From Kindlen (2003) with permission from Elsevier

process of muscle contraction is explained further in Chapter 6.

SELF-ASSESSMENT QUESTIONS

1. What are the names and main functions of the cranial nerves?
2. What are the intracellular and extracellular concentrations of sodium and potassium ions when the neurone is at rest (i.e. not firing an action potential)?
3. What ionic changes/movements take place during the course of the action potential? Your answer should also indicate the relevant changes in the membrane potential.
4. Make a drawing of the neuromuscular junction.
5. From memory, draw an overview of the brain, and indicate each of the three primary regions and their key components.

Further reading

Diamond, M.C., Scheibel, A.B., Elson, L.M., 1985. The Human Brain Coloring Book (Coloring Concepts Series). Harper Collins, London.

Drake, R., Vogl, A.W., Mitchell, A.W.M., 2004. Gray's Anatomy for Students. Churchill Livingstone, UK.

Hughes, M., Miller, T., Briar, C., 2007. Crash Course: Nervous System, third ed. Mosby, UK.

Kindlen, S., 2003. Physiology for Health Care and Nursing. Churchill Livingstone, UK.

Lifespan changes in the nervous system

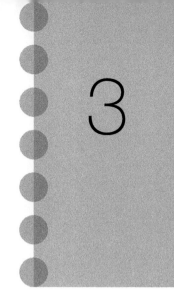

3

CHAPTER CONTENTS

LEARNING OUTCOMES

At the end of this chapter you should be able to:

- identify the key changes and time points in the process of neurulation
- explain what is meant by the term 'cell differentiation' and what is thought to influence this process in the early stages of neurodevelopment
- describe the cause of the condition known as spina bifida and outline the defects found in the three types of spina bifida: occulta, meningocoele and myelomenigocoele
- discuss the basic ideas behind some of the general theories of ageing
- highlight the main physiological, biochemical and pathological changes associated with ageing.

Introduction

Allied health professionals (AHPs) who work in rehabilitation encounter people across the lifespan; from babies with cerebral palsy, children with brain damage following meningitis, young adults with spinal cord lesions, to older people with Alzheimer's disease. AHPs need to have a sound understanding of the normal development and ageing of the nervous system in order to understand the impact of developmental disorders, injury, illness and degenerative conditions.

A significant amount of neuroscience is targeted at trying to gain further understanding as to how the system operates and what contribution is made by all of the component parts. There is much interest in both ends of the spectrum, i.e. the *in utero* development and the age-related deterioration of the system. It is hoped that by gaining a more detailed understanding of how the system developed at the beginning, we may gain further insight into what happens as the system starts to break down during the process of normal ageing, and vice versa. As a result of this interest this chapter will focus on the two extremes of lifespan changes – neurodevelopment and ageing of the nervous system.

Neurodevelopment

Approximately 12 hours after the moment of fertilisation of the female reproductive tract the zygote divides in two, followed by further divisions every

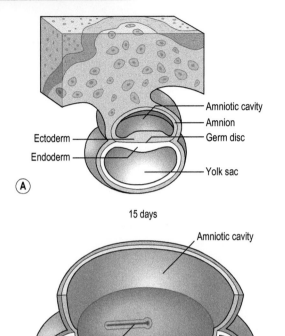

Fig. 3.1 • Embryonic day 15 (E15). With permission from the Open University

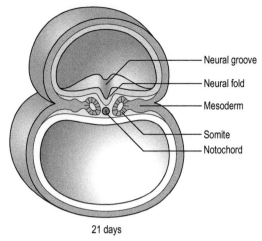

Fig. 3.2 • Embryonic day 21 (E21). With permission from the Open University

12 hours or so into four cells, then eight, etc. This process of division continues with little increase in size, until about day 7 when implantation of the embryo occurs. By embryonic day 15 (E15) the structures necessary to sustain the embryo are in place, i.e. the placenta, amniotic cavity and yolk sac (see Fig. 3.1).

At this stage the embryo is a flat germ disc comprising two layers of cells known as the endoderm (from the Greek words *endo* and *derma*, meaning *inner skin*) and the ectoderm (from the Greek for *outer skin*). At about E15 these two layers begin to separate and form a cavity between them into which ectodermal cells flow to create the mesoderm (*middle skin*).

Neurulation

Around day 22 the process of neurulation begins roughly halfway along the neural plate and in the early stages of the process the cranial and caudal ends stay open. The process then spreads along the groove with

the cranial neuropore closing around day 25 and the closure of the caudal neuropore taking place around day 27. The closure in both directions occurs in a segmented way and this segmental arrangement is retained in the spinal cord (see Figs 3.2, 3.3 and 3.4).

The cells just above the neural tube form the neural crest and these cells will migrate from the neural tube to form the neurones and glia of the sensory and sympathetic ganglia, the neurosecretory cells of the adrenal gland and the enteric nervous system (a subdivision of the peripheral nervous system controlling the gastrointestinal system).

Embryology of the spinal cord

The spinal cord develops from the part of neural tube caudal to the 4th pair of somites (paired blocks of mesoderm) segmentally arranged on either side of the neural groove. After neurulation, the lateral walls of the tube thicken and are covered by neuroepithelium, which will ultimately form the neurones and glia of the spinal cord. The cells form two plates on each side:

• the anterior **basal** plate
• the posterior **alar** plate

and these plates are separated by a shallow groove known as the sulcans limitans.

By week 10 the lumen of the neural tube starts to form a small central canal. It is at this point that the alar plate cells develop into the ascending projection neurones and interneurones that will subsequently

22 days

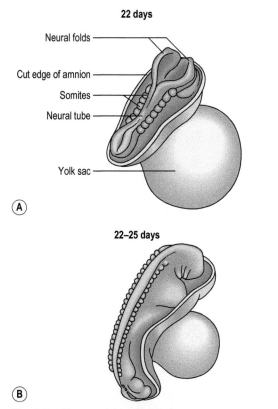

Neural folds

Cut edge of amnion

Somites

Neural tube

Yolk sac

(A)

22–25 days

(B)

Fig. 3.3 • Closure of the neural tube. With permission from the Open University

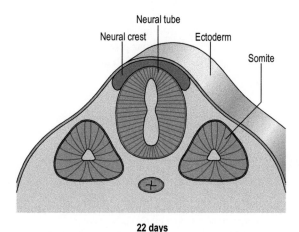

Neural tube

Neural crest   Ectoderm

Somite

22 days

Fig. 3.4 • Embryology of the spinal cord. With permission from the Open University

form sensory pathways and reflex circuits. Simultaneously, the basal plate cells differentiate into the motor neurones and interneurones that will transmit information out of the spinal cord down to the muscles (i.e. the descending projection neurones). The cells

in the thoracic segment develop into the sympathetic preganglionic neurones, while the cells in the sacral segment develop into the parasympathetic preganglionic neurones – thereby forming both parts of the autonomic nervous system (see Chapter 1).

Development and role of the meninges

The brain and spinal cord are surrounded by three connective tissue layers, the meninges. These three layers are:

- the dura mater
- the arachnoid mater
- the pia mater.

The **dura mater** (dura meaning *tough*) is a tough, inelastic membrane which is actually composed of two layers, one round the spinal cord and brain and the outer fused with the periosteum (or lining) of the cranium. The inner layer of the dura is fused to the outer one except over the dural and venous sinuses. This structure allows the venous blood to drain into these sinuses on the return journey to the heart. The dura is separated from the periosteum of the vertebral canal by the epidural space (i.e. the space into which an epidural anaesthetic would be injected). If the blood vessels in the dura were to rupture and bleed into the space between the dura and the arachnoid mater layers, this would result in a subdural haemorrhage or haematoma. The **arachnoid mater** (arachnoid meaning *spiderlike*) is a very delicate, highly vascularised layer. In fact it is the density of the vasculature that gives the arachnoid its 'cobwebby' appearance. The space between the arachnoid and underlying pia is the subarachnoid space and it is through this space that the cerebrospinal fluid (CSF) flows. This would also be the location of the type of stroke known as a subarachnoid haemorrhage. The **pia mater** (pia meaning *gentle*) is the most fragile and highly vascularised of the meningeal layers and it adheres to the surface contours of both the brain and spinal cord. The pia extends into the main body of the brain alongside the blood vessels that penetrate the brain surface.

The meningeal layers around the spinal cord develop from the mesenchymal tissue surrounding the neural tube. A membrane is formed with the inner layer becoming the pia mater and the outer layer becoming the dura mater.

Developmental malformations

The information about normal neurodevelopment in the previous section is essential in order to understand what may go wrong in this highly complex process – and what may be the consequences for the child affected. Failure of the caudal neuropore to close causes the disruption of the lumbar and sacral segments of the spinal cord. The structures superficial to the cord (i.e. the meninges, vertebral arch, paravertebral muscles and skin) also become involved since development relies on closure of the neural tube. Box 3.1 explains the condition associated with this developmental disorder, known as spina bifida.

Cell differentiation

Cell differentiation, in terms of the developing nervous system, is the process by which vertebrate cells acquire neural properties. In order to understand what is going on, one has to identify what controls the formation and regional identity of the neural plate. The definitive research in this area was published in 1924 by Spemann and Mangold when they produced evidence that the differentiation of the neural plate from the ectoderm was induced by the mesodermic cells. Their work involved transplanting cells from a region of the embryo destined to form mesoderm into a ventral area that would normally give rise to skin. They showed that the transplanted cells developed normally, but the surrounding ectoderm cells formed a second neural tube – this led to the identification of the specialised region of the mesoderm known as the organiser. Two proteins have been identified with neural-inducing properties – noggin and chordin.

Following induction by signals from the organiser region, the neural plate cells differentiate into either neurones or glial cells. The neural crest cells are a transient and migratory group of cells which come from the dorsal neural tube and disperse along various pathways. The groups migrate to various peripheral locations where they coalesce, or come together, to form the neurones and Schwann cells of the sensory and autonomic nervous systems, the neuroendocrine cells of the adrenal medulla, the melanocytes of the skin and the tissue of the face and skull.

The neural crest cells have the potential to become one of a number of cell types and their fate is dependent upon the signals coming from the migratory environment. Their development options, however, become increasingly restricted by the environmental changes which occur during migration. A number of different 'environmental' molecules controlling the fate of the crest cells have been identified, including the glucocorticoid hormones which activate nuclear receptors that function as transcription factors. A transcription factor is a protein that binds to DNA sequences, thereby controlling the transcription of the genetic information from the DNA to mRNA. This alters the protein synthesis carried out by the cell. Since every cell in the body has the same genetic material they all have the capacity to make the same proteins. However, the aforementioned 'environmental' molecules alter the particular proteins that each specific cell type makes, thereby changing the function and type of the cell.

Box 3.1

Spina bifida

Spina bifida means cleft spine and comes about due to the incomplete closure of the spinal column. There are three main types: spina bifida occulta (from the Latin word *occultus*, meaning *hidden*); meningocoele; and myelomeningocoele

Spina bifida occulta is a common, but relatively minor, defect of one or more spinal arches. The condition, which may affect up to 10% of the population, is usually only found incidentally through a radiological exam for another disease. In this condition, although the spinal cord is normally formed and in the normal position with normal function, occasionally there can be minor neurological defects.

Spina bifida meningocoele is fairly common and manifests itself as a simple herniation of the meninges through a defect in the neural arches. Due to this relative exposure of the meningeal layers the condition carries the risk of infection and it may be accompanied by some level of neurological disability.

The third and most severe form of spina bifida, *myelomeningocoele*, results in the herniation of the meninges and the spinal cord through a defect in the neural arches into a skin-covered sac. This condition accounts for about 75% of all cases of spina bifida and the rate of occurrence in the UK is somewhere in the region of 0.15 cases per 1000 births. As the nerve roots are abnormally situated there is usually paralysis (i.e. a reduction of muscle force) below the level of the defect, with meningitis occurring as a further complication which may lead to additional central nervous system damage.

A significant number of developmental studies have been carried out using glial cells, specifically glial cell development in the rat optic nerve. Three classes of glial cells in rat optic nerve cultures have been identified (oligodendrocytes, type 1 astrocytes, type 2 astrocytes) which all differentiate postnatally from a common precursor, the O-2A progenitor cell. Growth factors play an important role in the differentiation of the glial cells, namely platelet-derived growth factor (O-2A cell proliferation) and ciliary neurotrophic factor (CNTF; astrocytes). The neuroblasts (neuronal precursors) and neurones also migrate from their site of formation.

The peripheral nervous system neurones also derive from the neural crest cells. These cells migrate throughout the body while completing their differentiation into the autonomic, sensory and enteric neurones. The eventual location of the central nervous system neurones is achieved by the migration of the aforementioned neuroblasts from their proliferation site. Different neuroblasts migrate at different stages, i.e. some before and some after extending their axons. The migration of the neuronal precursors has a dual function. Firstly, it has a role in establishing the identity of the neurones, and, secondly, it has a role in defining the functional properties and future connections.

Synapse formation

The formation of the synapse is a key event in the establishment of functional neuronal connections. Our understanding is probably most advanced at the special synapse that is found between motor neurones and skeletal muscle fibres.

The developing motor axon approaches the skeletal muscle fibre and at this early stage neither is well equipped for synaptic transmission. The axon growth cone does not resemble a presynaptic terminal and the postsynaptic muscle mass has not yet cleaved to form individual muscles, however, primitive synaptic transmission does exist. Full neuromuscular transmission requires two important features: the presynaptic axon must be able to release the neurotransmitter acetylcholine (ACh) and the postsynaptic membrane of the muscle fibre must be able to respond to ACh. When the motor neurone and muscle fibre make contact, this results in the formation of endplates (specialised receptor zones) in the muscle fibre. When this happens the postsynaptic potential amplitude increases markedly. In order to get the increased

transmission required for full contact and transmission, a number of pre- and post-synaptic changes have to occur. These include changes in the distribution and stability of the ACh receptors, changes in the functional properties of the receptors and increases in the number of nerve/muscle contacts.

Before innervation, the ACh receptors are spread evenly over the muscle fibre surface, but when the motor axon reaches the muscle, the ACh receptor density increases at the sites of innervation, with the ACh receptor density decreasing at the extrasynaptic sites. This is achieved by the receptors already present in the muscle membrane being redistributed as they diffuse within the plane of the membrane before becoming immobilised at the synaptic site. There is also an increased synthesis of new receptors which are then inserted into the muscle membrane at or near the synaptic site. At the end of the distribution process the endplate receptor density is several thousand times greater than the extrasynaptic receptor density.

The nerve terminals control both the synthesis and the distribution of the postsynaptic receptors on the muscle fibres through the actions of proteins released from presynaptic terminals. Agrin causes the clustering of pre-existing receptors, while ARIA (AChR inducing activity) increases the total number of ACh receptors on the muscle. Calcitonin gene-related peptide (CGRP) causes an increase in intracellular cyclic AMP (adenosine monophosphate) in skeletal muscle and an increase in the synthesis of ACh receptor subunits. As ACh receptors cluster at the synapse, extrasynaptic receptors disappear. This loss is controlled by electrical mechanisms.

Many neurones die in the normal course of development. This neuronal death is a perfectly normal, widespread occurrence during embryonic development and it may result in a loss of up to 50% of all of the neurones initially generated. This process of overproduction followed by drastic reduction occurs in almost all regions of both the central and peripheral nervous systems and is known as **programmed neuronal death**.

Several genes appear to be involved in programmed cell death. The overexpression of the bcl-2 protein can suppress the death of sensory and sympathetic neurones that occurs after the removal of neurotrophic factors. These neurotrophic factors have a role in neuronal survival and may act by suppressing the cell death programme in postmitotic cells. Several neurotrophic factors have been identified (nerve growth factor, brain-derived neurotrophic factor, neurotrophin-3 and ciliary neuro-trophic factor) and each is thought to support the survival of distinct neuronal groups. Administration of large amounts of nerve growth factor (NGF) to embryonic or newborn animals will prevent neuronal death.

Having discussed the key changes taking place in the nervous system during development, we are now going to move ahead to the other end of the lifespan spectrum and discuss the key changes found as the system starts to age.

Ageing and the nervous system

The increased life expectancy of humans is con-tributing to an epidemic of 'old age' and this is providing us with more opportunities to investigate the readily observed consequences of the deterio-ration of the nervous system that occurs with age. We understand significant amounts about how neurones develop, how they reach their targets, how they modify synaptic inputs and how they re-generate/refunction after injury. What we need to do now is address the mechanisms whereby neu-rones age. An understanding of this normal ageing process is essential, again, for health-care pro-fessionals to understand how healthy ageing may be promoted – and how to differentiate between 'normal' ageing and degeneration or disease of the nervous system.

There are numerous theories proposed for why and how we age. Rather than try and discuss them all in this chapter, we shall discuss some of the theory groups. It is possible to combine the various theories into three proposed theories of neuronal ageing: the redundant message theory, the pre-programmed ageing theory and the mutational DNA theory.

Redundant message theory

Many gene sequences can be classified as non-functional or redundant. These redundant sequences are held in 'reserve' to be utilised if required. Chro-mosomal anomalies/mutations occur naturally from time to time and it is proposed that the aforemen-tioned redundant genes, with similar sequences, may take over the function of the dysfunctional gene. As we age, anomalies accumulate to a point where all the redundant genes are used up and this situation results in genetic abnormalities that are subsequently expressed as abnormal proteins which may compro-mise neuronal function.

Pre-programmed ageing theory

This particular theory proposes that just as pre-programmed neuronal cell death (apoptosis) occurs in development, so too may neuronal death be pro-grammed in later life. The 'biological clock' theory assumes that deterioration of ageing neurones is the normal expression of a genetic programme that begins at fertilisation and ends with death. That said, it is not known whether the mechanisms of death evident in development are the same as those found in ageing.

Apoptosis has several properties which may be examined in the ageing nervous system. It has been shown that neurotrophins (e.g. NGF) and afferent electrical input, along with macromolecular synthesis inhibitors (e.g. cycloheximide), can prevent death. When DNA fragmentation occurs, the neurones change morphology. Recent evidence suggests that these properties are also expressed by neurones both in the ageing nervous system and also in degenerative diseases associated with ageing, e.g. Parkinson's/Alzheimer's disease. Ageing may involve specific gene products designed to kill cells when 'switched on' by pre-determined signals.

Mutational DNA theory

This theory proposes that the ageing of neurones is the result of errors in DNA duplication, which result from random damage (e.g. wear and tear, ex-posure to low-level radiation). As we age, these errors accumulate with increased expression of abnormal mRNA protein, resulting in senescence.

Physiological consequences of neuronal ageing

Probably the main change in the nervous system that is found with ageing is that of the rapid decline in brain weight (e.g. by age 80 the brain loses approxi-mately 15% of its weight), when compared to a young adult brain. This reduction in size is evident by a decrease in bulk of the gyri and a widening of the sulci (grooves). There is also evidence of a marked increase in size of the ventricles brought about by tissue loss.

As well as the physical changes in brain size and weight, there are also a number of biochemical changes. The total brain protein declines with age, with a reduction of over 30% by the age of 80, which would manifest itself as a reduction in enzymes, ion channels, receptors, etc. Interestingly, although protein content and cell number fall with age, there is an increase in total DNA content brought about by increased glial cell proliferation.

Another major change observed in the ageing brain is the marked change in neurotransmitter function. Not only is there a decrease in the levels of the enzymes synthesising dopamine, noradrenaline (norepinephrine) and acetylcholine, but there are also decreased receptors for the transmitters. Both of these effects will have a significant impact on neuronal function. Decreased levels of neurotrophic factors can also be found.

In order for the brain to function properly there has to be a constant blood supply linked directly to metabolic demand. This coupling of flow to metabolism ensures that each brain area receives an adequate supply of substrates to support the metabolic demand. However, in the ageing brain, blood flow to the brain and capacity for O_2 consumption are both reduced.

As well as the above changes, which could be considered internal changes, there are a number of more obvious signs of ageing which are indicative of a change in neuronal function. These include altered sleep patterns, changes in mood, irritability, apathy, loss of appetite, loss of memory, dementia, reduced motor control and impaired sensation, perception and motor commands.

Postmortem analysis of the ageing brain can reveal further 'hidden' changes. In general, ageing leads to a progressive loss of neurones (up to 90% in some areas), a swelling and distortion of neurone cell bodies by infiltration, a retraction of dendritic spines and a resultant loss of synaptic input. **Neurofibrillary tangles**, which are only found in ageing humans and are most evident in the hippocampus, consist of paired helical filaments. These abnormal fibrils accumulate in the axoplasm and tangle up into knot-like clusters to form a neuronal lesion. **Neuritic (senile) plaques** are again most densely concentrated in the hippocampus, but unlike the axoplasmic tangles they are found in the extracellular matrix. The plaques are composed of a central core of amyloid protein surrounded by a dense mass of degenerating neurones and infiltrating glia. **Lipofuscin granules** are pigmented subcellular organelles found in aged brains as green, yellow or brown granules and are thought to be large, end-stage lysosomes mopping up debris from neuronal degeneration. The **granulovascular organelles** found in the ageing brain are vacuoles or holes forming within the cytoplasm and dendrites of neurones.

SELF-ASSESSMENT QUESTIONS

1. What are the main events taking place between day E15 and E27 of neurodevelopment?
2. What factors control the formation and regional identity of the neural plate?
3. What events take place during the processes leading to the establishment of a neuromuscular junction?
4. What causes spina bifida, and what physiological and functional problems can occur in each of the types of spina bifida highlighted in this chapter?
5. Which main theories have been proposed to describe and explain physiological changes associated with ageing?
6. How can the biochemical changes observed during the ageing process lead to a reduction in the function of the nervous system?

Further reading

Chudler, E., Neuroscience for kids. Available online at: http://faculty.washington.edu/chudler/neurok.html.

Greene, N.D.E., Copp, A.J., 2009. Development of the vertebrate central nervous system: formation of the neural tube. Prenat. Diagn. 29, 303–311.

Mora, F., Segovia, G., del Arco, A., 2007. Aging, plasticity and environmental enrichment: structural changes and neurotransmitter dynamic in several areas of the brain. Brain Res. Rev. 55, 78–88.

Toescu, E.C., Vreugdenhil, M., 2010. Calcium and normal brain ageing. Cell Calcium 47, 158–164.

Reference

Spemann, H., Mangold, H., 1924. Über
induktion von embryonalagen durch
implantation artfremder
organisatoren. Wilhelm Roux' Archiv
für Entwicklungsmechanik der
Organismen 100, 599–638.

An introduction to pharmacology

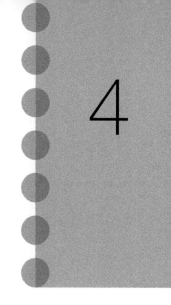

4

CHAPTER CONTENTS

> ### LEARNING OUTCOMES
>
> At the end of this chapter you should be able to:
> - identify the various cellular targets for drugs to work on
> - explain what is meant by the terms agonist and antagonist
> - identify the processes involved in the pharmacodynamics of a particular drug, namely absorption, distribution, metabolism and excretion.

Working in a rehabilitation setting, allied health professionals will inevitably be confronted with patients taking medication, whether this be to reduce pain, spasticity or seizures, or to lower blood pressure. Throughout the course of this book we will make numerous references to drugs working within various parts of the nervous system. It is, therefore, important that we have a basic appreciation of the area of science known as pharmacology. There are many pharmacology textbooks available and we have tried to give a short selection of appropriate texts in the further reading list at the end of this chapter. We are not trying to rewrite these texts, but simply give you an overview of the basic principles and concepts of pharmacology which we think are most relevant in clinical practice.

Introduction

Pharmacology can be defined as the study of chemicals (drugs), which can influence and, by this means, change the activity of living structures, i.e. the cells of the body. Consider three types of cell: (i) a typical human cell, (ii) a bacterial cell (as a representative of micro-organisms which may cause disease in humans) and (iii) a tumour cell (see Fig. 4.1). Drugs have been designed to influence each of these cells.

Drugs can manipulate the multitude of biochemical reactions which underpin the very life of cells. In the human cell we aim to use drugs to alter particular aspects of cell function to, in turn, improve the activity of body systems and thereby achieve the desired change in body health status. In the bacterial cell the aim of drugs is to kill the cell or at least disable it, in order to facilitate its destruction by our immune system. In this case we design drugs which are essentially damaging. They disrupt a process in the bacterial cell which is not found in human cells, e.g. the wall of a bacterial cell can be targeted. In this way we can damage the bacterial cells while leaving our own cells, in theory, undisturbed. In other words we aim for *selective toxicity* which, hopefully, minimises the side effects for us. Lastly, in the tumour cell, we can use drugs to target a crucial characteristic

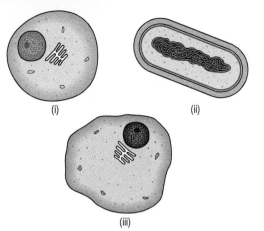

Fig. 4.1 • Basic cell types: (i) a typical human cell; (ii) a bacterial cell; (iii) a tumour cell

of this large, and somewhat metabolically greedy cell; its rapid rate of cell division. Drugs designed to inhibit the process of mitosis can be employed to reduce tumour growth. Unfortunately body cells, which are also normally dividing, are vulnerable, e.g. those lining the gut or hair root cells. In this situation selective toxicity is more difficult to attain.

Pharmacodynamics and pharmacokinetics

Pharmacology can be sub-divided into two topics of interest; firstly how drugs interact with our body cells – *Pharmacodynamics* – and, secondly, the factors we should consider when we want to find the best route of administration of a drug, how it is carried around the body, metabolised and then excreted – *Pharmacokinetics*.

We shall begin by considering pharmacodynamics and reconsider the structure of our human cell in order to describe more clearly the targets of drug action.

Our cells can be likened to highly organised factories contained within a barrier, the cell membrane. The internal organelles house the biochemical processes of the cell orchestrated by complex arrays of enzymes. Figure 4.2 shows a diagrammatic view of

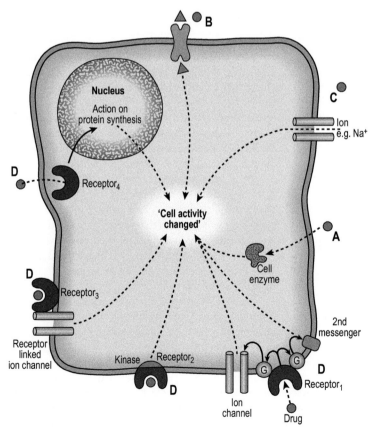

Fig. 4.2 • Diagrammatic representation of the human cell and drug targets

a human cell and the various targets of drug action detailed below.

The first potential cell target we will describe for drugs are the cell enzymes (labelled A on Fig. 4.2). It is possible for a drug to inhibit these biological catalysts to bring about a change in cell activity. For example, the liver cells of the body contain an enzyme responsible for the production of cholesterol. By inhibiting the enzyme in this cell using the statin drugs, less cholesterol is produced, the build up of cholesterol in blood vessels is reduced and the benefit for the individual is reduced cardiovascular disease risk.

Other drugs which influence enzymes in the body are aspirin and the ACE inhibitors – you may have heard of the latter in the context of the renal system and regulation of blood pressure.

You will also recall the role of the cell membrane. It acts as a selective barrier controlling what can and cannot enter the cell. Drugs can act on the cell membrane in several ways; firstly, by acting on structures within the membrane important to the passage of material in and out of the cell and, secondly, on structures called receptors.

In the first group we can include carriers (sometimes referred to as transporters) and ion channels. Carriers are often protein structures which the cell uses to transport material into the cell. Drugs can be used to block the activity of these structures, i.e. the compound is not taken into the cell (see Fig. 4.2 label B). Drugs are used in this manner to act on carriers in the membranes of nerve cells forming a synapse. The neurotransmitter released is not carried back into the cell that discharged it and instead accumulates in the synapse and, in this way, continually stimulates its target cell. An example of a drug which acts in this manner is cocaine.

Ion channels (labelled C in Fig. 4.2) can be viewed as small tubes through the membrane which permit the passage of certain small ions. One role of the cell membrane is to maintain an unequal distribution of two ions (sodium and potassium) across this membrane boundary. This arrangement plays an important role in the electrical signalling of cells in the body, for it is the phased disturbance of these ion concentration differences. This means that the movement of ions in and out of the cell through the channels leads to nerve impulses or, in the case of muscle cells, contraction. Again, it follows that if drugs are used to interfere in this process, i.e. prevent the movement of ions through channels and the consequent concentration disturbances, nerve signalling

can be stopped. This, very simply, is the action of local anaesthetic drugs. Lignocaine acts to block the channel which normally allows the movement of the sodium ion across the membrane. At the nerve cell level the nerve impulse is not carried, at the person level the sensation of pain is temporarily blocked.

The targets of the second group of drugs (labelled D in Fig. 4.2) are the receptors of a body cell. These are protein structures on the cell membrane or within the cytoplasm or nucleus which bind to body chemicals, e.g. hormones. Once this link is achieved there are 'knock on' effects within the cell for its activity is changed or regulated as a result. By this means these physiological chemicals ensure the smooth running of body functions and promote homeostasis. Therefore, it is important to appreciate that receptors are normal components of our cells. By designing and using drugs that act by binding to them, we are simply capitalising on this natural cell regulatory process, which has been present since before birth.

Our cells literally contain many different types of receptor which we can split into four main groups based on their action (see Fig. 4.2). Three of these are found in the cell membrane, the fourth type may be located in the cytoplasm or actually within the nucleus.

The **first** group comprises G-protein-coupled receptors. Once a drug binds to this membrane receptor an adjacent, i.e. linked, protein called a G-protein is activated. This G-protein can in turn activate either an ion channel that will cause ion movement across the cell membrane or an enzyme. If it is the latter, then a second molecule (called a second messenger) is produced which will promote some change in cell biochemistry activity. You may have heard of the second messenger cAMP (cyclic AMP). Ventolin, the bronchodilator drug, acts in this way.

The **second** group, the kinase-linked receptors, are proteins with enzyme (kinase) activity. Binding of a hormone or a drug causes the first of many enzyme reactions. The hormone insulin acts on receptors of this type.

Thirdly are receptors where their component protein is actually part of an ion channel. When a drug or hormone binds to this receptor the channel opens and ions flow through. These receptors are called ionotropic (pertaining to ions). This process of ion movement is extremely rapid. You will have heard this type of receptor mentioned when discussing the actions of acetylcholine on nicotinic receptors at the neuromuscular junction.

You may also hear these receptors referred to as ligand-gated. The ligand is the hormone or drug which when bound (ligated) to the channel opens (its gates) and allows ions to flow through. (This characteristic distinguishes them from 'voltage-gated' channels which open/close in response to a change of voltage across a membrane, not the presence of a drug or hormone.)

Thus ionotropic receptor, when activated, cause an immediate action in a cell by directly opening ion channels. Metabotropic receptor is a term used to describe receptors that influence the activity of a cell by first producing a metabolic change in the cell.

The **fourth** type of receptors comprises those that once a hormone or drug binds, regulate gene activity within the cell nucleus. Thus protein synthesis can result. Thyroid and steroid hormones are examples of hormones that bind to this type of receptor.

Drug classifications

Agonist drugs

The term agonist is used to describe chemicals, drugs, which bind and then activate cell receptors and thereby influence the cell (see Fig. 4.3). Most drugs show specificity, i.e. they have a relatively selective binding to one type of receptor. The ability of a drug, once it is bound, to activate the receptor and so cause a cell effect is termed its efficacy. Some drugs can be described as partial agonists because, although they can bind to a receptor, they cannot elicit full efficacy.

Antagonistic drugs

Antagonists bind to the receptor but produce no activation (see Fig. 4.4). They have no efficacy. The important point to appreciate is that antagonists, by

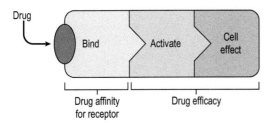

Fig. 4.3 • Diagrammatic representation of an agonist drug binding to a receptor

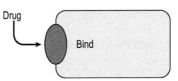

Fig. 4.4 • Diagrammatic representation of an antagonist drug binding to a receptor

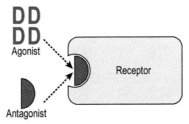

Fig. 4.5 • Binding of an antagonist drug to a receptor preventing access of the agonist

occupying the receptor, may prevent (block) an agonist from binding. You may hear the term 'blocker' used to describe an antagonist drug (see Fig. 4.5).

Antagonists may be further sub-divided into competitive and non-competitive antagonists. These terms reflect the strength of the link between drug and receptor. A strong link will be formed by a non-competitive (or irreversible) antagonist, while a competitive antagonist can be ousted from its binding site on the receptor by a higher concentration, greater numbers of agonist molecules.

'Families' of receptors can exist

The hormones adrenaline (epinephrine) and noradrenaline have widespread actions in the body and do so by binding to cell receptors. Investigation of the protein structure of these receptors has identified sub types, i.e. subtle differences in structure which distinguish them from each other despite the fact that they all bind with adrenaline. This finding has important implications.

For example, these slight variations in structure allow pharmaceutical companies to develop drugs that bind more effectively to one receptor sub type rather than another. When you also consider that receptors for adrenaline are widespread in the body, and that the various tissues tend to have a preponderance of a particular receptor sub type, you should predict that drugs which target more specifically one sub type should be associated with fewer side effects throughout the body.

The receptors of adrenaline/noradrenaline have been sub-divided into two sub types, alpha (α) and beta (β) and within these, further subdivisions are possible, e.g. β_1, β_2 and β_3 receptors. This sub-division can also be applied to other well-known body transmitters, e.g. histamine and acetylcholine. For acetylcholine the two subclasses of receptors are distinguished on the basis of whether they interact more with the plant alkaloid nicotine (N, nicotinic receptors) or muscarine (M, muscarinic receptors).

Finally, it is worth noting that the name of a transmitter is often used to name the receptors it interacts with. For example, adrenaline acts on adrenergic receptors, acetylcholine on cholinergic receptors, dopamine on dopaminergic, etc.

Pharmacokinetics

This process can be summarised as having four phases; absorption of the drug, its distribution around the body, its metabolism and, finally, its excretion.

All these processes involving the movement of the drug within the body are captured within the term pharmacokinetics.

Consider each of the phases briefly.

Absorption

Drugs can be administered to the body in many ways, e.g. by injection (intravenously, intramuscularly, subcutaneously, etc.), inhalation, swallowing, patches and suppositories. The term parenteral is used when the gut is avoided. Factors which influence the route selected may be the chemistry of the drug (e.g. it is destroyed by the enzymes in the gut, it is not fat soluble) or other factors (e.g. the patient hates needles, the patient has difficulty swallowing tablets). How quickly an effect is required (e.g. injection may be favoured over the oral route) or perhaps one route minimises side effects (e.g. the use of the inhaled route to deliver corticosteroid drugs in the prophylactic treatment of asthma reduces the dose required compared with that of the oral route) are additional points to be considered.

Two relevant and important terms are 'bioavailability' and 'first-pass metabolism'. Bioavailability is the proportion of the dose which reaches the blood in an active form. For example an intravenous injection should ensure high bioavailability. First-pass metabolism describes the effect of body enzymes on drugs taken in by the oral route. This process can occur in the gut wall, but particularly in the liver. (Remember that all absorbed components from the diet pass through the portal vein to the liver before reaching the general circulation.) During this time the drug chemicals are exposed to a large array of hepatic enzymes. Often these enzymes destroy the drug and greatly reduce the amount entering the general circulation. In this case the bioavailability of the drug would be low. However, note, this is not always the case and sometimes the drug is converted to a more active compound by liver exposure, e.g. some beta blockers. You should now appreciate the important implications of liver damage, immaturity or infection on the handling of drugs by the body and thereby the safe dose which is to be prescribed.

Distribution

Distribution denotes the process of the drug travelling round the body and coming into contact with the tissues where a beneficial action may occur. Structures in the body with good blood flow should receive the drug rapidly; however, areas with poor flow, e.g. the skin, or pathologically induced poor flow, e.g. the gut in cardiovascular shock, may receive very little drug. Again the chemistry of the drug molecule will influence how readily it passes through cell membranes, etc. Most drugs travel in the blood attached to plasma proteins, e.g. albumin, and it is important to note that it is only the unbound drug that is biologically active. This is important to consider when you administer a second drug that is also transported bound to plasma protein. The second drug may displace the first drug from plasma protein binding sites. The level of free, biologically active drug is suddenly raised and a much exaggerated response to drug one can result. Similarly in infection the amount of plasma protein can change in the blood and again the amount of biologically free drug may change.

Metabolism

The metabolism of a drug occurs mainly (but not exclusively) within the liver, where a vast array of enzymes are located. The purpose is to transform the drug chemical into a water-soluble product that can be eliminated in urine. Metabolic efficiency will be decreased in the elderly, the very young and in cases of liver damage, e.g. hepatitis, etc. Finally, it is worth remembering that the levels of enzymes in the liver can be induced. Continual exposure of liver cells to a chemical can cause the liver to become more effective at dealing with the chemical. Greater doses of drug may be required to achieve a therapeutic effect.

Excretion

Drugs can be excreted from the body by a variety of routes, e.g. the breath (alcohol and general anaesthetics), sweat, saliva, through the bile and then the faeces, in breast milk and in urine. The last named is a very important route. Water-soluble drugs are excreted in this fashion and, as noted above, lipid-soluble drugs can be converted by the liver to achieve this transformation. Again it is worth stressing that the immature, damaged or older kidney will have decreased ability to excrete drugs from the body, blood levels may remain high and a greater than anticipated response may result.

Half-life is a term used to describe the time taken for the plasma concentration of a drug to fall to half its initial value. Drugs vary greatly in this regard, for some it may be 1 hour, for others 200 hours. When drug dosing stops, it is usual to estimate that it will take 4–5 half-lives to eliminate the drug from the body.

Drug names

Drugs can be known by their generic name, which is an officially agreed chemical name, and also by a brand (trade or proprietary) name. The latter is devised by the pharmaceutical company that produces the drug and is usually written with a capital letter, e.g. the analgesic tramadol (generic name) is manufactured as Zamadol (trade name).

SELF-ASSESSMENT QUESTIONS

1. What are the main differences in the way that an agonist and antagonist drug interact with a particular receptor?
2. What is meant by the term 'first-pass metabolism'?
3. What is meant by the term 'half-life' when used in the context of pharmacology?

Further reading

Rang, H.P., Dale, M.M., Ritter, J.M., et al., 2007. Rang & Dale's Pharmacology, sixth ed. Churchill Livingstone, Edinburgh.

Waller, D.G., Renwick, A.G., Hillier, K., 2009. Medical Pharmacology & Therapeutics, third ed. Elsevier Saunders, London.

Wecker, L., Watts, S., Faingold, C., et al., 2009. Brody's Human Pharmacology, fifth ed. Elsevier Mosby, London.

The brain–behaviour relationship: an introduction

5

LEARNING OUTCOMES

At the end of this chapter, you should be able to:

- describe main afferent and efferent pathways and key functions of the main anatomical regions of the central nervous system in terms of behaviour, cognition and emotion.
- explain the main effects of lesions to these regions.
- compare and contrast three methods for mapping the relationship between the brain and behaviour:
  - Projection maps
  - Functional maps
  - Cyto architectonic maps

- identify key principles of functional organisation of the cortex and explain the processes mediating neuroplasticity
- provide a coherent summary of the relationship between the brain and behaviour.

Introduction

As described in Chapter 1, it is now widely accepted that the brain is the centre for behaviour, thinking and emotion, but how does it govern these functions? What is the relationship between the brain and behaviour? Can knowledge about the site of a brain lesion help to explain difficulties with behaviour, thinking and emotion? Is the relationship between the brain and behaviour fixed, or does it change? Does therapeutic input, aimed at improving behavioural outcomes, have any influence on the brain?

These and other interesting questions will be explored in this chapter. We will build on Chapter 2, which introduced the main anatomical subdivisions of the brain. In particular we will expand on the cerebral cortex and explore how various regions within the cortex are involved in behaviour, cognition and emotion.

The aim of this chapter is to present a summary of current thinking about the relationship between the brain and behaviour, which will be expanded upon in subsequent chapters. The purpose of this information is to enable a deeper understanding of the potential impact of brain lesions, affecting different areas of the brain, on a range of behaviours. A sound knowledge of the relationship between the brain and behaviour may also prepare health-care professionals working with people with conditions affecting the brain, to be alert to signs and symptoms of emotional, cognitive and behavioural difficulties, and to help interpret these difficulties.

Anatomical organisation of the brain: a brief revision

You will remember the main anatomical subdivisions of the brain, which were presented in Chapter 2. Table 5.1 expands this table by adding a column with the main functional roles of each area of the brain. In this chapter, we will focus primarily on the role of the cerebral cortex in behaviour (Fig. 5.1). During the process of evolution, this part of the brain in particular has undergone a considerable expansion, which

is thought to be related to skills and abilities that make humans stand out in the animal kingdom, i.e. the ability to use sophisticated language, reasoning, planning and problem solving, judgement, and…humour.

Information highways: neural connectivity within the brain

Following the overview of the major subdivisions of the brain and their key roles in human behaviour, we will consider the connections between these areas.

Association fibres are neurones that connect different areas *within* each hemisphere (Fig. 5.2a). For example, the parietal lobe receives visual and acoustic information from the occipital and temporal lobes respectively. Association fibres serve to combine the information from those areas with somatosensory information from within the parietal lobe itself. This confluence of information enables different sources of sensory information to be associated and integrated into a coherent percept about the body in space. This information is then relayed to the frontal lobe, which is responsible for preparing and executing action. In turn, any action planned by the frontal lobe is relayed back to the parietal lobe to enable it to interpret sensory feedback correctly, as the action unfolds. This reciprocal communication, evidenced by extensive white matter connections within each hemisphere, is found throughout the brain.

Commissural fibres provide connections *between* the two hemispheres by the corpus callosum (Fig. 5.2b). It has been estimated that there are around 200 million of such fibres, which illustrates the importance of integration of information between the left and right sides of the brain. For example, consider the ease with which you open a jar; one hand grasps the jar while the other manipulates the lid. Usually, the action is fluid and effective. Now try and undertake this action with another person; one holds the jar while the other opens the lid. Why was that so difficult? In the latter situation, the left hand did not know what the right hand was doing! The ease with which we normally undertake bimanual activities can be attributed to the extensive communication between the two hemispheres, in this case with respect to the position and forces applied to the object by each hand. In rare cases, e.g. of intractable epilepsy, the connectivity between the two hemispheres has been surgically disrupted to prevent electrical abnormality spreading from one hemisphere to the other. This

Table 5.1 Anatomical subdivisions of the brain and their main functions

Forebrain	Telencephalon	**Cerebral cortex**	Voluntary control of movement Perception Language Cognition (e.g. organisation and planning, thinking, decision-making)
		Basal ganglia	Coordination and modulation of movement
		Limbic system	Learning and memory Emotion and motivation
	Diencephalon	**Thalamus**	Relay station for all sensory input Motor control
		Hypothalamus	Key role in survival; regulation of homeostatic functions (e.g. fluid and food intake, temperature control) by controlling the autonomic nervous system and the endocrine system. Organisation of fright, fight, flight reactions, feeding and reproductive behaviour
Midbrain	Mesencephalon	**Tectum**	Mediation of visual and acoustic behaviours (e.g. orienting)
		Tegmentum	Reward, cognition, motivation
Hindbrain	Metencephalon	**Cerebellum**	Regulation of tone Balance and posture Coordination of skilled actions Eye movements, eye–limb coordination
		Pons	Regulation of attention; sleep and arousal
	Myelencephalon	**Medulla**	Integration of input from spinal cord Arousal and activation Sleep–wake rhythm Cardiovascular control Respiratory control Digestive control Modulation of pain Regulation of postural and equilibrium reflexes; muscle tone

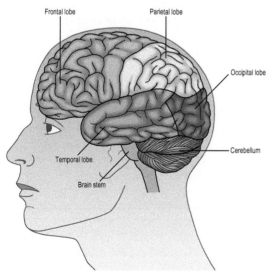

Fig. 5.1 • Gross anatomy of the brain, showing the occipital temporal, parietal and frontal lobes

results in the so-called 'split brain' syndrome, which gives rise to peculiar symptoms, as each hemisphere is independent and restricted to perceiving information from, and controlling action of, the contralateral side only. More about this syndrome can be read in Kolb and Whishaw (2008).

Projection fibres provide connectivity *between higher and lower* areas by formeing connections between end points of a neurone (Fig. 5.2c). For example, there are projection fibres from the primary motor cortex to the anterior horn in the spinal cord, or from the eye to the primary visual area in the occipital lobe.

In summary, there is extensive connectivity within the brain; both within and between the hemispheres, as well between higher and lower areas of the nervous system. This connectivity enables extensive, simultaneous and reciprocal communication between different areas to take place. This type of

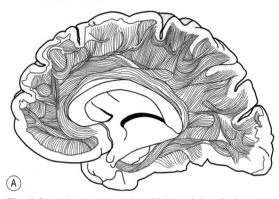

(A)

Fig. 5.2.a • Interconnectivity within each hemisphere: association fibres.

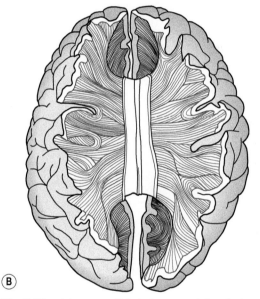

(B)

Fig. 5.2.b • Interconnectivity between each hemisphere: commissural fibres.

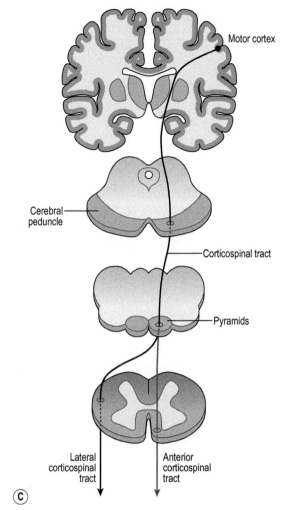

Motor cortex

Cerebral peduncle

Corticospinal tract

Pyramids

Lateral corticospinal tract

Anterior corticospinal tract

(C)

Fig. 5.2.c • Interconnectivity higher and lower stations: Projection fibres.

information processing is known as parallel distributed processing (PDP) – examples of which we will point out as we go through this chapter.

Functional organisation of the cortex

Having established the various brain areas and their extensive connectivity, we are ready to explore the relationship between brain areas and behaviour. But first, we will explain how this relationship has been mapped. There are three main maps that describe the brain–behaviour relationship.

Projection maps

Projection maps are *anatomical* maps, which have been derived from following projection fibres from their origin to their destination. For example, one can follow the optic nerve emanating from the eye to the primary end station for visual information at the back of the occipital lobe. Or, starting from the primary motor cortex in the frontal lobe, one can identify neurones that connect with the anterior horn of the spinal cord and hence with motor end plates of skeletal musculature. Thus, projection maps chart the various areas of the brain in terms of the type of information they receive or disseminate.

Functional maps

Functional maps are *behavioural* maps, which have been devised by charting connections between brain areas and specific behaviours or experiences. There are three main methods for producing a functional map:

- By relating specific deficits to known brain lesions. A good example of this is Paul Broca's identification of the speech production area in a patient with a localised lesion of the left frontal lobe (see Chapter 11 for more detail). The case study of H.M. has resulted in recognition of the role of the medial temporal lobe in memory (Chapter 9), while the case study of Phineas Gage placed the frontal lobe on the map in terms of its role in executive function (Chapter 12). As you can see, maps of the brain–behaviour relationship of this kind are primarily based on case studies. However, illuminating and fascinating these may be, it is important to consider the possible problems with this approach. For example, H.M.'s medial temporal lobes were removed because of severe epilepsy. How confident can we be that H.M.'s brain was otherwise normal, and that findings based on this case study can, therefore, be generalised to a normal population?
- Functional maps can also be constructed by noting behaviour(s) elicited during electrical stimulation of the cortex. A well-known contributor to this body of research was Wilder Penfield (1891–1976), a pioneer in neurosurgery in the treatment of epilepsy, who was introduced in Chapter 1. Surgical interventions for epilepsy are usually only undertaken if pharmacological interventions are ineffective, and/or where side effects are prohibitive. Surgical interventions aim to disconnect the source of epilepsy, thereby preventing the abnormal electrical activity from spreading. However, it is crucial of course that areas with normal function are preserved. The surgical procedure requires patients to be alert and interacting with the surgeon. The surgeon electrically stimulates different areas of the cortex and observes the patient's responses. These may range from specific movements, to sensations, to the experience of emotions or memories. By noting these observations and collating the responses from numerous patients, Wilder Penfield was able to draw up what is now

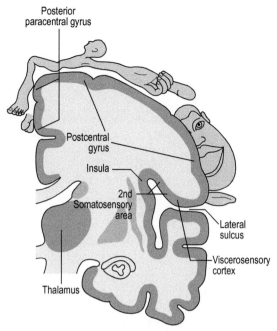

Fig. 5.3 • The sensory homunculus. Fig. 17.12 from Haines (2005) with permission from Elsevier.

known as the 'homunculus' (Latin for 'little man'), of which there is a motor and a sensory variation, each identifying the brain areas involved in movement and sensation, respectively (see Fig. 5.3).

- Finally, functional maps of the brain–behaviour relationship can be devised by recording activity of the cortex during a specific activity. With the advent of neuroimaging technology (Chapter 2), this area of research has seen a virtual explosion. Groundbreaking research into the neural correlates of chronic depression was published by Drevets et al. (1992), using PET scans to identify areas of abnormal activity, compared to controls. This work identified, among other areas, the left frontal cortex and the amygdala to be abnormally active. Another example is the discovery of the mirror neurone system in monkeys, using single-cell recordings, which demonstrated the involvement of the frontal lobe in observational learning – the so-called mirror neurone system (Chapter 8). Since the original discovery, the mirror neurone system has also been found in humans and theories on its potential role in empathy have been expanded.

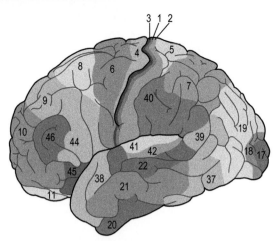

Fig. 5.4 • Brodmann's areas. From: http://thebrain.mcgill.ca/flash/capsules/outil_jaune05.html

Cytoarchitectonic maps

These maps are based on architectural properties of brain cells, such as size, shape and arrangement (Fig. 5.4). Brodmann, who pioneered this approach, used different stains to identify different types of cells. Although continually being updated and refined, the Brodmann map is still useful as the main areas correspond with functions, identified through functional or projection techniques. Brodmann's areas and their key functions that allied health professionals (AHPs) should be familiar with are listed in Table 5.2.

In summary, there are three main maps that have helped to chart the relationship between the brain and behaviour, i.e. projection, functional and cytoarchitectonic maps.

Current understanding of the brain–behaviour relationship

Synthesising the information emerging from the brain–behaviour maps, what is our current understanding of the brain–behaviour relationship? A pioneer in this area was Aleksandr Romanovich Luria (1902–1977) who laid the foundation for neuropsychology, through numerous scientific as well as case study publications. Luria was a Russian neuropsychologist and much of his work is based on his experiences with war victims, affected by bullet wounds to the head. Luria's talent was to integrate his expertise as a neuropsychologist with the experiences of his patients in his writings, crafting a unique insight into the impact of certain brain lesions on an individual's life. A recommended read is *The Man with a Shattered World* (Luria 1987), which brings to life the impact of brain injury on a person's behaviour, thinking and emotion, through years of naturalistic observation and conversation between Luria and Zasetsky, his patient.

Although the details of Luria's model have been updated with emerging experimental findings, his global interpretation is still of value. Luria proposed that the brain was broadly divided into two units, i.e. the motor unit (all brain area ventral of the central sulcus) and the sensory unit (all brain areas rostral to the central sulcus) (Fig. 5.5). Let's use the example of stopping before a red traffic light. The information process would commence with visual information being relayed from the eyes to the primary sensory area (i.e. the first port of call for raw visual sensory information such as light, colour or shape), where this

Table 5.2 Brodmann's areas relevant for allied health professionals and their main functions

Brodmann's area	Name	Main function
1, 2, 3	Primary sensory cortex	Somatosensory function
4	Primary motor cortex	Movement execution
6	Pre-motor cortex	Movement planning
8	Frontal eye field	Eye movement
17	Primary visual cortex (V1)	Vision
22	Wernicke's area	Speech and language: comprehension
41	Primary auditory cortex	Audition
44	Broca's area	Speech and language: expression

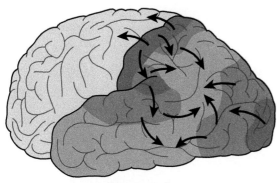

The sensory unit

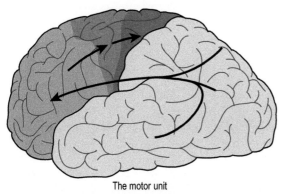

The motor unit

Fig. 5.5 • Luria's model of the brain. This model comprises the sensory unit (top) and the motor unit (bottom). Dark areas are primary areas, medium shaded areas indicate secondary areas, and light areas indicate tertiary areas. The arrows indicate the flow of information within the brain from, from primary sensory areas eventually to primary motor areas that initiate an action. See text for details. From Kolb B, and Whishaw IQ (1996), with permission from W.H. Freeman & Co./Worth Publishers.

information is integrated into the percept of 'traffic light'. The secondary area would elaborate on this information, by taking in the traffic scene as a whole, while in the tertiary area, this information is further integrated with memories and emotions of past experiences, prompting with a sense of urgency the recollection that this signal implies a 'stop'. Next, this information is relayed from the sensory unit to the action unit, where the appropriate action is prepared. In the tertiary area of this unit, different plans may be considered (e.g. to speed up/stop) from which one is selected, based on the visual information, memory and emotion. The plan is further prepared in the secondary area, which is responsible for planning the action. The actual initiation of the action is the responsibility of the primary area, which issues motor commands through the dedicated motor

pathways – resulting in the final action of operating the brake. Luria's model – the first comprehensive model explaining the relationship between the brain and behaviour – is now considered to be simplistic, however the legacy of this pioneering work is evident in that some of his original terminology (e.g. primary and secondary (or association) areas) are still in use today:

- Primary sensory areas are brain areas that receive raw sensory information, which is processed in secondary – or association areas into meaningful percepts (see Chapter 10).
- Primary motor areas are cortical areas involved in issuing motor commands, which are planned in secondary – or association areas (Chapter 7).

A more contemporary model of the brain was suggested by Felleman and van Essen in the 1990s, whose work has highlighted the following key principles of brain function:

- The organisation of the brain is hierarchical.
- Information is processed in a parallel-distributed manner:
  - Many (sub)cortical areas process information simultaneously
  - Connections are often reciprocal.

To explain the above in more detail: the brain operates in a hierarchical manner, which means that some areas are essential for particular functions. An example is Brodmann's area 17 (known as V1 or primary visual area), where all visual sensory information converges. If a person has a lesion that has affected this entire area, then the person will experience what is known as 'cortical blindness'. This means that, although the visual system proper (i.e. eyes and optic nerves) is intact, the person acts as if they are blind as the processing of visual information is impaired. Cortical blindness is an interesting phenomenon, for which the interested reader is referred to Kolb and Whishaw (2008).

Information is processed in a parallel-distributed manner, which means that information is usually processed by more than one brain area at the same time. As explained earlier, parallel-distributed processing (or PDP) is enabled by the extensive neural connectivity within and between different areas of the brain. An example is a speech and language therapist examining a patient, integrating acoustic information (about speech sounds) with visual information (e.g. about non-verbal communication) and memories involving previous patients with a similar condition, while considering plans for intervention.

A key phenomenon of brain function is plasticity, also known as neuroplasticity.

Neuroplasticity

Neuroplasticity[1] is the capacity of the nervous system to adapt itself to a change in input. For example, learning a new language, a new musical instrument, or learning to walk with crutches. There are several aspects to neuroplasticity: anatomical, physiological and pharmacological. This section will discuss neuroplastic responses to injury and compare processes in the peripheral nervous system with those in the central nervous system.

How modifiable are the connections made during development?

By birth we possess a full complement of neurones within our nervous system. However, this 'rough' pattern, which developed *in utero*, does not bear comparison to the settled pattern of neuronal connections in the fully formed adult nervous system. The first question we really need to ask ourselves is; what happens to allow such refinement? The refinement has nothing to do with the growth of additional new neurones (i.e. neurogenesis), but is brought about by the process of plasticity. Neuroplasticity is defined as the ability of the nervous system to adapt or modify in response to imposed change, either **physiological** or **pharmacological**.

Anatomical change

Redundancy refers to the ability of the brain to recruit intact, surplus substrate in order to recover function. Work on primates by Nudo et al. (2000) has shown that specific portions of the motor map (e.g. of the hand) contain connections with a considerable amount of overlap. This implies that if some connections have been damaged, others can be recruited to support the original function (Kleim and Schwerin 2010).

Initially it was thought that cortical representations (e.g. the motor and sensory homunculus) were static once adulthood had been reached. However, more recent studies have shown that these representations are dynamic; their size changes depending on how much the area is being used. Studies on healthy primates (Nudo et al. 2000) have shown that after practising a new skill (e.g. using fingers to retrieve food pellets from small wells), the cortical motor representation of the fingers expanded significantly. Conversely, studies involving animals with experimental brain damage showed shrinkage of cortical maps of affected extremities, with parts of the representations of the hand being replaced by those of more proximal limb segments. These animals did not receive any training after the brain damage however, whereas in cases where training was provided, this shrinkage did not occur (Nudo and Milliken 1996, Nudo et al. 2000). In people with stroke, studies examining neuroanatomical changes following interventions aimed at improving arm function suggest that the motor map of the affected upper limb may increase following the intervention (Koski et al. 2004, Wittenberg et al. 2003).

A further thought-provoking finding from animal research has shown that neuroplastic changes in cortical representation of the hand only emerged after learning *new* skills – but not after repetitive movement (Nudo et al. 2000, Nudo 2003a, b).

Taken together, these studies show that cortical maps are dynamic, with changes depending on learning experiences. However, mere repetitive movement does not seem to instigate these neuroplastic changes. The implications from these and other studies for rehabilitation are that therapeutic input has the potential to prevent shrinkage and mediate recovery of cortical representations of affected parts of the body. It appears also that therapeutic input needs to be of sufficient intensity and novelty to forge these neuroplastic changes. Determining the optimum levels of these parameters for individuals with different skill levels and cognitive abilities is a challenging question for future studies.

Physiological change

This type of change involves the refinement of synaptic connections by activity-dependent mechanisms modulated by experience after birth. This experience may be sensory (e.g. being exposed to music), physical (e.g. learning to swim), emotional (e.g. being loved and made to feel safe) or social (e.g. belonging to a group). This type of change is also known as functional plasticity and forms the basis of our

---

[1]Plasticity: from Greek πλασσειν: to mould (Chambers English Dictionary,1990)

cognitive, memory and learning processes. In simple terms, the more we experience and do, the better the connections become.

Pharmacological change

This involves the adaptation of synaptic connections after damage, injury or toxic insult to nerves resulting in abnormal activity/recovery of function. This is also known as adaptive plasticity and forms the basis of recovery after injury. It is this type of adaptive change that we are going to investigate in more detail, both peripherally and centrally.

What can we learn from early developmental processes that helps us to understand recovery after injury?

To understand adaptive plasticity we have to understand the neuronal changes that accompany injury to neurones.

Effect of injury in the peripheral nervous system

Injury to peripheral nerves results in both motor loss (plegia, paresis, atrophy) and sensory loss (subjective loss of sensation – pain, numbness, tingling; objective loss of sensation – 2 point discrimination, analgesia, anaesthesia). All symptoms relate to a loss of the integrity of both anatomical and functional synaptic connections. If damage to a peripheral neurone results in a transection injury, two separate types of damage processes occur at opposite ends of the neurone (see Fig. 5.6).

Wallerian degeneration

Wallerian degeneration takes place at the terminal end of the neurone. The transection injury prevents the transport of proteins, lipids and neurotransmitter to the axon terminal. As a result, the terminals retract and the muscle fibre atrophies. Macrophages then invade and phagocytose the myelin sheath of the 'dying' neurone, producing a layer of scar tissue. The compensatory proliferation of Schwann cells underneath the scar tissue creates a banded appearance, known as the bands of Bünger.

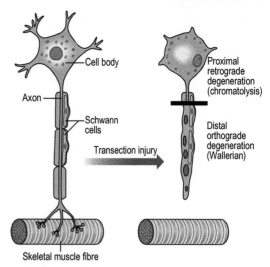

Fig. 5.6 • Peripheral neurone damage following a transection injury

Chromatolysis

Proximal degeneration at the cell body end of the damaged neurone produces an axon reaction which manifests cell body swelling, displacement of the nucleus (eccentric), dispersion of the rough endoplasmic reticulum, the detachment of the presynaptic terminals and the resetting of the biosynthetic and metabolic activity.

If the cell body/cut axon is displaced by injury, this leads to degeneration and death of the neuron. However, if they remain spatially close there is a possibility of regeneration of axotomised neurones (see Fig. 5.7).

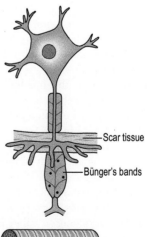
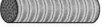

Fig. 5.7 • Non-displaced transection injury

Non-displaced transection injury

If the cell body/cut axon is non-displaced at 1 to 3 days post injury, the tip of the proximal 'stump' forms a growth cone under the influence of neurotrophic factors, such as nerve growth factor (NGF), neurotrophin-3 (NT3) and brain-derived neurotrophic factor (BDNF). The cone sends out many exploratory pseudopodia. If they force their way through the scar tissue they enter the bands of Bünger, where the proliferating Schwann cells are bound by basal lamina and form a 'cord' or 'guide tube' for the regenerating axon to follow toward the target tissue. There is an over-production of branching in the early recovery stage, and most degenerate after the successful synaptic contact of one. After re-innervation of the target cell, which occurs at a rate of approximately 1 to 4 mm per day, the injured axon always remains thinner and less myelinated than before. This results in the new contact being less efficient as both axon diameter and level of myelination are directly related to the speed of action potential propagation. Since injured motor axons never re-innervate sensory structures and injured sensory axons never re-innervate motor structures, it is likely that there are chemical cues from the damaged target cells.

Effect of injury in the central nervous system

Axonal regeneration almost never occurs in the central nervous system as it is limited by the inhibitory influences of the glial cells and the extracellular environment, and this is the basis for degenerative neurological disease and ageing. This then leads to the question: why does axonal regeneration not occur? The answer to this question is linked to the myelin sheath, or rather the cells responsible for myelin production in the central nervous system.

In the peripheral nervous system the myelin is produced by Schwann cells, of which there are large numbers associated with each neurone. Following injury, these Schwann cells can proliferate (rapidly increase in number), leading to the production of the regeneration tube. However, in the central nervous system the myelin is produced by oligodendrocytes, of which there is only one cell per neurone. As a consequence, there can be no injury-induced proliferation and, consequently, no regeneration tube. If there is no regeneration tube, how does adaptive neuroplasticity/functional recovery occur in the central nervous system?

Mechanisms of central nervous system plasticity

There are known to be two main mechanisms of central plasticity:

- Latent synapses
- Collateral sprouting.

Latent synapses

There are over 1000 trillion unused synapses in the brain. These 'latent' synapses may be activated following injury/lesion, possibly as a result of the removal of tonically inhibitory influences from a pre-existing pathway (i.e. the one damaged by the injury). This 're-modelling' allows potential alternative pathways to open-up, which is especially important for restructuring important functional connections after stroke.

Collateral sprouting

During development, many CNS neurones naturally produce axon collaterals, a process which is believed to be non-functional in normal circumstances. After injury to the main axon, a collateral may extend or grow towards the target cell, once again under the influence of various chemical cues, e.g. brain-derived growth factor (BDGF). The establishment of the new synapse ensures that the new projection will survive. The axon collaterals have fewer ion channels, therefore the new projection is not as efficient as the original. This is caused by the fact that the reduction in ion channel density will reduce the number of Ca^{2+} channels. This will, in turn, reduce the amount of Ca^{2+} that can enter the cell in response to an action potential, thereby reducing transmitter release.

Denervation supersensitivity

Injury to a central nervous system neurone prevents synaptic transmission at the presynaptic terminal. The process of denervation supersensitivity allows the post-synaptic terminal to respond to the little neurotransmitter that it still receives. The consequences of this are illustrated in Figure 5.8:

1. An induction or receptor up-regulation at post-synaptic target terminal – giving more targets for the limited number of neurotransmitter molecules to work on.

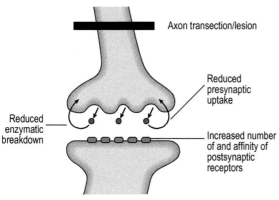

Axon transection/lesion

Reduced presynaptic uptake

Reduced enzymatic breakdown

Increased number of and affinity of postsynaptic receptors

Fig. 5.8 • Denervation supersensitivity

2. The damaged axon has a reduced ability for re-uptake of the released transmitter, which results in increased transmitter in the synaptic cleft.

3. The amount of transmitter degradation decreases as more transmitter collects in the cleft.

As a consequence of these more immediate changes, any new axon sprouts are ensured of evoking post synaptic potentials, and, as a result, the new functional pathway is maintained.

Clinical consequences of plasticity in the central nervous system

There is now a considerable body of evidence to indicate that therapeutic exercise can bring about changes in brain function (e.g. Buma et al. 2010, Calautti and Baron 2003, Hodics et al. 2006). Probably one of the longest lines of research in this field is constraint induced movement therapy (CIMT), also known as forced use therapy. Research Box 5.1 provides an overview of research in this area, showing that the brain is plastic, and that structure and function can change with experience.

Neuroplasticity is not always conducive to recovery, however. Nudo et al. (2000, p. 190) stated that long-term neuroplastic changes may be 'adaptive, maladaptive or epiphenomenal'. Some latent synapses activated after neuronal injury may target other afferent pathways as well as the damaged one. This may lead to some degree of functional abnormality, such as abnormal synergies. Following injury-induced synaptic degeneration, the axon collaterals that sprout to fill the vacant synapse may be haphazard, i.e. many neurones of diverse origin may sprout. As a result, some abnormal reflexes may be seen

following stroke injury (e.g. Babinski the reflex). Supersensitivity within the affected target site may contribute to an exaggeration of normal nerve function (e.g. hyperreflexia). We can now understand how the phenomenon of spasticity, characterised by abnormal sensori-motor control (Chapter 6), can be interpreted as neuroplasticity 'gone haywire'. Additionally, there are several reports of adverse effects in rodents following rehabilitation that was too intensive too early (Grotta et al. 2004, Schallert et al. 2000), hence the timing and intensity of therapeutic input need to be carefully considered to avoid adverse effects on neuroplastic processes.

Summary and overview of plasticity

The lack of neurone-to-neurone communication results in the death of injured neurones. In order for damaged nerves to recover function successfully, new synaptic connections have to be made and these must respond to afferent stimulation. No matter what the recovery mechanism, or if damage is in the peripheral or central nervous system, the final outcome is the establishment of new, but abnormal, synaptic pathways. These abnormal pathways may be inappropriate or non-specific, but, with good therapeutic management, they can be 'harnessed' to function in a broadly similar manner to before. It has been suggested that for good functional recovery to occur, adaptive plasticity has to be encouraged in the early phase post injury – provided that the patient is medically stable.

All in all, the challenge increasingly lies with the therapist to be aware of adaptive plasticity and to ensure that the beneficial sprouting/regeneration/supersensitivity, etc. (via target cell stimulation), are achieved as soon as possible – and safe – after a neurological event.

The brain and behaviour: an overview

Introduction

Having discussed the general principles of how we currently think the brain works, we will now explore brain function, and how it adapts to change, in more detail. This section will give an overview of the main functions of the occipital, parietal, temporal and

Research box 5.1

Constraint-induced movement therapy (CIMT): can practice change the brain?

Constraint induced movement therapy (CIMT), also referred to as forced use of the affected upper extremity in hemiplegic patients, is a therapeutic strategy that combines two key ingredients: firstly, the primarily affected arm is engaged in intensive training for prolonged periods of time each day. Secondly, the non- (or less-) affected arm is constrained by a mitt, sling or splint, for a period of up to 90% of 'waking hours' (Taub and Uswatte 2003). This strategy forces the patient to use the primarily affected arm in functional activities for most part of their day. To ensure safety, patients normally need to have a certain degree of active wrist (and sometimes finger) movement to be eligible for this type of treatment.

The idea for CIMT was originally based on observations of monkeys after experimentally induced deafferentation (Taub et al. 1993). Deafferentation is a surgical technique whereby transsection of the dorsal root (i.e. dorsal rhizotomy) prevents sensory information from the limb reaching the dorsal horn. Interestingly, following deafferentation, it was observed that the animals avoided using their affected arm – despite the fact that the efferent system had been left intact. So in principle, the monkeys should be able to move their affected arms – but they didn't. Initially, this was explained by spinal shock following the acute injury, but as several weeks or months passed, this was no longer a plausible explanation. Instead, the behaviour was interpreted as a form of **'learned non-use'**, to which three processes are thought to contribute (Taub and Uswatte 2003). Firstly, the animal experiences punishment for using the affected limb (e.g. it falls when trying to climb). Secondly, it receives positive reinforcement for using the non-affected limb, as this is more effective and efficient. Thirdly, changes in brain organisation were observed, which will be discussed in more detail below. Thus, following initial spinal shock, the animal learns to cope with just the use of the non-affected limb, and may not even be aware of any recovery taking place in the affected limb.

In an attempt to force the animals to use the affected limb, researchers then experimented with constraining the non-affected limb, which resulted in the animals starting to make use of their affected limb more frequently.

From these initial animal experiments, the theory emerged that 'learned non-use' could develop after any type of CNS shock, including stroke (Taub et al. 1993). Research then focused on the question as to how stroke patients could be encouraged to make more use of their affected upper limb.

The first report on CIMT in humans was published by Ostendorf and Wolf in 1981, a single case study of a hemiplegic patient, showing promising findings. This was followed by a number of cohort studies and randomised controlled trials (RCTs) of patients with hemiplegia (e.g. Taub et al. 1993, van der Lee et al. 1999, Wolf et al. 1989), and the extremity constraint-induced therapy evaluation (EXCITE) trial, a multi-site randomised controlled clinical trial involving a total of 222 patients (Wolf et al. 2006). A Cochrane systematic review (Sirtori et al. 2009) involving 19 randomised controlled trials with 619 participants with stroke evaluated the effects of CIMT. The authors concluded that CIMT had significant and moderately positive effects on disability, arm motor function and arm motor impairment at the end of the intervention. However, long-term effects were more difficult to establish because of the few studies including long-term follow-up, loss to follow up and small sample sizes. There was no evidence at the time that CIMT had a positive effect on disability at 6-months after completing the intervention. The authors therefore recommended further studies with larger sample sizes and longer follow-up periods in future.

In addition to studying the *behavioural* effects of CIMT, an interesting line of enquiry explored the *neural correlates* of changes in upper limb behaviour. Using neuro-imaging techniques, a number of studies have provided evidence of neuroplastic changes occurring as a result of CIMT. For example, Liepert et al. (2001) used focal transcranial magnetic stimulation (TMS) to investigate changes in motor output areas of the paretic m. abductor pollicis brevis following CIMT. Associated with improvements in dexterity, increased motor cortex excitability was found, as well as recruitment of adjacent brain areas within the affected hemisphere. Using functional magnetic resonance imaging (fMRI), Levy et al. (2001) found an increase of activation nearer the lesion site in two stroke patients as a result of CIMT. Although such studies were typically small and lacked a control group, the results were, nevertheless, groundbreaking.

In summary, research on CIMT has sparked a fascinating line of enquiry into neurological rehabilitation, associating changes at a behavioural level with those at a neuronal level. In particular, the neuroimaging results indicate that the cortical representation of a particular part of the body is not fixed, but dependent on the amount of use. This suggests that training may change the way in which the brain is organised.

---

frontal lobes of the brain. In order to understand the effects of conditions affecting the brain, we will follow the afferent and efferent pathways, main functions and, finally, the effects of lesions on each of these brain areas.

Occipital lobe

Location

The occipital lobe is situated at the back of the brain (Fig. 5.1).

Input and output

The occipital lobes receive their input, or afferent information, from the eyes. The visual pathways are - illustrated in Figure 5.9. Note how the information pertaining to each visual field (i.e. visual information pertaining to either the left or right half of each retina) is represented in the occipital lobes: the left visual field in each eye is projected onto the right occipital lobe, while the right visual field is projected in the left occipital lobe. From the occipital lobes, three main visual pathways emanate: the dorsal stream, which connects with the parietal lobe; the ventral stream, which goes to the temporal lobe; and a middle pathway to the superior temporal sulcus.

Main functions and effects of lesions to the occipital lobe

The main function of the occipital lobe is **vision**. Given the dominant role of visual information in our lives, it is perhaps not surprising that a considerable part of the brain is dedicated to visual processing; compare the proportion of the cortex taken up by the occipital lobes with that by the parietal and temporal lobes. All visual information, conveyed through the optic tract, arrives in V1, the primary visual area. (Fig. 5.4, Table 5.2) From there, this information is 'sorted' and relayed to specialised brain areas, each of which is responsible for processing a specific type of visual information. There are areas designated to colour, motion and shape detection. This raw sensory information is then relayed to the secondary (association) areas, which are involved in perception by integrating this information into concepts that are meaningful (e.g. a person's face, or a stethoscope). As mentioned above, three main visual pathways originate from the occipital lobe.

The dorsal stream to the parietal lobe conveys visual information about the location of objects in space, which is used for visually guided reaching (i.e. visual information detailing 'how' an action should be carried out).

The ventral stream to the temporal lobe is thought to be primarily involved in the visual recognition of objects (i.e. detailing 'what' the visual information represents).

The middle stream is thought to be engaged in interaction between the dorsal and ventral stream.

There is a certain extent of **cerebral asymmetry**, or **hemispheric specialisation**, involving the occipital lobes, meaning that one hemisphere plays a more dominant role in a particular function compared to the other. The left occipital lobe is more involved in the visual recognition of words, whereas the right one plays a dominant role in the visual recognition of faces.

Lesions to the occipital lobe affect vision, depending on the side and site of the damage (see Fig. 5.10). A common problem after stroke, brain injury or a tumour to this part of the brain is **homonymous hemianopia**. *Homonymous* refers to the fact that the same side of the visual field has been affected in both eyes (i.e. both left or right), *anopia* refers to the inability to obtain visual information, while *hemi* stands for half-sided. Taken together, homonymous hemianopia refers to a condition whereby the person is unable to obtain information about one of the visual fields from both eyes. Note that this has nothing to do with 'blindness' as such, as the eyes and optic nerves are intact. Instead, the problem of homonymous hemianopia is located in the brain area responsible for processing visual information.

It may have a considerable impact on a person's life, as visual information pertaining to one side of their body and space may be left undetected. People with this condition may bump into obstacles they have not seen, fail to greet others appearing on the affected side, or have difficulty seeing food on one side of a plate. **Homonymous hemianopia** may

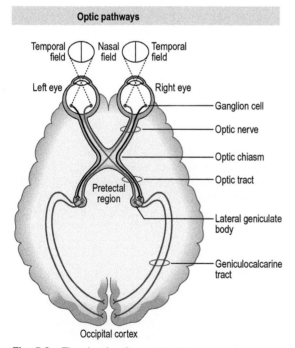

Optic pathways

Temporal field · Nasal field · Temporal field

Left eye · Right eye

Ganglion cell

Optic nerve

Optic chiasm

Optic tract

Pretectal region

Lateral geniculate body

Geniculocalcarine tract

Occipital cortex

Fig. 5.9 • The visual pathway. From Costanzo, with permission

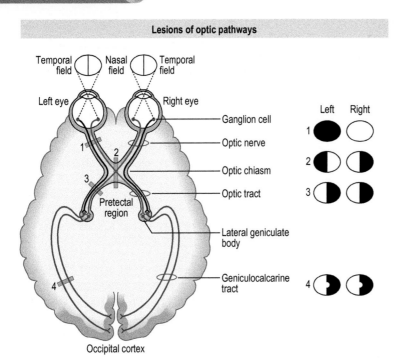

Lesions of optic pathways

Temporal field — Nasal field — Temporal field

Left eye — Right eye

Ganglion cell
Optic nerve
Optic chiasm
Optic tract
Pretectal region
Lateral geniculate body
Geniculocalcarine tract

Occipital cortex

Left   Right

1
2
3
4

Fig. 5.10 • Lesions of optic pathways. The impact of a lesion at point 1 to 4, indicating where visual loss would be experienced (black). Lesions at point 3 and 4 result in homonymous hemianopia (with macular sparing in the latter case). From Costanzo, with permission

contribute to hemi-inattention or neglect, which is a syndrome whereby the patient fails to attend to the affected side of the body and space. More detail about this syndrome can be found in Chapter 9.

Other visual deficits arising from lesions affecting the occipital lobes are problems with **visually guided movements** and **visual agnosias**. Problems with visually guided movement (e.g. reaching to grasp an object) may occur if visual information about the object and/or its location in space is not captured correctly, or in time for the action to occur. If visual information is absent or corrupted in the occipital lobe, it fails to correctly inform other areas of the brain, including the frontal lobe involved in planning the movement.

Visual agnosias are conditions where the patient is unable to identify an object (from the Greek a-gnosia, meaning 'having no knowledge of'). People may be able to *see* but be unable to *identify* a hairbrush or an apple – let alone distinguish different brushes or pieces of fruit. There are different types of visual agnosia, including object agnosia and face agnosia (or prosopagnosia). The latter may have a particular impact on the lives of patients and their family, as the patient may be able to see *a* face, but

unable to identify *whose* face it is. Education of the patient and their family is of particular importance to avoid misinterpretation of this situation, and possible detrimental impact on relationships. Using alternative strategies (e.g. one's voice) may be a useful strategy to compensate for prosopagnosia.

Parietal lobe

Location

Situated ventrally to the occipital lobes, and just rostral to the central sulcus, are the parietal lobes. Each parietal lobe comprises an anterior zone (including Brodmann's areas 1, 2, 3 and 43), and a posterior zone, which takes up the majority of space in this lobe.

Input and output

The afferent information into the parietal lobe comprises visual information from the occipital lobe through the dorsal stream, as well as information from the auditory and vestibular systems. Information from the parietal lobes is relayed to the frontal lobe, which prepares action on the basis of this information. More specifically, the combined visual/somatosensory information is relayed to motor areas, including the primary motor cortex (area 4), the frontal eye fields (area 8) to control eye movements, to the premotor and supplementary motor cortex (area 6), which are both involved in planning movement (see the section on the Frontal Lobe below). Information is also relayed to the prefrontal region (area 46), which is involved in short-term memory for events in space. From the frontal lobes, afferent pathways are routed back to the parietal lobes, thus providing reciprocal connections.

Main functions and effects of lesions to the parietal lobe

The main functions of the parietal lobe, part of what Luria labelled as the 'sensory unit', can be summarised as follows:

(1) somatic sensation and perception;
(2) integration of sensory information (i.e. cross-modal matching);
(3) using perception for action in viewer-centred space;
(4) attention,
(5) spatial cognition and
(6) symbol recognition.

More specifically, the anterior zone of the parietal lobe is involved in **processing somatosensory information**, i.e. tactile and proprioceptive feedback from the body (remember that the sensory homunculus is located in this region).

The posterior zone is involved in integrating sensory information, known as **cross-modal matching**. This means that information from different modes of sensation (i.e. visual, tactile, proprioceptive, acoustic) are matched to yield a meaningful, multimodal construct (e.g. your dog, with its unique look and way of moving, feel and sound). An important role of the posterior parietal lobe is also integrating somatosensory and visual information (via the dorsal stream from the occipital lobe) into a coherent concept of the body in space. This information can then be shunted to the frontal lobe, which plans movement based on this information, particularly visually guided action in user-centred space. Examples of this are reaching for a phone, cutting vegetables, or putting on a shoe: what these diverse actions have in common is that they rely heavily on matching visual information about the object and where it is in space, with proprioceptive information about

the body and the space in its immediate vicinity (i.e. user-centred space).

The posterior parietal lobe plays an important role in **attention;** it is involved in disengaging, moving and re-engaging attention to a particular location. This explains the connection with the frontal eye field (area 8 in the frontal lobe): the eyes follow the commands from the brain's attentional system. For reasons further explained in Chapter 9, the right parietal lobe is more involved in attention than the left. **Spatial cognition** is another role of the posterior parietal lobe, and involves the construction of a coordinate system of space in relation to the body, resulting in a 'body schema' with its distinction between left and right, front and back, and up and down, as well as different body parts.

The posterior zone of this lobe is also involved in symbol recognition, such as reading, **writing and arithmetic**. Although this appears to be disparate from spatial cognition mentioned before, symbol recognition does involve a distinctive spatial element. Consider reading; you need to be able to distinguish between a 'b' and a 'd', which comprise similar components (i.e. an 'l' and an 'o') – but the relative location of the components determines the meaning of each symbol as a whole. Similarly, in arithmetic, the relative spatial locations of components determine the meaning of each symbol, e.g. compare 31 with 13.

Given the diverse and complex functions of the parietal lobe, it is perhaps not surprising that lesions to this part of the brain can manifest themselves in very different ways. Lesions to the anterior zone are likely to cause **deficits in sensation**, e.g. hypesthesia (i.e. a reduced level of sensation), allodynia (i.e. normal sensations are experienced as painful), or errors in proprioception.

Lesions to the posterior parietal lobe may be apparent through deficits in **attention**, including difficulties shifting attention towards the affected side. This condition, known as 'hemi-inattention' or '**neglect**' will be further explained in Chapter 9.

Deficits in **spatial orientation** and **body schema** may also result from lesions to the posterior parietal lobe: patients may demonstrate confusion between left and right, up and down, front and back, their own body parts, other people's body parts and even between body parts and items of clothing. An activity in which body schema confusion may be particularly apparent is dressing; patients may get confused in identifying which part of a top goes where, or confuse their arm with yours – a form of **apraxia**, a disorder of learned skilled movement that is not caused by impaired movement, sensation, comprehension or intellect per se (see Chapter 9 for more detail). The problem with apraxia appears to be integrating relevant information about objects (if applicable), one's body and space, in planning and executing a purposeful activity. An excellent case study is described in *The man who mistook his wife for a hat* (Sacks 1985).

Interestingly, although the frontal lobe has often been associated with intellect, it is damage affecting the parietal lobe that may show up in IQ tests as errors in reading, writing and arithmetic – symptoms of **impaired symbol recognition**.

Temporal lobe

Location

The temporal lobes are situated ventrally to the occipital lobe, rostral to the central sulcus and underneath the temporal bones of the skull. The temporal lobes comprise a range of regions, including the primary auditory cortex, the secondary auditory and visual cortex, the limbic cortex and amygdala, as well as the hippocampus.

Input and output

The temporal lobes receive a wide range of input from many sensory systems, including the visual, auditory, gustatory and olfactory systems. Output from the temporal lobes is relayed to the parietal and frontal association areas, the limbic system and basal ganglia, with numerous interconnections between these areas.

Main functions and effects of lesions to the temporal lobe

The temporal lobe may be loosely considered as one's 'multimedia system', including all the memories that images, music or smells may evoke. The main roles of the temporal lobes in behaviour can be summarised as follows:

(1) processing auditory information;
(2) processing visual information;
(3) adding emotional experience to sensory information; and
(4) long-term memory.

It follows that lesions to this part of the brain may affect any or a combination of these functions.

Problems with **processing auditory information** may be apparent in difficulties with selecting sounds. Typically, patients may complain that they have problems listening to a conversation in a group. This problem is aggravated if there is additional background noise. In this scenario, some information needs to be selected and attended to, while other information is to be ignored. The clinical implication of this phenomenon is that practising a new skill in a noisy environment may not be the best place for such patients.

Damage to the temporal lobes may also result in problems with **perceiving speech and music**. Lesions to the left temporal lobe are likely to result in deficits in **language comprehension** (see chapter 11 Communication). Speech production may appear to be relatively intact, but patients tend to have difficulty processing feedback from speech sounds – including their own. A lesion affecting the right temporal lobe usually does not affect language comprehension per se, but may impact on **music perception**. It is important to be aware of this, as the meaning of a communication is conveyed not only through actual words, but also through our tone of voice ('c'est le ton qui fait la musique'). For example, there are a number of ways in which you could say 'I told you so', including an accusatory and a playful variation. If a person has problems perceiving the tone in which this statement was made, they may misunderstand the meaning entirely. The dominant role of the left temporal lobe in speech and the right temporal lobe in music is another example of hemispheric specialisation.

Processing visual information is another important role of the temporal lobe. In contrast to the parietal lobe, which processes visual information primarily in relation to action ('how'), the temporal lobe processes visual information primarily for the purpose of recognition (e.g. recognising a tooth brush and distinguishing this from a hairbrush). This information is relayed from the occipital lobe to the temporal lobe through the ventral stream. A deficit in object recognition is also known as **visual agnosia**.

The temporal lobe is also involved in recognising and using so-called 'contextual information', which means adjusting one's language and behaviour according to a specific situation. For example, compare the language you might use in a professional situation involving a patient, with a family occasion involving your siblings. People with temporal lobe lesions may have difficulty **using contextual information** and the result can have far-reaching effects on social relationships. Inappropriate language or gestures, or misplaced jokes may be interpreted by others as 'insensitive behaviour', 'altered personality' or 'social blunders'. It is essential for health-care professionals to understand the causes of such behaviours, and recognise that they may be the result of the brain lesion.

Finally, a key role of the temporal lobe is long-term memory. In-depth and longitudinal analysis of patient H.M. by Scoville and Milner (1957) has contributed much to our appreciation of the contribution of this part of the brain to memory. Chapter 9 tells the story of H.M. This showed for the first time that brain lesions affecting the temporal lobe may cause long-term memory loss **(amnesia)**. Again, there is some evidence of hemispheric specialisation, as damage to the left temporal lobe tends to result in loss of verbal memory, while damage to the right temporal lobe causes deficits in non-verbal memory (e.g. recognising music, or drawings).

Frontal lobe

Location

The frontal lobe is the part of the brain situated ventrally to the central sulcus. This lobe in particular has shown considerable expansion in the process of evolution. Long thought to be associated with intelligence (probably a myth stemming from the work by the phrenologists (Chapter 2)), converging evidence has shown that the frontal lobe is involved in action, from the initial planning stages through to issuing actual motor commands (remember that Luria coined this part of the brain the 'action unit'). The frontal lobe comprises the following main areas:

- Primary motor cortex (area 4)
- Premotor and supplementary motor area (area 6) with the frontal eye field (area 8)
- Broca's area 44
- Pre-frontal cortex.

Input and output

Input to the premotor areas comes from the posterior parietal lobe via the dorsal stream, and the prefrontal area, while output is issued directly to corticospinal projections or indirectly to the primary motor cortex. Output from the motor cortex is projected to the basal ganglia and spinal and cranial motor neurones for the control of limb, digit and facial movement respectively.

Input to the prefrontal areas includes both visual streams (i.e. the ventral stream from the temporal lobes and the dorsal stream from the parietal lobes), as well as other areas within the temporal and parietal lobes. Output is relayed back to the temporal and parietal lobes, the cingulate cortex, basal ganglia, red nucleus, hypothalamus and amygdala. In summary, the frontal lobes receive extensive information directly or indirectly from virtually all areas of the brain, and relay processed information back to an extensive number of brain areas, again demonstrating parallel, distributed and reciprocal connectivity.

Main functions and effects of lesions to the frontal lobe

The main functions of the frontal lobe can be summarised as executive in nature. More specifically, different regions within the frontal lobe are responsible for:

(1) movement;
(2) planning and thinking;
(3) executive control of behaviour and
(4) memory.

The following impairments and activity limitations may be observed as a result of a condition affecting the frontal lobes. Lesions to the primary motor cortex (area 4) may affect a range of **motor performance** parameters, including fine motor control, strength (i.e. paresis), speed, motor programming as in sequencing actions, gaze control (i.e. difficulty directing gaze to the contralateral side) and speech (i.e. Broca's **aphasia**).

Lesions to the premotor cortex are likely to affect the programming stages of action (see Chapter 7), including a more generic loss of **planning** and **behaviour**, such as divergent thinking, strategy formation and spontaneous behaviour. Divergent thinking is required in situations where an established behaviour turns out to be ineffective, e.g. your normal transport to university has been cancelled, and you need to find a different way to get to your destination. What do you do? You may find a range of different options to get to university, or you decide to work from home and change your plans altogether. A person with loss of divergent thinking may have difficulty coming up with such solutions, and may instead decide to run all the way along the usual bus route. Strategy formation is another form of problem solving, for example you decide to sacrifice a social evening with your friends in order to be fit for a triathlon the next day. People with impaired strategy formation may miss important goals in life, as they lack the strategic decision making needed to achieve their goals.

Lesions to the prefrontal cortex may affect more complex **executive functions**, and result in risk taking and rule breaking, difficulties following instructions or adjusting behaviour following feedback, disinhibition and impaired social and sexual behaviour, and in some cases pseudodepression – or pseudopsychopathic behaviour. Noteworthy are the connections between the prefrontal cortex and structures involved in the autonomic system (i.e. the hypothalamus) and emotion (i.e. the amygdala), mediating integration between decision-making and emotion. Taken together, this cluster of problems is known as executive dysfunction, which is more fully discussed in Chapter 12.

Finally, the frontal lobes play a role in **memory** – not so much the recognition of objects, or faces, but remembering the *sequence* of events. For example, imagine you need to find an answer to a question and decide to use the internet. While browsing, you may get diverted into all sorts of topics that are only peripherally related to the question of interest. You may also look up different sources of information, and accidentally revisit the same several times. Sequential memory, the ability to remember what you have just done, is essential for making progress in this kind of task. Impaired sequential memory may, therefore, result in a person getting lost in a task, repeating certain steps and omitting others, and, finally, failing to complete the task.

In summary, we have looked at each part of the brain, examined information coming into and emanating from the area, and explored the main roles in behaviour, thinking and emotion. Having a good understanding of this information enables you to reason what the effects of lesions to each part of the brain might be. Given the scope of this book, we have inevitably needed to simplify matters, so further reading is indicated for more in-depth and specialist information.

As a note of caution against over-simplifying matters, it is essential to appreciate that in real life, lesions to the brain are likely to cross anatomical boundaries and affect a number of areas at the same time. For example, a malignant brain tumour may directly affect several brain regions with its invasive growth, while pressure on surrounding tissues may have an even more extensive effect. Furthermore, everyone's neural network is wired in different ways, depending on both genetic and environmental factors, as well as experience. Therefore, considerable variation between individuals in the relationship between the brain and behaviour is inevitable.

Synopsis: the emerging brain–behaviour puzzle

Having explored the role of each cortical area of the brain in isolation, how can we summarise the big picture? This section provides an overview of the key principles of the relationship between the brain and behaviour:

- The brain is the most **complex** structure in the universe, so it is unrealistic to expect simple answers to anything about brain function!
- Function is **localised** in the brain, which means that the brain comprises neural networks that are dedicated to specific functions. Examples are networks specialised in motion detection or the production of consonants. This implies that discrete activities may be disrupted by local lesions. However, it would be incorrect to think that each function has a specific site in the brain, e.g. Chapter 13 will show that there is no single brain area devoted to 'emotion'. Many functions are complex and comprise numerous subroutines (e.g. consider writing a sentence, or finding a route to a destination), and rely on **integration** between dedicated networks for specific subroutines.
- Normal function requires **integration** between different brain centres and pathways. It is essential to appreciate that normal brain function relies on communication between various parts of the brain. This involves both brain areas AND the neural pathways within and between them. For example, consider a person with apraxia who brushes their hair with a toothbrush. Although this error manifests itself in action, the cause may not reside within the frontal lobe per se; it is possible that a lesion in the association area of the occipital lobe affects the person's object recognition. This information is then relayed, from the occipital to the frontal lobe via the temporal and the

parietal lobes. All that these brain areas have to work with is corrupted information. The end result is an error in action, but the cause is further down the information processing process.

- **Hemispheric integration and specialisation**. As demonstrated by the extensive number of commissural fibres, hemispheric integration plays an important role in behaviour. However, there are some behaviours where one of the hemispheres plays a dominant role (this does not mean that the contralateral side does not play a role). In general, the left hemisphere is more specialised in verbal activities (including recognition of text and numbers, production of speech and language) while the right hemisphere is more dominant in non-verbal tasks, such as recognizing music or musical components of speech and face recognition. This depends to some extent on hand dominance: in 96% of right-handed and 70% of left-handed people, the left hemisphere is dominant in speech and language.

- There is **plasticity**. The clinical relevance of neuroplasticity cannot be emphasised enough to health-care professionals. Plasticity is the ability of the nervous system to adapt and modify its responses to change, for example training in speech, dressing or walking. Although neuroplasticity reduces with age, it is never too late to learn! The challenge for health-care professionals is to establish the most

appropriate time, content and intensity of rehabilitation, to optimise the functionality and durability of ensuing neuroplastic changes.

SELF-ASSESSMENT QUESTIONS

1. Can you describe/draw the gross anatomical organisation of the brain with its four lobes, including the afferent and efferent pathways of each lobe?
2. Which methods have been used to investigate the relationship between the brain and behaviour and what information does each convey? What are the strengths and drawbacks of each method?
3. What is plasticity and how does it express itself? What are the differences in neuroplastic mechanisms between lesions of the peripheral and central nervous system?
4. For each of the four cerebral lobes:
   - What are its main functions in terms of behaviour, cognition and/or emotion?
   - What are the main effects of a lesion affecting each part of the brain?
5. Why is there no simple one-to-one relationship between brain area and function?
6. According to current knowledge and understanding, what are the key principles of the relationship between the brain and behaviour?
7. Discuss the relevance of knowledge of the brain–behaviour relationship for neurological rehabilitation.

Further reading

Bear, M.F., Connors, B.W., Paradiso, M.A., 2007. Neuroscience: exploring the brain, third ed. Lippincott Williams & Wilkins, Baltimore.

Chen, Z.L., Yu, W.M., Strickland, S., 2007. Peripheral regeneration. Annu. Rev. Neurosci. 30, 209–233.

Clark, D.L., Boutros, N.N., Mendez, M.F., 2010. The Brain and Behaviour. An introduction to behavioural neuroanatomy, third ed. Cambridge University Press, Cambridge.

Sacks, O., 1995. An Anthropologist on Mars. Picador, London.

Smith, E.E., Kosslyn, S.M., 2007. Cognitive Psychology. Mind and brain. Pearson Prentice Hall, New Jersey.

Tallis, R., 2008. The Kingdom of Infinite Space. A fantastical journey around your head, Atlantic Books, London.

Vargas, M.E., Barres, B.A., 2007. Why is Wallerian degeneration in the CNS so slow? Annu. Rev. Neurosci. 30, 153–179.

References

Buma, F.E., Lindeman, E., Ramsey, N.F., et al., 2010. Functional neuroimaging studies of early upper limb recovery after stroke: a systematic review of the literature. Neurorehabil. Neural. Repair. 24, 589–608.

Calautti, C., Baron, J.C., 2003. Functional neuroimaging studies of motor recovery after stroke in adults: a review. Stroke 34, 1553–1566.

Drevets, W.C., Videen, T.O., Price, J.L., et al., 1992. A functional anatomy of unipolar depression. J. Neurosci. 12, 3628–3642.

Grotta, J.C., Noser, E.A., Ro, T., et al., 2004. Constraint-induced movement therapy. Stroke 35, 2699–2701.

Haines, D.E., 2005. Fundamental Neuroscience for Basic and Clinical Applications. Churchill Livingstone Elsevier, London.

Hodics, T., Cohen, L.G., Cramer, S.C., 2006. Functional imaging of intervention effects in stroke motor rehabilitation. Arch. Phys. Med. Rehabil. 87 (12 Suppl. 1), 36–42.

Kleim, J.A., Schwerin, S., 2010. Motor map plasticity: a neural substrate for improving motor function after stroke. In: Cramer, S.C., Nudo, R.J. (Eds.), Brain Repair after Stroke. Cambridge University Press, Cambridge, pp. 1–10.

Kolb, B., Whishaw, I.Q., 1996. Fundamentals of Human Neuropsychology, fourth ed. W.H. Freeman & Co., New York.

Kolb, B., Whishaw, I.Q., 2008. Fundamentals of Human Neuropsychology, sixth ed. Worth Publishers, New York.

Koski, L., Mernar, T.J., Dobkin, B.H., 2004. Immediate and long-term changes in corticomotor output in response to rehabilitation: correlation with functional improvement in chronic stroke. Neurorehabil. Neural. Repair. 18, 230–249.

Levy, C.E., Nichols, D.S., Schmalbrock, P.M., et al., 2001. Functional MRI evidence of cortical reorganization in upper-limb stroke hemiplegia treated with constraint-induced movement therapy. Am. J. Phys. Med. Rehabil. 80 (1), 4–12.

Liepert, J., Uhde, I., Gräf, S., et al., 2001. Motor cortex plasticity during forced-use therapy in stroke patients: a preliminary study. J. Neurol. 248 (4), 315–321.

Luria, A.R., 1987. The Man With a Shattered World. The history of a brain wound. Harvard University Press, Cambridge, Massachusetts.

Nudo, R.J., 2003a. Adaptive plasticity in motor cortex: implications for Rehabilitation after Brain Injury. J. Rehabil. Med. (Suppl.), 7–10.

Nudo, R.J., 2003b. Functional and structural plasticity in motor cortex: implications for stroke recovery. Phys. Med. Rehabil. Clin. N. Am. 14, S57–S76.

Nudo, R.J., Milliken, G.W., 1996. Reorganization of movement representations in primary motor cortex following focal ischemic infarcts in adult squirrel monkeys. J. Neurophysiol. 75, 2144–2149.

Nudo, R.J., Barvay, S., Kleim, J.A., 2000. Role of neuroplasticity in functional recovery after stroke. In: Levin, H.S., Grafman, J. (Eds.), Cerebral Reorganisation of Function after Brain Damage. Oxford University Press, New York.

Ostendorf, C.G., Wolf, S.L., 1981. Effect of forced use of the upper extremity of a hemiplegic patient on changes in function. Phys. Ther. 61, 1022–1028.

Sacks, O., 1985. The Man Who Mistook his Wife for a Hat. Pan Books, London.

Schallert, T., Bland, S.T., Leisure, J.L., et al., 2000. Motor rehabilitation, use-related neural events, and reorganisation of the brain after injury. In: Levin, H.S., Grafman, J. (Eds.), Cerebral Reorganisation of Function after Brain damage. Oxford University Press, New York.

Scoville, W.B., Milner, B., 1957. Loss of recent memory after bilateral hippocampal lesions. J. Neurol. Neurosurg. Psychiatry 20, 11–21.

Sirtori, V., Corbetta, D., Moja, L., et al., 2009. Constraint-induced movement therapy for upper extremities in stroke patients. Cochrane Database Syst. Rev. 4, CD004433. doi:10.1002/14651858.

Taub, E., Uswatte, G., 2003. Constraint-induced movement therapy: bridging from the primate laboratory to the stroke rehabilitation laboratory. J. Rehabil. Med. 41, 34–40.

Taub, E., Miller, N.E., Novack, T.A., et al., 1993. Technique to improve chronic motor deficit after stroke. Arch. Phys. Med. Rehabil. 74, 347–354.

van der Lee, J.H., Wagenaar, R.C., Lankhorst, G.J., et al., 1999. Forced use of the upper extremity in chronic stroke patients; results from a single blind randomised clinical trial. Stroke 30, 2369–2375.

Wittenberg, G.F., Chen, R., Ishii, K., et al., 2003. Constraint-induced therapy in stroke: magnetic stimulation motor maps and cerebral activation. Neurorehabil. Neural. Repair. 17, 48–57.

Wolf, S.L., Lecraw, D.E., Barton, L.A., et al., 1989. Forced use of hemiplegic upper extremities to reverse the effect of learned nonuse among chronic stroke and head-injured patients. Exp. Neurol. 104, 125–132.

Wolf, S.L., Winstein, C.J., Miller, J.P., et al., 2006. Effect of constraint-induced movement therapy on upper extremity function 3 to 9 months after stroke: the EXCITE randomized clinical trial. JAMA 296, 2095–2104.

Movement and coordination

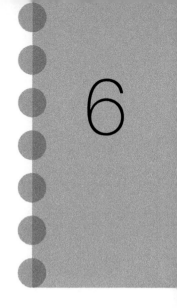

6

CHAPTER CONTENTS

> ### LEARNING OUTCOMES
>
> At the end of this chapter, you should be able to:
> - describe the different types of movement, i.e. reflex and voluntary
> - explain what is meant by the term spasticity and compare and contrast this with rigidity, hypertonia and contracture
> - explain the role of the various brain areas, highlighted in the text, in movement
> - describe the problems associated with cerebral palsy and the use of anti-spasmodic therapies to treat the motor symptoms of the condition.

Movement is fundamental to human life; not only is it essential for survival and self care (e.g. feeding, dressing), it is involved in expressing ourselves (e.g. through speech, gestures, music and art) and participating in society (e.g. by engaging in an occupation, or looking after a relative). When a health condition affects movement, it affects an essential body function, and it may also have far-reaching impact on engaging in functional activity and life roles. It is, therefore, essential that allied health professionals involved in neurological rehabilitation have a sound understanding of the neurophysiological processes involved in normal movement, as well as how different neurological conditions may impact on movement and functional activity.

Movement of our body, as well as aspects of support and control functions, usually involves the coordinated contraction and relaxation of the skeletal muscles. The most basic form of coordinated movement occurs in what are known as reflex movements involving, in the main, the spinal cord, the brainstem and the peripheral nerves. These basic reflex movements are different from the more complex controlled movements seen in voluntary activity, which bring into play other brain areas, including the motor cortex, basal ganglia and cerebellum. Before going on to discuss these types of movements in more detail, it is important to re-establish our understanding of the contraction process utilised by skeletal muscle.

The aim of this chapter is to provide you with a refresher of skeletal muscle contraction, before it goes on to explain the control of muscle contraction. We will start with the basic building block of movement, i.e. the reflex, and work up to increasingly complex movement. The role of key parts of the nervous system in motor control, in particular that of the motor cortex, basal ganglia and cerebellum, will be explained, alongside examples of clinical case studies. The neurophysiological basis of key concepts in disordered motor control, i.e. spasticity and rigidity, as well as disordered tone and contracture which are often encountered in clinical practice, will be explained. Finally, the chapter will explain the action of commonly used pharmacological interventions for spasticity.

Introduction

The contraction of the skeletal muscle involves the complex interaction of four specific proteins: actin, myosin, troponin and tropomyosin. Many individual skeletal muscle units (i.e. sarcomeres) fuse together to form the long fibres which have one end attached to the tendon, which is in turn attached to the skeleton. It is this connection that is responsible for muscle contraction resulting in skeletal movement. The structure of normal muscle can be seen in Figure 6.1.

Unlike cardiac and smooth muscle, which have regular contraction and relaxation patterns, skeletal muscle usually only contracts under the influence of neuronal stimulation. This stimulation occurs at the neuromuscular junction (Fig. 6.2), where the neurotransmitter involved is acetylcholine. The motor neurone releases acetylcholine which travels across the junction and interacts with nicotinic cholinergic receptors on the skeletal muscle fibres. This receptor stimulation results in the creation of a muscle action potential, brought about by the opening of voltage-gated sodium channels, which in turn causes the release of calcium from the sarcoplasmic reticulum (the intracellular store of calcium). Inside the skeletal muscle cell can be found a complex formed by two proteins, troponin and tropomyosin, which, on interaction, inhibits the interaction of the two contractile proteins, actin and myosin. The calcium which enters binds to the troponin and displaces the troponin–tropomyosin complex, thereby allowing the actin and myosin to interact. This leads to the contraction of the muscle via the sliding filament theory. As calcium levels fall, the troponin–tropomyosin complex is re-established, the actin–myosin interaction is again inhibited and the muscle relaxes (note that the muscle is only relaxed when neural transmission halts – it is unable to elongate (stretch) itself!).

Now that we have established how the muscle contraction comes about let us move on and look at the control of the different types of movement mentioned earlier.

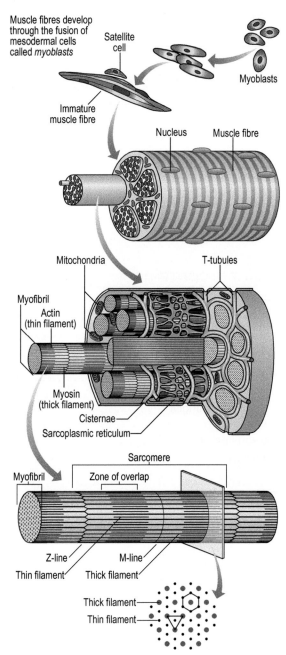

Fig. 6.1 • The structure of normal muscle. From Kindlen 2003, with permission

Types of movement

Probably one of the most straightforward ways to classify movement is to split it into either **reflex movements** or **willed (voluntary) movements**. The key brain areas involved in the control of voluntary movement include the motor cortex (and associated cortical areas), the basal ganglia and the cerebellum. What makes these areas so important is the fact that they are involved in the control and coordination of our movements and, as a result, play a key part in everyday functions that we take for granted: maintaining posture, moving around, using our hands.

Fig. 6.2 • The neuromuscular junction.
From Spina 2008, with permission

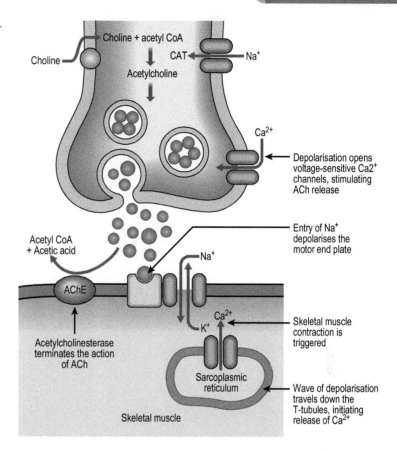

Think of this the next time you lean forward to pick up a watermelon in the supermarket and **don't** fall head first into the fruit and veg!

Reflex movements

You will recall from Chapter 1 that reflex movements were first described by Charles Sherrington, the eminent British pathologist and neurophysiologist, at the turn of the 19th century. Reflex movements are those automatic movements that happen without us even thinking about them. Probably one of the best-known examples of a reflex movement is the knee jerk that follows a tap on the patellar tendon just below the knee. This is a relatively straightforward example of a reflex and comes about following the reactive contraction of the quadriceps femoris (thigh) muscle in response to the tap (which had caused it to stretch). A more complex example of a reflex movement can be seen when there is a coordinated muscle response, allowing us to maintain our balance following a large push, for example.

Simple reflex movements, like the knee jerk, are obviously very localised and only involve a small number of sensory receptors linked to only a few muscle groups and just one synapse in the spinal cord; hence this is known as a **monosynaptic stretch reflex** (M1 response), which has a latency (lag) of around 30–50 ms. The more complex reflex movements arise following the integration of sensory information from more muscles, which results in a complex interaction of many muscle groups leading to a higher level of coordinated control. Reflexes involving more synapses are known as **polysynaptic stretch reflexes** (or M2 response), which have a latency of 50–80 ms. This is because the stimulus travels up to higher levels in the central nervous system, and the efferent commands may involve multiple muscle groups. M2 responses allow for more flexibility and modulation than the basic M1 response.

The basic structure of a reflex arc involves sensory input and motor output linked by small interneurones. The reflex movement initiated is very much dependent on the particular muscle mass stimulated. If we take the example of limb movements, contraction of the extensor muscles leads to extension of the limb, whereas contraction of the flexor muscles leads to withdrawal of the limb. It is the reflex withdrawal of our limbs and body that gives us a level of protection when we encounter potentially harmful stimuli, e.g. touching a hot surface. One other aspect of the reflex movement system is that there is also a level of variability of response within it. If your hand were to come into contact with a slight heat, producing a low level of pain, then withdrawal of the arm would be seen (Fig. 6.3). However, if the thermal stimulus was exceptionally hot, producing a high level of pain, then a withdrawal of the whole body would be seen. This variability in response can be achieved through so-called '**triggered reactions**', with a latency of 80–120 ms. These reactions can result in complex responses, involving a number of muscle groups which may be relatively remote from the area stimulated originally. Note that we are still within the domain of reflexes; **voluntary reaction time** (the M3 response) takes longer with a latency

of 120–180 ms, as various stages of information processing need to be dealt with (see Chapter 7).

In addition to this flexor reflex there is also the stretch reflex (Fig. 6.4), which occurs when, as the name implies, a muscle is stretched. The level of muscle activation observed can vary from individual to individual and can be altered under certain conditions, e.g. spinal injury, stroke, etc. The abnormal changes in muscle activation that are observed arise from a reduction in the level of neuronal impulses coming from the brain areas involved in movement. These efferent neuronal impulses are normally inhibitory and if they are removed, or reduced, a hyperexcitation of the α and γ motor neurones can be seen. This hyperexcitation may lead to muscle rigidity or spasticity.

Spasticity, rigidity, hypertonia and contracture

Spasticity is a common problem in neurological conditions and is considered as one component of the upper motor neurone (UMN) syndrome. The UMN syndrome is a constellation of symptoms that are traditionally divided into 'positive' and 'negative' (Barnes and Johnson 2001). Positive symptoms are associated with an exaggeration of motor activity, whereas negative symptoms arise from a lack of it (Table 6.1). A full discussion of positive symptoms of the UMN other than spasticity can be found in Sheean (1998, 2001).

Although the prevalence of spasticity is not precisely known across different neurological conditions, it has been estimated that approximately 38% of stroke patients develop this impairment in the first year after the acute event (Watkins et al, 2002). Particularly

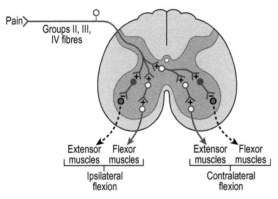

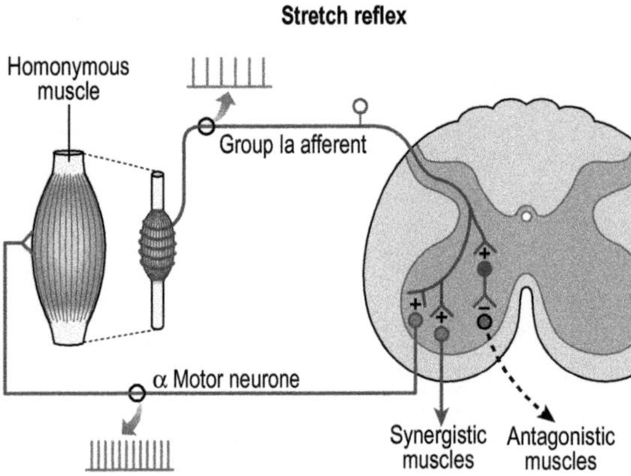

Fig. 6.3 • The flexor-withdrawal reflex. From Spina 2008, with permission

Fig. 6.4 • The stretch reflex. From Costanzo 2006, with permission

Table 6.1 Examples of 'positive' and 'negative' symptoms of the upper motor neurone syndrome. (Based on Barnes & Johnson, 2001)

Upper motor neurone syndrome	
Positive features	**Negative features**
Spasticity	Hypotonia
Rigidity	Paresis
Spastic dystonia	Loss of dexterity
Associated reaction	Fatigueability
Clasp-knife phenomenon	
Clonus	
Spasm	
Co-contraction	
Increased tendon reflexes	
Abnormal reflexes (e.g. Babinski)	

when it involves the upper limb, spasticity may cause pain and interfere with the patient's self-care and ability to carry out activities of daily living (Barnes & Johnson, 2001).

There is considerable confusion in the literature about the term 'spasticity', and, moreover, this term is often used interchangeably with the term 'high tone', 'hypertonia' or 'hypertonicity'. We will see further down that these two terms are not the same, however.

A traditional description of spasticity, put forward by Lance in 1980, is:

'a motor disorder, characterised by a velocity-dependent increase in tonic stretch reflexes (muscle tone) with exaggerated tendon jerks, resulting from hyper-excitability of the stretch reflex as one component of the upper motor neurone (UMN) syndrome'

Although very precise with its emphasis on the stretch reflex, this definition is perhaps too narrow to be clinically useful. Indeed, in clinical practice, the term 'spasticity' often refers to the UMN syndrome in its entirety (Edwards 2002). This can also be problematic, since different components of the UMN syndrome (e.g. paresis and spasms) may require quite different interventions (e.g. muscle strengthening and anti-spasmodic drugs respectively). To enhance the clinical applicability of Lance's ideas, and yet to acknowledge the clear distinction between positive and negative components of the UMN syndrome, a more recent definition of spasticity was put forward as follows:

'Spasticity is disordered sensori-motor control, resulting from an upper motor neurone lesion, presenting as intermittent or sustained involuntary activation of muscles.'

(Pandyan et al 2005, p. 5)

You can see that, in contrast to the traditional Lance definition, this more recent definition suggests that 'spasticity' is an umbrella term for all of the active, positive symptoms of the UMN syndrome. Please note that spasticity is about the *active* (as well as positive) symptoms of the UMN – we will come back to this when we introduce the term 'muscle tone'. In this book, we will use the more recent definition.

Thus, spasticity is identified by the presence of exaggerated reflexes, resulting in an increased resistance to passive movement (RTPM) of the limbs. RTPM means that, if a clinician passively moves the affected limb through its range of movement (e.g. from elbow flexion to extension), they will feel a certain level of stiffness. In the case of spasticity, this will be higher compared to normal. In the case of flaccidity, this will be lower than normal. Additionally, the movement may not be smooth; in the case of spasticity, there may be a 'catch' where the stiffness suddenly increases. In line with Lance's definition, spasticity is velocity dependent, which means that the faster the passive movement, the higher the resistance encountered.

With **rigidity** (which is often seen in Parkinson's disease), however, the muscles are tensed in the absence of any form of movement, active or passive, while agonists and antagonists of the limbs are similarly affected (Rothwell 1994). The differences in muscle activation which are observed under both of these conditions are due, in the main, to the specific brain areas affected, as we will see later in this chapter.

Earlier, we mentioned that 'spasticity' and '**hypertonia**' are different phenomena. Both are commonly assessed in the clinic by testing RTPM. Let us examine more closely what happens when we test RTPM: which tissues are being stretched? Indeed, both muscle and non-contractile soft tissue are being elongated. It follows then that both 'neurogenic' (i.e. reflexes) and non-neurogenic (i.e. biomechanical) factors contribute to RTPM (Johnson 2001, Katz and Rymer 1989). Figure 6.5 gives an overview of these two distinct contributions to RTPM.

It is important to remember that the clinical phenomenon of 'muscle tone' is a *combination* of both neurogenic and non-neurogenic factors (Fig. 6.5),

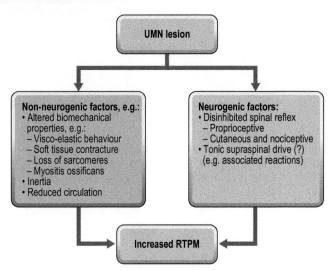

Fig. 6.5 • A dissection of resistance to passive movement (RTPM) following an UMN lesion: neurogenic and non-neurogenic factors. Based on Johnson (2001) and Sheean (1998)

i.e. muscle activation and biomechanical factors, and careful examination is required to differentiate between these two. Why? In theory, patients may present with increased 'tone', but little or no increased muscle activation. This may be the case in patients in whom soft tissue adhesions and shortening are the primary causes for reduced joint range of motion, and muscle activation is absent following long-standing inactivity and atrophy. In more extreme cases, lack of voluntary muscle activity may result in fixed joint positions, known as **contractures**. Such patients, however, would not be indicated to benefit from pharmacological interventions aimed at reducing spasticity. Ideally therefore, EMG (electromyographic) examination should be carried out prior to administering such drugs.

An interesting discussion on the role of biomechanical factors in RTPM can be found in Walsh (1992). Walsh debunked – elegantly and effectively – the commonly held belief that resting tone is the manifestation of minuscule activation of skeletal musculature. Walsh's arguments are based on data from Basmajian (1957), who reported a complete absence of electrical activity in relaxed muscles of normal subjects. In his own work, Walsh (1992) found no change in tone following the administration of anaesthetics and nerve blocking agents in non-impaired subjects. These findings indicate that 'resting tone' in non-impaired people has no neural input but represents a biomechanical property of soft tissue instead.

Having introduced the term 'spasticity' as an expression of abnormal motor control, let us now look at a selection of the brain areas involved in the initiation, control and coordination of movement.

Motor areas of the brain

When we choose to initiate any form of willed movement (e.g. turning a page of a book to see what wonders lie on the next page – as you will be doing shortly!) the control of the muscles required to make that movement is coordinated using three key areas:

- Motor cortex
- Basal ganglia
- Cerebellum.

The initiation of the command originates in the cortex, with the basal ganglia and the cerebellum involved in refinement and adjustment.

The motor cortex

The primary motor cortex lies in the frontal lobe of the brain and its location can be identified in Figure 6.6. In order to initiate a movement, signals are passed from the association areas of the cortex which are involved in perception and thinking. The motor cortex, in turn, passes the information on to the upper motor neurones required to process the movement. This control that the motor cortex has over muscle contraction (and hence movement) can occur either directly or indirectly as seen in Figure 6.7.

If the motor cortex was to be damaged (e.g. following a stroke) our voluntary movement would obviously have the potential to be significantly impaired. In this situation – although the voluntary movements would be weak (paresis) – the muscles

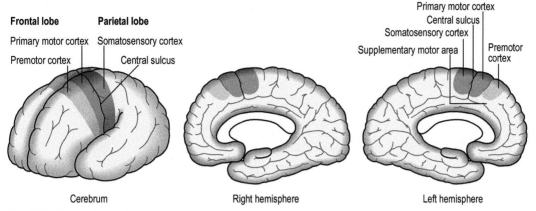

Fig. 6.6 • The motor cortex. From Kindlen 2003, with permission

Fig. 6.7 • Direct and indirect motor pathways

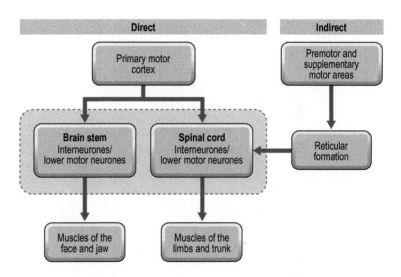

could still be activated reflexly (as mentioned earlier). Not only is it the case that the reflex activity could still be present, in some cases they could even be exaggerated. This is due to the fact that the upper motor neurones of the motor cortex play a role in inhibiting reflexes such as the knee jerk. Therefore, if the cortex is damaged the inhibitory influence of the cortex is removed, leading to an exaggeration – or even alteration – of reflexes. If this enhancement occurs with the stretch reflex, spasticity can occur. Following an upper motor neurone lesion, new and abnormal reflexes may also be observed, e.g. the Babinski reflex. This change in reflex activity could be seen as a **maladaptive form of neuroplasticity**. The occurrence of spasticity in cerebral palsy will be discussed later in this chapter.

The basal ganglia

The basal ganglia is the name given to the cluster of interconnected subcortical nuclei which lie deep within the cerebral hemispheres. In addition to being linked to each other, the nuclei are also connected to the thalamus (see Fig. 6.8).

As the basal ganglia receives input from the various parts of the association areas of the cortex it is, therefore, supplied with information about our thoughts (you could say our intended movements). The neuronal information 'spins' round the basal ganglia before passing to the thalamus and then on to the motor cortex. Much of the information on the role of the basal ganglia has been obtained from studies involving patients with damage to the area. The most obvious

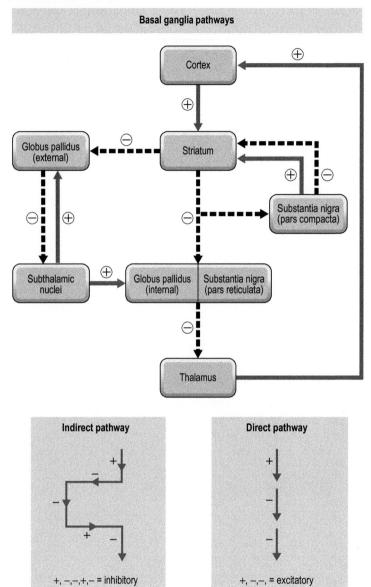

Basal ganglia pathways

Fig. 6.8 • The basal ganglia pathways.
From Costanzo 2006, with permission

of the problems associated with basal ganglia 'damage' is the lack of ability to control skilled/learned movements. The exact nature of these movements is dependent upon the nuclei affected, e.g. damage to the nigrostriatal pathway results in Parkinson's disease. Another key feature of basal ganglia damage is abnormal muscle activation, but unlike the spasticity seen following motor cortex damage, there is actually a rigidity found. Chapter 7 on motor control includes

a case study on a patient with PD and the typical motor control problems found in this population.

Cerebellum

The cerebellum (or 'little brain') sits at the base of the brain at the back of the brain stem (see Chapter 2). The afferent and efferent fibres of the cerebral peduncles are responsible for the connections between the cerebellum and the brain stem. In addition to these connections, there are also links between the cerebellum and the vestibular system – not surprising given the importance of balance in so much of our movement. The cerebellum, like the cerebrum itself, is divided into specific areas each with a particular area of specialty in terms of movement:

- Flocculo-nodular lobe:
  - balance
- Vermis/paravermal regions:
  - walking/gait
- Lateral hemispheres:
  - skilled movements (e.g. drawing, speaking).

As well as receiving inputs from all of the areas of the brain involved in movement, the cerebellum also receives information from the proprioceptors and the vestibular system. As a result, the cerebellum has the ability to compare the actual movement carried out with the intended movement. In making this comparison the cerebellum can identify any differences between the actual and intended and make suitable minor adjustments via the upper motor neurones. This system is used as a way of increasing the accuracy of our movements. You will see in Chapter 7 that this 'comparator' function is an essential component of motor control.

Any disorder of the cerebellum will result in inaccurate, uncoordinated movement, i.e. **ataxia**. To illustrate the problem of inaccuracy, we should think of an individual reaching to pick up an object such as a pen. They may over- or under-shoot, then under- or over-correct, until eventually the object is secured. People with ataxia have difficulty producing smooth, accurate movements. For example, when a non-impaired person reaches for an object, the velocity profile of their wrist shows a classic 'bell-shaped' profile with one phase where speed increases followed by one where it decreases (Jeannerod, 1984). In people with ataxia however, this profile is often fragmented, showing a number of accelerations and decelerations. The lack of accuracy and smooth coordination also has an impact on, for example, walking or speech. Multiple sclerosis, a disease caused by demyelination of the nervous system, may first become apparent by signs and symptoms of cerebellar dysfunction: a person's gait looks unsteady, their speech sounds slurred and they appear clumsy, unintentionally knocking things over or bumping into objects.

Cerebral palsy

Cerebral palsy (CP) is described in the International Classification of Diseases (ICD-10, WHO 1996) as 'difficult to define but is conventionally described as a group of motor disorders with or without associated sensory and intellectual deficits where the cause is injury to the immature brain'. The brain damage may have been caused by asphyxia (i.e. oxygen deprivation), infection, trauma or metabolic disorders, but in most cases, the cause is unknown. In some instances, CP occurs due to a lack of oxygen during a difficult birth, although, conversely, a difficult birth may result when the baby has already developed CP in the ante-natal period.

The most common symptoms of cerebral palsy include problems with fine motor skills (e.g. writing), difficulty with walking or balance and, in some types of CP, involuntary movements. The motor symptoms of CP may also be manifest in difficulties with speech, eating and swallowing, or in impaired continence. Although these symptoms are the most common, they do differ from individual to individual and may change over time. In addition to the motor impairments, a considerable proportion of children also experience sensory impairments, in particular visual impairment, which further compounds problems with visually guided movement (e.g. avoiding obstacles). There are different types of CP, about which more can be found in clinical texts, e.g. Pountney and Green (2004).

Although the brain damage associated with CP does not change per se, the manifestations of CP may change as the child develops, e.g. he/she may fail to thrive as a result of difficulties with eating and swallowing, one of the hip joints may become subluxed due to abnormal biomechanics of the muscles around it, or developmental delays may occur as the child is unable to move around and explore the world around him. Box 6.1 describes a case study of a child with CP.

One common characteristic of cerebral palsy, as explained earlier, is spasticity. This can interfere with a number of everyday functions including walking and speaking, and if the situation is untreated, contractures may develop, resulting in fixed joint positions (i.e. contractures). The spasticity occurs as a result of damage to the brain areas involved in the control of voluntary movement that were mentioned earlier.

Box 6.1

G and her twin sister B were born prematurely, following a complicated pregnancy. G was in respiratory distress during the birth and had to be taken into neonatal intensive care. B's development was normal, but G's motor development was delayed and she was eventually diagnosed with spastic diplegic cerebral palsy (CP). In this type of CP, the main problem is spasticity affecting both lower limbs, while the upper limbs are usually not affected. G is now aged 10, goes to her local primary school with her sister, and enjoys horse riding for the disabled. The spasticity mainly affects the flexors, internal rotators and adductors of both hip joints, as well as knee and ankle flexors. As a result, G walks on her toes with flexion in her knee and hip joints (a pattern known as 'crouch gait'), and requires two sticks for support and balance. Although G manages to walk independently, she finds it increasingly tiring. G's physiotherapist has made an appointment with the orthopaedic surgeon to see how they can improve G's gait to optimise the biomechanics and reduce the energy expenditure of G's gait pattern, and prevent any future musculoskeletal complications.

Box 6.2

Antispasmodic therapies

The key requirement for an antispasmodic agent is that it has to interfere, somewhere, with the pathway carrying the neuronal signal from the central nervous system to the muscle fibre. This can be brought about in a variety of ways and some examples are given next. It may be useful at this point to refer back to Chapter 4 for some basic discussion on pharmacological concepts.

Baclofen

Baclofen is a chlorophenyl derivative of γ-aminobutyric acid (GABA). GABA is the principal inhibitory transmitter of the central nervous system, but as it is a lipophobic compound it is not able to cross the blood–brain barrier if given systemically. Baclofen, however, is a lipophilic agent, which readily crosses the blood–brain barrier and gains access to the presynaptic GABA$_B$ receptors on the spinal cord. As an agonist at the receptor, baclofen inhibits both the monosynaptic and polysynaptic activation of the motor neurones.

Dantrolene

Dantrolene is a muscle relaxant that acts by blocking the release of intracellular calcium from the sarcoplasmic reticulum of the skeletal muscle cells. This action on the sarcoplasmic reticulum decreases the elevation of intracellular calcium levels required for contraction, thereby leading to relaxation. As a result of this, dantrolene is often used to treat the muscle spasms observed in cerebral palsy.

Botulinum toxin

Botulinum toxin is the same toxin responsible for certain types of food poisoning, i.e. botulism. It is also the same agent used in cosmetic surgery procedures to relax muscle contraction to make wrinkles disappear. Clinical studies have shown that the injection of botulinum toxin into muscles affected by spasticity blocks neural transmission, which leads to paresis and causes the muscles to relax. The mechanism of action of botulinum toxin involves the inhibition of acetylcholine (ACh) release from the presynaptic terminal. Botulinum toxin is comprised of two subunits. One subunit binds to a membrane receptor, thereby allowing the toxin to enter the cell. Once inside the cell the second subunit produces the toxic effect of blocking ACh release. The toxin comprises several peptidases, which break down the specific proteins involved in the exocytotic release of ACh. If ACh release is reduced, then there will be a reduced postsynaptic stimulation of the muscle fibre at the neuromuscular junction – resulting in muscle relaxation. Following this chemical denervation, axonal sprouting and gradual reinnervation take place, resulting in full recovery of the neuromuscular junctions, usually after a period of 2–6 months (Davis and Barnes 2001). This explains why patients who are treated with botulinum toxin often require repeat injections.

A number of different therapeutic approaches can be utilised to manage the symptoms of cerebral palsy, but it should be noted that no standard therapy works for all patients. Potential approaches can be seen in Box 6.2 and include:

- drug therapy – known as antispasmodic therapy (see Box 6.2)
- braces/mechanical aids to compensate for imbalance
- surgery

- counselling (for psychological impact of the condition)
- therapy (physio, occupational, speech, orthotics).

Summary

Having used this chapter to lay out the basic aspects of movement and coordination, it is now appropriate to move on and gain a deeper understanding of two key aspects of movement: perceptuo-motor control (Chapter 7) and motor learning (Chapter 8).

SELF-ASSESSMENT QUESTIONS

1. What is meant by the term spasticity?
2. What are the factors contributing to hypertonia?
3. What role do the following brain areas have in the control of movement?
   a. Motor cortex
   b. Basal ganglia
   c. Cerebellum.
4. Describe the mechanism of action of the following anti-spasmodic therapies:
   a. Baclofen
   b. Dantrolene
   c. Botulinum toxin.

Further reading

Barnes, M.P., Ward, A.B., 2000. Textbook of Rehabilitation Medicine. Oxford University Press, Oxford.

Edwards, M., Quinn, N., Bhatia, K., 2008. Parkinson's Disease and Other

Movement Disorders (Oxford Specialist Handbooks in Neurology). Oxford University Press, Oxford.

Miller, F., Bachrach, S.J., 2006. Cerebral Palsy: A complete guide for

caregiving, second ed. The John Hopkins University Press, USA.

Stevenson, V., Jarrett, L., 2006. Spasticity Management. Informa Healthcare.

References

Barnes, M.P., Johnson, G.R. (Eds.), 2001. Upper Motor Neuron Syndrome and Spasticity. Clinical management and neurophysiology. Cambridge University Press, Cambridge.

Basmajian, J.V., 1957. New views on muscular tone and relaxation. Can. Med. Assoc. J. 77, 203–205.

Costanzo, L.S., 2006. Physiology, third ed. WB Saunders, UK.

Davis, E., Barnes, M.P., 2001. The use of botulinum toxin in spasticity. In: Barnes, M.P., Johnson, G.R. (Eds.), Upper Motor Neuron Syndrome and Spasticity. Clinical management and neurophysiology. Cambridge University Press, Cambridge, pp. 206–222.

Edwards, S., 2002. Abnormal tone and movement as a result of neurological impairment: considerations for treatment. In: Edwards, S. (Ed.), Neurological Physiotherapy. A problem-solving approach. Churchill Livingstone, Edinburgh, pp. 89–120.

Jeannerod, M., 1984. The timing of natural prehension movements. J. Mot. Behav. 16, 235–254.

Johnson, G.R., 2001. Measurement of spasticity. In: Barnes, M.P.,

Johnson, G.R. (Eds.), Upper Motor Neuron Syndrome and Spasticity. Clinical management and neurophysiology. Cambridge University Press, Cambridge.

Katz, R.T., Rymer, W.Z., 1989. Spastic hypertonia: mechanisms and measurement. Arch. Phys. Med. Rehabil. 70, 144–155.

Kindlen, S., 2003. Physiology for Health Care and Nursing. Churchill Livingstone, UK.

Lance, J., 1980. Pathophysiology of spasticity and clinical experience with baclofen. In: Lance, J.W., Feldman, R.G., Young, R.R., et al (Eds.), Spasticity: disordered motor control. Year Book, Chicago.

Pandyan, A.D., Gregoric, M., Barnes, M.P., et al., 2005. Spasticity: clinical perceptions, neurological realities and meaningful measurement. Disabil. Rehabil. 27, 2–6.

Pountney, T., Green, E., 2004. The cerebral palsies and motor learning. In: Stokes, M. (Ed.), Physical Management in Neurological Rehabilitation. Elsevier Mosby, London, pp. 313–332.

Rothwell, J., 1994. Control of Human Voluntary Movement. Chapman & Hall, London.

Spina, D., 2008. The Flesh and Bones of Medical Pharmacology. Mosby, UK.

Sheean, G. (Ed.), 1998. Spasticity Rehabilitation. Churchill Communications Europe Ltd, London.

Sheean, G., 2001. Neurophysiology of spasticity. In: Barnes, M.P., Johnson, G.R. (Eds.), Upper Motor Neuron Syndrome and Spasticity. Clinical management and neurophysiology. Cambridge University Press, Cambridge.

Walsh, E.G., 1992. Muscles, Masses and Motion. The physiology of normality, hypotonicity, spasticity and rigidity. Mac Keith Press, London.

Watkins, C., Leathley, M., Gregson, J., et al., 2002. Prevalence of spasticity post stroke. Clin. Rehabil. 16, 515–522.

World Health Organisation, 1996. ICD-10 guide for mental retardation. World Health Organisation, Geneva. Available online from: http://www.who.int/mental_health/media/en/69.pdf (accessed 05.09.2010).

Perceptuo-motor control

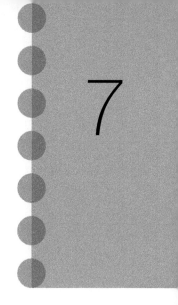

LEARNING OUTCOMES

At the end of this chapter, you should be able to:

- describe the concept of 'coordination' and explain the 'degrees of freedom' problem
- define motor control and explain motor control from an information-processing approach, critically evaluating the strengths and weaknesses of this approach
- compare and contrast the information-processing approach to motor control with a direct perception and dynamical systems approach
- explain the interaction between perception and action and explain the relevance of this interaction for rehabilitation
- explain how motor control is influenced by factors related to the individual, the task and the environment
- discuss the implications of the information presented in this chapter for health-care professionals working in rehabilitation in general, and neurological rehabilitation in particular.

Introduction

Having introduced the basic building blocks of the nervous system in Chapter 2 and explained the role of different neural circuits involved in movement in Chapter 6, the next two chapters focus on how we control and learn more complex, voluntary movements and activities.

Motor control involves the planning, initiation, execution, monitoring and adaptation of movement. Whether you are a physiotherapist, occupational therapist, speech and language therapist or orthotist, you will often play a key role in designing interventions to improve motor control, e.g. a patient's ability to move around, engage in sporting activities, express themselves through speech or music, and participate in occupation and leisure activities. An important aim of rehabilitation is to facilitate long-term improvement in an individual's functional activity within their own environment. The question is: how can we help patients to improve their motor control – not just within therapy sessions in the clinic – but out there, in the 'real world', and long after rehabilitation has ceased? A sound working understanding of motor control and learning is, therefore, essential for health-care professionals. Let us begin by considering a case study (7.1) about a person with Parkinson's disease that illustrates a particular motor control problem and the impact this may have.

The case study above is representative for many people with Parkinson's disease and poses the general question as to how to provide the most effective interventions for the motor control problems commonly seen in this condition. But before one can provide any solutions, one needs to understand the problem.

The ensuing two chapters are, therefore, linked; the aim of the current chapter is to introduce the topic of motor control and explain basic concepts related to coordination and the interaction between perception and action in skilled movement. This forms the foundation for the next chapter, which explores the role of health-care professionals in facilitating skill acquisition and focuses on motor learning.

Coordination

Introduction to coordination

You have just picked up this book, sat down and opened it – an activity that is so automatic to most of us that we don't give it any thought unless an injury or other health condition disrupts the process. Most activities of daily living are automatic;

Case study 7.1

Mrs B., a 67-year-old retired music teacher, was diagnosed with Parkinson's disease (PD) approximately 8 years ago. PD is a degenerative condition of the substantia nigra, which are part of the basal ganglia. PD is associated with a range of different signs and symptoms (see Chapter 6). This case study concentrates on Mrs B.'s particular problems with balance and gait Mrs B. has recently referred herself for domiciliary physiotherapy as she finds it increasingly difficult to move around the house, while she has also experienced an increasing number of falls. She is beginning to lose her confidence and is becoming more fearful of falling. During your history taking, Mrs B. tells you that she has particular difficulty walking across her sitting room. In contrast, moving across her kitchen seems to be much easier. You are curious to find out why Mrs B. has such difficulty in one situation, but not in the other.

During your observation of Mrs B.'s walking, you observe the typical signs and symptoms of PD: bradykinesia (slowness of movement), tremor, difficulty changing movement (i.e. difficulty with starting/stopping), shuffling gait and rigidity, expressed in reduced stride length, arm swing and trunk rotation. When you ask Mrs B. to walk across the sitting room, she makes a few small steps and then 'freezes': her feet appear to get 'stuck' to the floor and, although she shuffles her feet, she fails to make an adequate step forward. Due to the continuing forward motion of the rest of her body, her balance is challenged and she has to stabilise herself by holding onto a chair. Next, you ask her to walk across the kitchen. She performs this almost fluently. Mrs B. explains that the floor surface seems to make all the difference; the sitting room has carpet of the same colour and texture throughout;

instead, the kitchen floor is made up of large black and white tiles. Mrs B. explains that by putting each foot on the next tile, she is able to walk across the kitchen without 'freezing'. How can this be explained?

Well, Purdon Martin (1967) in his remarkable book was the first to demonstrate the effect of horizontal floor markers on stride length in people with PD. Since then, many studies have demonstrated that visual cues can improve speed of walking, stride length and reduce 'freezing' in people with PD (Lim et al. 2005, Rochester et al. 2010). Cueing, which is defined as using 'external temporal or spatial stimuli to facilitate movement (gait) initiation and continuation' (Nieuwboer et al. 2007 p. 134), may involve visual (e.g. stripes, upturned walking sticks), acoustic (e.g. rhythm) or proprioceptive stimuli (e.g. vibration). Exactly how these cues affect walking is not entirely clear. Azulay et al. (1999) compared gait parameters in people with PD and normal controls under different conditions, including no stripes and transverse stripes on the floor, both under normal and stroboscopic illumination. They found that people with PD relied more than normal controls on visual information during walking, and specifically appeared to use visual information about the *motion* of the stripes. The authors postulated that by relying more on dedicated visuo-motor pathways people with PD were able to involve the cerebellum and bypass the affected basal ganglia circuitry during gait.

How may this research inform your practice? The implications for therapy are that the therapist can use 'cueing' as a therapeutic strategy to try and improve the person's gait. Chapter 8 will present further detail from a study investigating the effects of cueing in motor learning in PD.

by the time we are adults, we will have undertaken them thousands of times. However, this does not make them any less complex; think, for example, about the processes involved in making a cup of tea. Even just the component of pouring boiling water into a cup requires precise regulation of the forces required to grip and lift the kettle, as well as eye–hand coordination to ensure the water does not spill – while stabilising one's posture. In the ensuing sections, we shall explain – in broad terms – how movement and activities are thought to be coordinated. A sound understanding of this process will enable therapists to analyse the coordination problems they encounter in clinical practice and design rational treatment plans to address these problems.

Defining 'coordination'

'Coordination' is a complex concept, which has fascinated scientists and clinicians for centuries (Latash 2008, Latash and Zatsiorsky 2001). Hence, unsurprisingly, the term 'coordination' has been defined in numerous different ways. A ground-breaking definition was articulated by Nikolai Aleksandrovich Bernstein (1896–1966), the famous Russian physiologist and founder of motor control science, whose legacy you can read more about in Bongaardt (2001). Bernstein (1984/1935, p. 355) stated that:

> 'The coordination of a movement is the process of mastering redundant degrees of freedom of the moving organ, in other words the conversion to a controllable system. More briefly, coordination is the organization of the control of the motor apparatus'.

Several points within this definition are worth considering; let us begin with 'the conversion to a controllable system'. The human skeleton is inherently unstable; it requires muscles and other soft tissue to control its posture and movement against gravity and other forces; without these, the structure collapses. Muscle force must be controlled in terms of timing and level of activity in order to avoid excess, insufficient or uncontrollable force. Controlling force production over a single joint is complex enough, but this problem is compounded by the number of ways in which we can use our joints to undertake an activity. For example, bringing a cup to one's mouth can be done using a number of different joints in different configurations; have a look around you, the next time

you are in a coffee shop. This refers to the 'degrees of freedom problem'; the next important point in Bernstein's definition.

In the context of motor control, a **degree of freedom** can be described as the smallest number of coordinates required to describe the state of a system. For example, the proximal interphalangeal (PIP) joint of the 4th digit has one degree of freedom, as it has one axis of movement, around which it is 'free' to move (i.e. flexion/extension). Therefore, just one coordinate (e.g. 45° degrees flexion from the anatomical position) is sufficient to describe the position of this system. The knee joint has two degrees of freedom, as it has two axes, (being a pivotal hinge joint, it permits flexion and extension as well as a slight medial and lateral rotation), while the hip joint has three – and so on. As each joint has a number of degrees of freedom, which can be configured in different ways with other joints to undertake an activity, a vast number of options are created. In fact, it can be shown that the number of options is in principle infinite (Latash 2008). And so far, we have only referred to position, but we should also include velocity to describe the state of a system! The question is how all these options can be coordinated, and not just in any haphazard way, but in a way that is effective, efficient and reproducible to such an extent that we can recognise people's gait, voice or hand writing? Taken together, 'coordination' is quite a considerable engineering problem, which is known as 'the degrees of-freedom problem', 'the Bernstein problem' or 'the problem of motor redundancy' (Latash 2008, Turvey 1990).

According to Bernstein, coordination involves the control of redundant degrees of freedom, turning it into a system that can be controlled. Clinical application box 7.1 may help to clarify what is meant by this idea.

In case study 7.1 on Parkinson's disease (PD) at the start of this chapter, the situation is quite the opposite from the case study on ataxic cerebral palsy below; PD induces rigidity, which pathologically reduces the number of degrees of freedom available below what may be required for normal functioning. Interestingly, there is a much higher incidence of falls in PD compared with age-matched controls (Bloem et al. 2001), rising even further in studies with longer follow-up times. Could the degree-of-freedom issue provide an explanation for the high incidence of falls in PD?

Think about what happens when your own balance is challenged, e.g. when walking on ice. In this situation, your base of support may slide away from

Clinical application box 7.1

Mastering degrees of freedom

The neurological condition of cerebral palsy (CP) was introduced in Chapter 6. CP may have wide-ranging effects on a child's development, and include motor, psychological and social difficulties. One particular motor impairment that may result from CP is **ataxia**, whereby the coordination of movement is disorganised. Children with CP may be unable to control their sitting position and have profound difficulty with eye–hand coordination. Lacking an adequate base of support, the control of head, eye and upper limb movement is even further compromised. Butler (1998) and Major et al. (2001) devised an intervention known as 'targeted rehabilitation', utilising a frame to immobilise different body segments (e.g. ankles, knees, hips, pelvis and/ or trunk) while leaving others free to move – depending on the child's level of coordination. The reasoning is that, due to the cerebral palsy, children are unable to intrinsically control the numerous degrees of freedom associated with an upright position. Targeted rehabilitation utilises a supportive device in which the child can sit or stand, using supports in specific locations. Control of head position in space is the first target, as this comprises the important sensory systems of vision, balance and hearing that play a key role in posture and movement. Once this has been achieved, support will be adjusted downward, leaving just one or two joints free above the support. In this way, targeted rehabilitation systematically reduces the number of degrees of freedom by imposing external constraints on various body segments and reduces the complexity of the motor control problem. Using this method, positive findings were reported in case studies, in terms of achieving sitting balance (Butler 1998) and gait (Farmer et al. 1999).

underneath your centre of gravity at any moment, threatening a fall. Therefore, you constantly need to compensate by involving a greater number of joints, sometimes in unusual planes of movement, compared to walking over normal ground. So what happens when your freedom to adapt has been reduced, as in PD? You are more likely to fail in keeping your centre of gravity over your base of support – resulting in a (near) fall.

In summary, organising the 'motor apparatus' involves complex control processes. On the one hand, having numerous degrees of freedom in the motor system is an asset, as it allows for substitution and compensatory strategies in situations where usual strategies are not possible, and for learning new patterns of coordination. For example, consider the situation where your shoulder is immobilised against your body with a sling and you want to reach for a pen in front of you. In this case, it is likely that you use hip and trunk flexion to compensate for the lack of shoulder flexion. However, on the other hand, the existence of numerous degrees of freedom in the motor system presents a challenge for the control system.

Controlling degrees of freedom: modelling motor control

The previous section introduced the degrees-of-freedom problem and explained how this is intrinsic to (human) movement. Equally, this problem is an unavoidable challenge for motor control scientists! Any theory that purports to explain the coordination of movement must offer a valid explanation for how the degree of freedom problem is to be resolved. There are numerous theories and models of motor control, which purport different solutions to this problem.

Before the degree-of-freedom problem had been identified in the Western world, an influential theory known as the **reflex-hierarchical theory** of motor control was widely accepted. This model integrates Sherrington's work on reflexes (see Chapter 6), with a model proposed by Hughlings Jackson, according to which the brain comprises a hierarchy of levels, each higher one capable of generating more sophisticated behaviours. For example, compare the stereotypical monosynaptic stretch reflex that operates at spinal level with a voluntary complex action such as drawing, initiated from the motor cortex. This model, in which fairly autonomous reflexes were incorporated into a hierarchical control structure, had a profound influence on ideas about motor control, child development and rehabilitation. For example, early work by Bobath (1990) who revolutionalised rehabilitation for people with neurological conditions, initially focused primarily on normalising reflexes and postural tone as a prerequisite for normal movement. With the benefit of hindsight, it would have been surprising if this approach had been effective in terms of improving functional activity, as we now understand that reflexes are only one part of the complex interaction between the various body

systems, environmental constraints and task requirements that play a role in functional activity – and this
has been incorporated in a more modern interpretation of Bobath (Raine 2009). A full discussion of
the reflex-hierarchical theory of motor control, and
implications for clinical practice are beyond the
scope of this book and readers are referred to Gordon
(2000) and Kamm et al. (1990).

More contemporary motor control theories can be
categorised by dividing them into two broad frameworks: '**motor systems theories**' and '**action systems
theories**' (Meijer and Roth 1988):

- 'Motor systems' theories (also known as the
  motor programming or information
  processing approaches), comprise the more
  traditional approach to motor control.
  Stemming from the background of cognitive
  psychology, this approach proposes that
  movement is controlled by programme that have
  been stored in memory. These theories
  concentrate on what information is necessary
  to control movement, and the role of cognition in
  this process.
- 'Action systems' theories are in direct contrast
  with the former as they question – if not reject –
  the role of cognition in motor control. They
  argue instead that the information required to
  control movement is directly available to the
  organism (the ecological approach to perception,
  or direct perception approach) or that movement
  is subject to laws of physics and thereby largely
  self-organising (the dynamical systems or natural-
  physical approach).

Both frameworks continue to be debated but both
are supported by an abundance of evidence. Hence
the question is not so much–'which model is best?' –
but rather – 'which model is most appropriate for
a specific question?'

Within the context of this book, there is only
scope to introduce the theoretical frameworks mentioned above and, in fact, we will focus mostly on one
model, i.e. the 'motor programming' approach. The
rationale for selecting this approach is that we feel
it is probably most compatible with the problem-
solving approach used in clinical practice, and has
been further developed in terms of its application
to practical settings – although these are predominantly physical education and sports settings.
However, we wish to emphasise that this approach
is not without limitations and these will be discussed
as we proceed.

Motor control: a motor programming approach

A hierarchical model of motor control: an introduction

We will start our discussion with the motor programming approach to motor control. For a potted history of the science of motor control, the reader is
referred to a particularly illuminating account by
Meijer (2001).

The motor programming approach to motor control represents a group of methodologies including
those that study the role of information processing
in motor control, modelling the nervous system as
a virtual neural network through computer simulations, or signal processing in the actual nervous
system. Central to this approach is the concept of
information processing. The first person to propose
that the human brain can be compared to a computer,
as they both receive and process sensory information
and produce output, was Craik in 1948 (in Summers
2004). This metaphor was hugely influential in
psychology and inspired information processing theories of a wide range of human behaviours, including
motor control and skill acquisition.

Among the first psychological theories about
motor behaviour based on this metaphor, those postulated by Adams (1971) and his student Schmidt
(1975) have been and continue to be particularly
influential (Summers 2004). Both came from a background of physical education and were interested in
increasing their understanding of human motor
control to enable them to design effective training
programmes. A historical overview of the development
of this approach to motor control and learning can be
found in Schmidt (1988) and Summers (2004).

The model of motor control, currently proposed
by Schmidt and Wrisberg (2008), is outlined in
Figure 7.1. This model presents the subsequent
stages of information processing, involved in generating motor output. Let's go through this model by
using the example from the PD case study: stepping
onto a stepping stone.

Starting with Input, you begin by gathering visual information, which comprises raw visual data about the
target and its environment. In the Stimulus
Identification stage, this raw sensory information is
processed into a meaningful percept, where you recognise what you see (i.e. square black and white tiles on

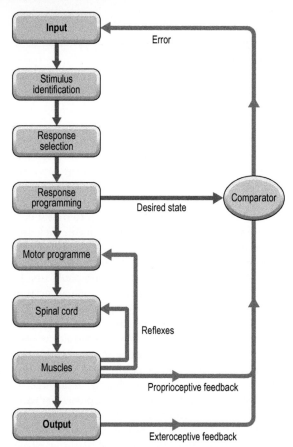

Fig. 7.1 • A motor programming model of motor control, according to Schmidt and Wrisberg (2008), with permission from Human Kinetics.

the floor). In general, this stage comprises processing sensory information about the nature of the object (i.e. what it is), as well as its location in relation to you (i.e. where it is).

In the Response Selection stage, you decide which action to take, e.g. taking a step forward, changing direction, jumping over, etc. Once the intended action ('desired state') has been decided, the response programming stage can begin.

The Response Programme stage is the preparation of the motor programme, where a basic template for a specific class of action (in this case walking) is fine-tuned to the specific action (i.e. stepping onto stepping stones). This template specifies the basic sequence and 'rhythm' of the action – a more detailed account of this stage will follow below.

When completed, the desired state is fed forward to the Comparator, to update it on the intended action. Having a plan of the intended action will later enable the comparator to match the intended with the actual action and generate an error signal should there be any discrepancy between the two. As we will see in Chapter 8, this stage is essential for skill acquisition.

So far, we have introduced the so-called 'executive' in the model, which comprises the stimulus identification, response selection, and response programming stages. The model then proceeds with the 'effector', including the motor programme, spinal cord and muscles.

Once compiled, the Motor Programme is then fired off via the final common path to the spinal cord, alpha motor neurones and the motor end plates, activating muscles – with motor output as a result. Following Chapter 6, this part of the process will now be familiar to you. Although the motor programme is finally realised through muscle activations, the controlling parameters used by the central nervous system are not necessarily expressed in terms of muscle parameters initially, as will be explained later (Section 3: Response programming: invariants and parameters).

Several forms of feedback ensue from this process: muscle reflexes are likely to be evoked; monosynaptic stretch reflexes (M1), longer duration functional stretch reflexes (M2) and voluntary reactions (M3) are all elicited to regulate posture and balance during the intended action (see Chapter 6). Proprioceptive feedback from muscle spindles, tendons and ligaments is also generated, providing information about posture and movement. Finally, exteroceptive feedback emerges, which is feedback about the environment (e.g. vision tells you that you have reached/ missed your target). This actual output is then fed into the comparator which, as explained above, compares the actual state with the intended state. If the two signals match, this indicates that all has gone to plan, and no error signal is generated. However, if there is a difference between the two, an error signal is fed back into the system as Input. If there is sufficient time for the action (e.g. self-paced stepping), this information is used by the organism to re-adjust its action as this unfolds. Going round the entire loop (i.e. from input, via exteroceptive feedback, and onto further input) takes around 300 ms. However, as we shall see, some actions (e.g. jumping) are too fast and feedback may not be processed in time for the current action. This means that you need to store the information and wait until the next try.

Note that an action may also arise from an internal – as opposed to an external – stimulus. Try to apply the motor programming process described above, using the example of being thirsty and deciding to walk across the room to get a drink from a water fountain. What visual information would be gathered, what would be in the plan of intended action, what would the basic template for the motor programme and how would this be fine-tuned for the specific action?

Open and closed loop control

Following this outline, we shall now examine the model in more detail. As Figure 7.1 suggests, the model comprises two components; an Open Loop (blue) and a Closed Loop component (grey). The Closed Loop component was proposed by Adams in the 1970s (Adams 1971). This component represents a full loop through all stages of the model, utilising *feedback* during and following the movement. Provided that an action is sufficiently slow, exteroceptive and proprioceptive feedback can be utilised to 'steer' the activity as required. The minimum time needed for a response to this visual and proprioceptive feedback is estimated at about 100 ms (Jeannerod 1988). For example, handwriting tends to be a slow and deliberate activity. The position of the pen in relation to the paper is carefully monitored on-line and adjustments can be made as the activity proceeds. This way, errors that are too small to be detected consciously, can be corrected. However, closed loop control on its own does not suffice for ballistic movements (e.g. kicking, jumping, punching) or ballistic components of a movement (e.g. initial phase of reach-to-grasp) that are faster than this.

Schmidt argued that Closed Loop systems are too slow for ballistic movements and that they would need to be pre-programmed. He, therefore, proposed to extend Adams' model with an Open Loop (or *feedforward*) component, which starts with Input and finishes at Output. This component, which is programme-driven, enables fast movement to be 'run off' without the need for feedback. An example of such a movement is a punch: Mohammed Ali's left jab was famously noted to take only 40 ms (Schmidt 1988). Exteroceptive and proprioceptive feedback is generated, but this arrives too late to benefit the current action which, by the time it reaches Input, will already have been completed. We have probably all experienced situations where we have set off to kick a ball, to discover we have made a terrible mistake but find there was nothing we could do to alter its course! Evidence for movements being pre-programmed and 'run off' comes from a number of classical studies (see Schmidt 1988 for an

overview). An example of an action involving Open Loop control is walking straight ahead over a flat, even ground without any obstacles. Once you have decided your endpoint, the activity can be run off automatically. This automaticity is challenged, however, in cases where this is affected by pathological conditions such as PD, unexpected changes in environmental conditions or in the task. Thinking back to our case study of Mrs. B., can you now explain why she has difficulty walking over evenly coloured and textured carpet – and why she does not experience these problems on a surface with clear visual cues? According to Schmidt's model of motor control, how may the presence of the large, black and white tiles influence the control of gait? We will return to this case study later in this chapter.

Together, by having a higher order Open Loop with a Closed Loop mode of motor control nested within, Schmidt's hierarchical model (Schmidt and Wrisberg, 2008) is able to describe how fast, as well as slow movements are controlled, and explain how errors can be corrected – depending on the amount of time available.

In summary, a motor programme is a template for motor control; a set of motor commands that prescribes the essential characteristics of a skilled action (Schmidt and Wrisberg 2008).

The generalised motor programme

It is important to highlight at this point that, rather than each movement having its own dedicated motor programme, Schmidt proposed that **classes of action** may be discerned (e.g. walking, reaching, rising from sit to stand). Each class of action is purported to have its own kinematic 'signature', or pattern, and all movements within the same class of action are controlled by the same motor programme, known as a **generalised motor programme** (GMP). So for example, the GMP for reaching comprises certain key components, as Research box 7.1 below explains.

In order to understand how GMPs may be fine-tuned for specific actions, we need to look at how the GMP is purported to work.

Response programming: invariants and parameters

If you were an engineer, tasked with building a robot that simulates human movement, how would you go about it? A daunting task – not least because of the

Research box 7.1

Example: Motor programme for reach-to-grasp

In healthy subjects, for a given reach-to-grasp movement the hand follows a characteristic path and trajectory as it moves towards an object, described as the 'transport' component (change over time of the position of the wrist (Jeannerod 1984)) and the hand opens and closes on the object, the 'grasp' component (change over time of the distance between the index finger and thumb (Jeannerod 1984)). Neurophysiological evidence supports separate but interdependent visuomotor control channels for these two components (Ungerleider and Mishkin 1982, Goodale and Milner 1992). The velocity profile of the hand is typically asymmetric, with the peak velocity achieved within 50% of movement duration. The time to PV is often described as 'ballistic' meaning it is assumed to be driven by force commands that have been planned and activated prior to the beginning of the movement (open loop control) (Nagasaki 1989). The time *after* PV is thought to be controlled in a *feedback* manner whereby part by visual or proprioceptive information made available to the central nervous system after the movement begins is used to correct the movement according to task goals and environmental demands. The time after PV is also described as the 'deceleration' phase, while the hand slows in readiness to grasp the object.

When the task requirement for the grasp is changed by making an object smaller, or by requiring a more accurate task to be performed with then object, peak velocity occurs earlier, resulting in a longer deceleration phase (Marteniuk et al. 1987), allowing time to process the various sources of sensory feedback.

When the task requirement for the transport is changed by increasing the speed of the reaching movement, the maximum amount of hand opening increases (Wing et al. 1986).

Thus the general motor programme for reaching and grasping is operating in these examples and being fine-tuned for different task requirements.

degree-of-freedom problem discussed above – that has challenged engineers and scientists all over the world. But let's start with getting a single joint to move. The only tools you have at your disposal to produce movement are contractile tissue (i.e. muscle), attached to two rigid levers (i.e. bones), which articulate through a linkage (i.e. a joint). You will probably find that the only options you have are: which muscles to use; the amount of force they generate; and the time at which they are to be switched on and off. This, in a nutshell, is the 'impulse-timing hypothesis' proposed by Schmidt (1988). In summary, this hypothesis postulates that movement is controlled by specifying the amount of force over time (i.e. impulse) by selected muscles.

So how is impulse-timing programmed? This process involves two main elements: **invariants** (i.e. those movement parameters that remain constant) and **parameters** (i.e. those movement parameters that may change, depending on the specific nature of the movement).

The invariants together represent the 'signature' of the class of action, i.e.:

- The sequence of events (i.e. the order of actions but not muscle contractions, e.g. the elbow flexes to lift the hand off the lap and then extends to move the hand towards the object)
- The relative force (i.e. the proportional force between agonists, antagonists and synergists)

- The relative timing (i.e. the temporal order of the muscle contractions, e.g. for relative force and relative timing-biceps brachii turns on to lift the hand off the lap, then relaxes while triceps brachii turns on to extend the elbow, then biceps brachii takes over to slow the movement as the hand approaches the object.)

The parameters comprise:

- The specific muscles involved
- The absolute amount of force
- The absolute amount of time a muscle is activated.

Based on the invariants that form the 'signature' of an activity, it can be seen how this can be adjusted for specific variations. A classic experiment by Raibert (1977) compared writing the same sentence with one's dominant hand, non-dominant hand, pen gripped between teeth, or pen attached to the foot, all resulting in a strikingly similar writing pattern. The similarity in handwriting was seen as providing clear evidence for the existence of a generalised motor programme. However, the parameters of this required quite a bit of fine-tuning, given the diversity of the effectors!

By changing the absolute amount and duration of force production, a movement can also be slowed down or speeded up. In summary, the combination of invariants and parameters that can be varied within a GMP enables a class of movement to be programmed efficiently (as the invariants already provide the template) and adjusted through the parameters.

Having introduced a motor programming approach to motor control, it is time to go back to our degrees of freedom problem. We emphasised that any valid theory on motor control should offer a solution for this problem. So how does Schmidt's hierarchical model of motor control fit in – and what are the challenges?

A key concept in Schmidt's model of motor control is the assumption of the GMP, which is a blueprint that specifies the invariants for each class of movement. Returning to the motor programme for reach to grasp, one of the invariants of this programme is that the start of transport of the hand toward the object occurs at the same time (within 60 ms) as the start of hand opening. This invariant reduces the possible degrees of freedom. Once a response has been selected, this blueprint only has to be fine-tuned to the specific movement. A parameter of the reach to grasp motor programme that can be fine–tuned is the timing of the peak velocity, which varies according to the accuracy requirements of the task. Rather than starting 'from scratch', the GMP offers a ready-made solution that constrains the degrees of freedom. Some theorists, however, are not convinced by the assumption of the GMP and their arguments will be discussed at the end of this chapter.

Schmidt's model of motor control is not the only one within the cluster of 'motor theories'. Another seminal body of literature stems from Jeannerod's work on neural models for action, which has made a major contribution to our understanding of motor control, as well as how strategies such as observational learning and mental practice can improve motor control. A research box including some of the findings from Jeannerod's work is included above (Box 7.3), while we will come back to this body of work in Chapter 8 on motor learning.

Perception–action coupling

The previous section attempted to explain how movements are controlled by motor programmes. However, this should not be taken to mean that movement is controlled by motor programmes alone; sensory information also has an important role to play, as will be explained further below. Taking the example of picking up a cup of coffee from your desk, what information is required in order to complete this action safely and effectively?

- Prior to the action, you need information about where you need to reach towards, i.e. the position of the object in relation to you. Information about the dimensions of the cup, its weight, type of surface and other factors, such as temperature and amount of liquid, are essential to complete the action. In other words, in order to be able to programme a movement or action, *prospective* information is required about the initial conditions of the situation. In humans, prospective information for motor control is often of a visual nature; we tend to look where to place our feet, or where to move our hand to.

- During the action of reaching, picking up the cup and bringing it to your mouth, automatic reflexes will be at work to stabilise your posture. This reflex activity is a coordinated response to proprioceptive stimuli from soft tissue and skin, as explained in Chapter 6. Additionally, you need to check that you don't knock things over on your desk and take the hot liquid to your mouth without under- or overshooting. You are likely to use visual information about other objects, as well as proprioceptive information when picking up and guiding the cup to your mouth. In general, provided there is sufficient time to process the information, sensory information is used to guide the movement on-line. The movement may have to be slowed down in order for the information to be processed.

- Following the action, information is fed back about the success of the movement. In the case of this example: did you knock anything over? Did you spill any liquid? Did you manage to bring the cup to your mouth in a controlled manner? In general, exteroceptive feedback (e.g. visual or acoustic information) and proprioceptive information (i.e. what the movement felt like) are fed back into the system and compared with the intended action (i.e. the desired state). Any errors will be fed back and used for a subsequent action. If you reached too fast the last time, you will probably attempt to slow down the next time. This feedback information can be broadly categorised as follows:

  ○ **Knowledge of results**: this is information about the *outcome* of an action, e.g. to what extent it was on target, either in terms of space or time (e.g. overshooting your coffee cup and spilling liquid).
  ○ **Knowledge of performance**: this is information about the movement *pattern*, i.e. what it looked or felt like (e.g. whether the movement was smooth, or whether there were any compensatory movements).

In summary, you can see how tightly perception is linked with action. Rather than using the term 'motor control', 'perceptuo-motor control' may do more justice to the coupling between the two.

Returning to the case study of Mrs. B., we can see how she uses perceptuo-motor coupling to improve her walking difficulties; contrasting tiles in the kitchen (visual sensory information) facilitate her walking. The tiles provide a visual 'rhythm' for the action of stepping. This 'cueing' strategy, whereby sensory information acts as a prompt for action, has been widely researched in PD (Lim et al. 2005). Other forms of cueing may also be visual (e.g. lines on the floor), acoustic (e.g. a metronome or music at the rhythm of the preferred cadence) or proprioceptive (e.g. shoulder tap). Schmidt's model of motor control could help us interpret some of the problems in PD: according to this model, the open loop mode of motor control appears to have been affected; the automaticity of learned movement has been impaired at the level where motor programmes should be 'run off'. Motor programmes can still be compiled (there is evidence that, under certain circumstances, Mrs B. is able to demonstrate a near normal gait pattern), but the difficulty lies in initiating the action. This explains the difficulty with starting, stopping and adjusting movement. Substituting internal triggers with external cues may compensate for this loss. However, the question is whether patients can only perform while using a cueing device, or whether they can eventually learn to perform without it. Also, since most of the studies in the review by Lim et al. (2005) were performed in laboratory settings, the question is whether similar effects can be achieved in more natural environment. Chapter 8 will explore this question further in the context of motor learning.

Strengths and limitations of the motor programming approach

So far, we have used a motor programming model to explain how movements are coordinated. The strengths of this particular model are that it is generic (i.e. it applies to any class of movement) and provides a broad information-processing framework for understanding motor control. This, in turn, may be used to understand disorders of motor control in more depth (see Clinical application box 7.2) and provide a rationale for designing interventions.

In principle, however, models can only present a simplification of reality. So what are the limitations and weaknesses of this particular model of motor control?

A key challenge is the assumption that GMPs exist in the first place. This elicits the question about the origin of this construct. How do these programmes come into being? This refers to the notion of a **homunculus** (Latin for 'little man', or executive) that governs behaviour from within the head. This is a classic philosophical conundrum which is debated in depth elsewhere (e.g. Dennett 1997). The problem of the 'explanation' that movement is controlled by programmes only shifts the problem to another level, and a legitimate question would be: who controls the programmer? You can see the emergence of a Russian doll-like scenario, but the problem does not actually get solved. It is clear that such a 'loan on intelligence' (Dennett 1997, pp. 123–124) cannot provide a satisfactory explanation; the homunculus merely displaces the problem to another level of analysis.

Another challenge to this model is what is happening when one tries an action that is entirely new – and it is successful the first time round. Where did the GMP for this action come from so suddenly? Or, if it is based on other, familiar actions, how was it compiled so quickly?

A further question pertains to the ability of the model to explain transitions from one movement pattern to the next, e.g. shifting from walking to running. How do these transitions occur, does the GMP suddenly switch, and if so: how (and does this require a programme for switching)? There are other models of motor control (e.g. the Dynamical Systems model – see below), which have more robust explanations for this common phenomenon in movement.

In conclusion, the motor programming model of motor control, introduced above, has some important challenges. However, as a generic model it offers a useful framework for health-care practitioners who need to be able to analyse problems with perceptuo-motor control, in order to design interventions.

Other approaches to motor control

Ecological/direct perception approach

The ecological approach to perception and action was pioneered by James Gibson (1904–1979), a

Clinical application box 7.2

Apraxia

Mr J. has had a right-sided parietal stroke 2 weeks ago. He has made a good recovery and has been discharged from the acute stroke unit. However, upon assessment, his occupational therapist has decided that he is not ready to be discharged home: despite Mr J. being fully compus mentus, motivated, able to move freely, having intact sensation and able to understand verbal instructions, when asked to put on his glasses (or any item of clothing), he does not know how to do this. Mr J. fumbles around, gets confused between front/back, up/down and left/right. He will try various ways, but does not succeed and eventually gives up, exhausted. Following further assessment, the occupational therapist concludes that Mr J has apraxia (or dypraxia) and will require intervention before discharge home, where he lives independently by himself.

The term apraxia comes from the Greek 'prassein' ('action', Chambers English Dictionary, 1990). A classic definition of apraxia is the following by Kolb and Whishaw (2009, p. G-3):

> 'inability to make voluntary movements in the absence of paralysis or other motor or sensory impairment; especially an inability to make proper use of an object'.

Clinically, apraxia is manifest in patients such as Mr J. who confuses objects with his body, or does not know which side is which, who have difficulty using objects in an intended way (e.g. they may use a toothbrush to comb their hair, or place tooth paste straight onto their teeth as they don't know how to use a toothbrush). They may have difficulty imitating gestures, or with constructing designs (e.g. they may be unable to copy a cube, drawn on paper). They may get a sequence of actions in the wrong order (e.g. when getting dressed), or they may attempt to get out of bed without having first removed the sheets, or place a teabag in the kettle when making a cup of tea. Actions may have missing components, finish before they have been completed, or continue when the task is actually complete. Movements may also be executed in abnormal ways, e.g.

in the wrong direction or with an inappropriate amount of force, leading to overshoot and knocking things over. Children with apraxia are often known as having **developmental coordination disorder (DCD)**.

How can we understand this perplexing array of problems – despite lack of movement, sensation, etc., to explain them?

Let's think for a moment about what is involved in completing a task such as making a cup of tea. We need to generate the idea, in which we use attention, memory and mental imagery of the action. In planning the activity, we may use language to talk ourselves through (especially if the task is unfamiliar or complex), and we need to obtain accurate sensory information about ourselves, the object(s) we will be using and our environment. Finally, we need to execute the actual task, producing the movements as planned.

These stages can be aligned with Schmidt's model of motor control. At different stages, problems may occur, leading to different expressions of apraxia. There are many different types of apraxia (e.g. 'dressing' or 'constructional' apraxia'), which are debated amongst clinicians and researchers, but here we will only consider a number of generic forms. Ideational apraxia involves difficulty understanding the goal of an action (Kolb and Whishaw 2009), which suggests there are difficulties at the first stage. In ideomotor apraxia, the person understands the goal but there are difficulties with the initiation and execution of planned movement sequences. Patients may be unable to imitate movement, or make gestures upon request (e.g. signal to stop). This form of apraxia would fit in with the final stage. Careful assessment, often by the occupational therapist, is required to determine where the main problem is located in this process from action ideation to execution, before interventions can be recommended. Having a framework to categorise this wide range of perception – cognition – motor problems may help to make sense of what is a seemingly diverse array.

---

psychologist who developed a theory to explain how organisms engage with their natural environment by coupling perception and action. He published his final book, *The ecological approach to visual perception* (1979), just before he died. The term *ecological* reflects Gibson's endeavour to understand meaningful interaction between organisms and their natural environment (van Wieringen 1989). This was in contrast to what he saw as the contrived behaviour in the psychology laboratory, where at the time much research focused on developing theories of perception based on visual illusions. Gibson criticised psychologists for using stimuli that were 'impoverished, ambiguous, or conflicting' (Gibson 1963, p. 11) and argued

that such artificial situations were not ecologically valid (i.e. representative) for perception in general. In contrast, he argued, in a natural environment, people move in order to perceive, and perceive in order to move (Gibson 1979). Just consider crossing a road: one uses eye movement, head movement and sometimes whole body movement to 'see' if the road is clear; an example of action for perception. Once in the middle of the road, the image of a fast approaching car makes us speed up; an example of perception for action. Crucial to Gibson's theory is the notion that the coupling between perception and action is highly specific. He argued that light illuminates an observer's environment – not in some general manner, but in a way that is structured and specific. Light is reflected by the surfaces (i.e. walls or trees, the floor and ceiling) around us, creating structure; an *optic array* (defined as 'the projection of an environment to a stationary point', Gibson 1958, p. 185, Fig. 7.2). Furthermore, this structure is specific to our position within this environment; it tells us whether we are upright, tilting or upside down with regards to the horizon. If we now change our position in this environment, the light reflected into our eyes changes accordingly; a phenomenon he called *optic flow* (defined as 'the projection of an environment to a moving point' (Gibson 1958, p. 185).

In the optic array, there are a number of invariants (i.e. constants) for the observer. For example, if you are standing in a long corridor with black and white tiles on the floor, the person standing in front of you looks larger than the person standing much further away. However, the proportion of the size of the person and the size of the textured floor remains the same. This invariant (known as size constancy) was a conundrum that posed a challenge to cognitive psychologists for a long time. But rather than presuming intricate cognitive processes, Gibson argued that this invariant can be 'picked up' (as opposed to 'processed', a term used by cognitive psychologists) directly. Hence the label *direct perception* that came to indicate Gibson's theory. Similarly, the optic flow specifies movement through the environment in such a way that the observer can pick up this information directly. Movement is

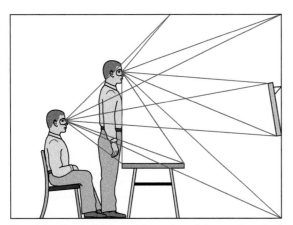

Fig. 7.2 • Perspective transformation of the patchwork of an optic array due to change of viewpoint (Gibson, J.J. 1963. The useful dimensions of sensitivity. American Psychologist; 18: 1-15. American Psychological Association, adapted with permission.)

essential, Gibson argued, for picking up the invariants, as only by changing one's position can one pick up what is constant (Gibson 1963). With vision playing such a distinctive role in specifying movement in the environment, Gibson allocated a proprioceptive function to vision ('visual kinaesthesis', Gibson 1958).

Gibson's theory proposed that organisms use visual information to pick up information relevant for action. A key concept in Gibson's work is the term '**affordance**', which he defined as follows: 'the affordance of anything is a specific combination of its substance and its surfaces taken with reference to an animal' (Gibson 1977, p. 67). In other words, an affordance offers possibilities for action within a specific environment or with a specific object for a specific organism. For example, water affords floating to a duck but not to a human being. A set of stairs affords stepping to adults but crawling to toddlers. Warren (1984) also included the kinetic properties of mass and work in the concept of 'affordance'. In an interesting study on the affordance 'climbability' of stairs, participants judged whether stairs with different riser heights were climbable or unclimbable. All participants – deliberately chosen to be short or tall – judged stairs to be unclimbable beyond a critical ratio of stair riser height to leg length. This ratio was also associated with the least amount of energy expenditure during actual climbing of the same stairs and – remarkably – this ratio was identical for all participants, i.e. irrespective of their absolute height. Based on these and other studies, Warren proposed that organisms perceive affordances in terms of action-scaled – as opposed to absolute – metrics to determine critical and optimal points for action (Warren 1984, 1988).

The concept of 'affordance' is important for therapists, as it implies that properties of objects and the environment can provide useful information to facilitate the organisation of action.

For example, a china cup affords a precision grip, but this is not an action afforded by a plastic cone. Referring back to the case study of Mrs. B with PD, a tiled floor (provided that the tile dimensions match a person's stride length) affords 'stepping' – an action not so clearly afforded by an unstructured carpet. In rehabilitation settings, therapists may use objects (e.g. a plastic cone instead of a cup) and provide treatment in environments (e.g. an empty hospital corridor instead of an outdoor environment) that are thought to simplify motor control. While this can be helpful in the initial stage of rehabilitation, therapists also need to consider that such objects and environments are in a sense 'impoverished' from an affordance perspective, rendering motor control more challenging in some cases. Carefully choosing objects and environments is therefore an important aspect of designing effective interventions.

Inspired by Gibson's ground-breaking work, Lee (1976) set out to develop a mathematical theory on visual control of movement. His endeavour was to explain how organisms utilise visual information to move around safely and effectively in their environment. Lee and colleagues studied a range of actions, including balance, steering and driving, walking, long-jumping and intercepting moving objects, with study participants representing human adults and infants, gannets, humming birds, bats

and amoebas (Lee 2009). Lee's classic experiment of the 'moving room' (Lee and Aronson 1974) is summarised in Research box 7.2 below.

Lee argued that animals, including small insects, are highly skilled in moving around complex environments – without having large central nervous systems available to undertake complex cognitive processing. The control processes involved in movement were, therefore, likely to be based on simple principles (Lee 1998).

Based on the paradigm of an object moving straight towards the stationary eye of an observer at a constant velocity, Lee elegantly demonstrated that the time at which this point would contact the plane through the nodal point of the lens can be expressed as the inverse rate of the expansion of the object's image on the

Research box 7.2

How do infants control their posture?
The role of proprioceptive and visual information

If you were asked which types of sensory information you use for controlling your posture, what would your answer be? You are probably thinking of vestibular and proprioceptive, and possibly acoustic and visual information. Would any of these be more important than the others? How would you design an experiment to find out?

In a pioneering study, Lee and Aronson (1974) set out to investigate the role of vision in the control of posture. At the time, the predominant view was that posture was controlled by proprioceptive information from the vestibular organs, muscle fibres and joint capsules. Although there were some suggestions that vision might play a role, there was no conclusive evidence. Lee and Aronson designed an experiment where proprioceptive and visual information would contradict each other. As part of their methods, they designed the ingenious (and since famous) 'moving room'. This room (3.6 m long x 1.8 m wide x 2 m high) was open at one end and suspended, just above the floor. The room could be swung horizontally from a lockable position 47 cm in front to 47 cm behind the long wall of the room but – and this is the crux – the actual floor on which participants were standing remained stationary.

The time taken for one 'swing' to complete from one position to the other was around 2.5 s, with a maximum velocity of 0.4 m/s. The researchers chose infants as their study participants, as they had less experience with standing than adults, so any intervention aimed at changing their standing posture was expected to have a more pronounced effect. The experiment involved one infant at a time, standing inside this room (together with its mother and an experimenter), with its back towards the open end. The room would then be moved, and the child's postural sway would be observed.

What would you expect to happen if one's posture was entirely under proprioceptive control? Remember that there was no movement of the floor, so in terms of proprioception, nothing was really changing compared to when the room was motionless. But what if vision dominated the control of posture? Lee and Aronson hypothesised that, if the infant used predominantly visual information, it would demonstrate abnormal body sway – in the direction *in which the room was being moved*. The researchers reasoned that a forward motion of the room would create an optic flow similar to a backward movement of the body (i.e. the person would think they were moving backward), and vice versa. (You may be familiar with the scenario where a neighbouring train speeding forward gives you, seated in a stationary train, the illusion that you are speeding backward.) In order to compensate for perceived backward motion, the person would instigate a movement in the opposite direction, i.e. in the same direction as that of the moving room.

Seven healthy infants took part, with ages between 13 and 16 months and walking experience ranging from 1 to 22 weeks. The results were unambiguous: 82% of all trials included in the analysis were 'positive', i.e. the infant demonstrated abnormal body sway in the direction in which was room was being moved. In 1/3 of the trials, they even fell over.

Lee and Aronson interpreted this evidence as supporting the notion that, in infants with limited experience in standing and walking, visual information is the dominant source of information for controlling postural sway.

Clearly, this was a small trial with infants in different stages of development. Additionally, modern methods of recording postural sway are more robust, but these methodological issues do not detract from the groundbreaking impact of this study.

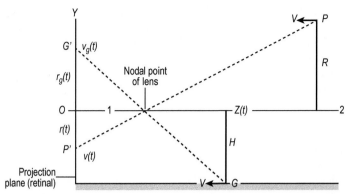

Fig. 7.3 • Schematic representation of the environment moving straight towards the stationary eye of an observer at a constant velocity V in the direction Z to O (e.g. a bicycle coming straight towards a seated person). P and G represent texture elements on surfaces in the environment, e.g. P being the top of the cyclist's helmet and G being the contact point of the wheel on the ground. H represents eye height. Light reflected from P and G passes through the nodal point of the lens, and elicits the moving optic texture elements P' and G' on the projection plane, which represents the retina. Springer and Springer-Verlag, Experimental Brain Research Series 15, 1986, p. 221. Gearing action to the environment, Lee, D.N. and Young, D.S. 1986, fig. 5, with kind permission from Springer Science+Business Media B.V. from Springer Science+Business Media B.V.

observer's retina (Lee 1976, 1986, Fig. 7.3). This optic variable, which specifies 'time to contact', was labelled *tau* (τ). As this information is available directly from the eye's retina, Lee argued that the observer did not need detailed information such as distance or velocity, or complex calculations based on these variables (Lee and Young 1986). Time to contact is an essential variable for controlling actions such as catching a ball, adjusting stride length when jumping from a take-off board, and avoiding collisions when walking or driving. Since the original publications, the paradigm has been generalised to include non-linear movement trajectories and non-constant velocity, other forms of perception (e.g. echolocation in bats and electrolocation in fish), while tau theory has been expanded to comprise the notion of tau as the time-to-closure of a 'gap' (Lee 1998). An example of a 'gap' is that between a hand (the effector) and a cup on the table that it is reaching for (target), or between a foot and a stepping stone. The tau of a gap is defined as '*the time-to-closure of the gap at its current rate of closure*' (Lee 2009, p. 837). In studies where mathematical algorithms describing reach-to-grasp motor control are run off in computer simulations, and then compared to real live reach-to-grasp data to check their validity, time to contact with the object (Hoff and Arbib 1993), and distance to the object are both important explanatory variables (Rand et al. 2006).

In many actions, more than one gap needs to be closed. Think about reaching for a cup that is now handed to us; in this situation you need to consider the gap between your moving hand and the expected end point, and the moving cup and the same end point. Both gaps need to be zero at the same time, meanwhile controlling the impact to prevent spilling the content of the cup. Experiments have shown that movement control in a range of actions is achieved through 'tau coupling', i.e. keeping a constant ratio between the taus, resulting in arriving at the goal at the same time (Lee 1998). Moving in sync to a rhythm (as in cueing to facilitate walking in patients with PD) is an interesting problem, as this requires the coupling of a motor 'gap' (i.e. placing a foot on the ground) with a sensory 'gap' (i.e. the space between successive beats). But what if one just decides to reach somewhere without any visual cue? This brings us to the more recent concept of 'intrinsic tau guidance', which is an attempt to explain the control of movement in situations where there is no extrinsic sensory information to control the movement. Lee (1998, 2009) proposed that such actions are intrinsically guided and assumed that the nervous system would generate its own intrinsic tau guide – although the precise origin of this variable remains to be elucidated.

In terms of clinical applications of tau theory, Craig et al. (2000) measured tau coupling during sucking behaviour in six pre-term infants compared to normal controls. A lower correlation (i.e. poorer tau coupling) was found between the tau of the suction pressure and that of the intrinsic tau guide in the pre-term infants. Interestingly, when exploring whether poor suction control was indicative of motor delay 6 months later, there was some correspondence between rankings of sucking performance and those of motor function. These exploratory data suggested that intra-oral sucking pressure could provide a sensitive and objective measure of impaired motor control in newborns.

In summary, tau theory is about prospective control of movement, which involves initiating control prior to an event (Lee 1998). According to Lee (2009, p. 840), organisms *'fit actions into 4D slots'*. Prospective control concentrates on closing gaps between effectors (e.g. hands, feet) and their goals (e.g. a moving ball), which organisms achieve by picking up the tau of each gap involved in the action, and coupling these by keeping a constant ratio between them (Lee 1998).

One of the key strengths of this seminal body of work is that '**time-to-contact**', a variable involved in so many different motor acts in so many different species, is directly available from the retina (or other sensors) without the need for complex computations. However, the question is whether tau theory is the only explanation for motor control or whether there are alternative explanations (Land, in Lee 2009). For example, imagine yourself nipping out to the bathroom at night, trying to avoid waking up anyone else: without much visual or auditory feedback, you may rely to some extent on tactile feedback as you move along, but your direction is likely to be largely informed by an internal representation of your environment. Some experiments suggest that the nervous system is opportunistic and will use any valid information to solve a motor problem (Rushton and Wann 1999). In other words, tau theory may be a powerful explanation for a range of motor problems, while other theories may be more suited to explain other types of actions.

A full expose of tau theory is beyond the scope of this chapter, and readers are referred to Lee et al. (2009) for a more in-depth explanation of this theory and other clinical applications that are in development.

Dynamical systems/natural-physical approach

Having introduced the direct perception approach within the cluster of 'action theories' of motor control, we now turn to an approach that focuses on the action side of the same coin. Based on Bernstein's and Gibson's work, the dynamical systems (or natural-physical) approach to motor control seeks to explain how organised motor behaviour emerges from complex biological systems in terms of the laws of physics.

The notion of a complex system can be gleaned from Bernstein's definition of coordination, the process whereby a system with multiple degrees of freedom works together to produce orderly behaviour. This system is complex – not only because of the numerous degrees of freedom within the system itself, but also because of the requirement to interact with external forces to achieve an intended goal (think about surfing – the trick is to work with wind and wave power). Bernstein had shown that it is impossible for neural impulses to fully specify movement, thereby arguing against a so-called *'push-button control-board model of the cortex'* (a bit like an organ key board, Bernstein 1984/1935, p. 94). Instead, movement is the result of an interaction between muscle force and environmental forces, including gravity, friction and inertia (Turvey 1990). A good example of how muscle forces interact with external forces is the ground-breaking study by Thelen et al. (1984) on stepping in newborns (see Research box 7.3 below).

Research box 7.3

Newborn stepping

Thelen and co-workers explored infant stepping and kicking under different environmental conditions in three sequential studies. Newborn stepping was of interest, as at the time it was believed that this was a reflex-type behaviour that could be elicited in newborns until the age of about 4–6 weeks, after which it 'disappeared' – allegedly, as the brain matured. In their first study with infants between 2 and 6 weeks of age, they found that those who had gained weight most rapidly at week 4 stepped less. This suggested that body weight influences stepping and that the ability to generate muscle force was insufficient to counterbalance the amount of weight gained. In the second study, the researchers added small weights to the infants' legs, and noted the amount of stepping when the infant was held upright. In the weighted condition, infants stepped significantly less than in the unweighted condition. In the third experiment, researchers held the infants so that their legs were submerged in a bath of warm water, and again compared stepping behaviour between the submerged and on-land conditions. In the submerged condition, stepping rate was much higher, due to the buoyancy of the water. Together, these findings indicate that newborn stepping is not just a reflex (that miraculously disappears at some point in the child's development, to 're-appear' as more mature walking), but a complex motor behaviour that can be explained by the interaction between the infant's ability to generate muscle force and gravity acting on the body.

The study of motor control from the dynamical systems perspective commenced with the study of rhythmic (or periodic) movement – a striking feature of motor control shared by all living organisms (just think of breathing, shaking, tapping, walking, swimming, jumping and flying). Each of these organisms can be seen as a complex biological system, i.e. comprising many subsystems, such as the nervous, muscular and other systems – each of which comprise many subunits (i.e. neurons and muscle fibres, respectively). Given the complexity at microscopic level (e.g. the firing of individual neurons), how does ordered behaviour (e.g. walking) emerge at a macroscopic level? In trying to answer this question, Haken and colleagues drew parallels between biological and complex physical systems (Haken and Wunderlin 1990).

For example, in laser light, a coherent wave emerges from the movement of numerous individual electrons, as a function of pumping energy into the laser-active material (Haken et al. 1985, and Haken and Wunderlin 1990). This is an example where ordered behaviour at a macroscopic level emerges from within the system through **self-organisation**, i.e. without specific commands from a so-called executive structure (1990), as in the motor programming theory discussed above. Thus, Haken and colleagues set out to study motor control, using concepts from synergetics, a theory of self-organisation in complex systems. Let us conduct an experiment with yourself as an example of a complex biological system, and see how order may (or may not!) emerge (Research box 7.4).

According to the dynamical systems approach, the phase relationship between the two fingers (in this case: in- or out-of-phase), describes and organises the order of the system at a macroscopic level. Parameters (such as phase) that describe the order of complex systems are known as *order-parameters*. In the experiment above, we saw that the order parameter changed dramatically at a critical frequency of movement. Parameters that can change the order of a system in this way are known as *control parameters*. Phase transitions in complex biological systems are accompanied by certain characteristic phenomena, i.e. *critical fluctuations* and *critical slowing down*. Critical fluctuations indicate that order parameters undergo large changes. Critical slowing down indicates that, if the system is perturbed, it recovers more slowly when it is close to a transition point than when it is in a stable coordination pattern. Taken together, these phenomena indicate that the systems we are looking at are self-organising systems that behave in a non-linear way. This means that a gradual change in the control

Research box 7.4

Phase transitions in finger movement

Sitting at your desk, place your forearms on the table and point both index fingers forward. Keeping the rest of your hands and arms in this position, slowly move both index fingers so that flexion in the metacarpophalangeal (MCP) joint on one side occurs together with extension in the MCP joint on the other side, i.e. anti-symmetrical (or out-of-phase). Slowly increase the frequency of movement and note the pattern of coordination between the two fingers. What happened? As your frequency increased, suddenly your fingers 'flipped' from an anti-symmetrical (out-of-phase) pattern to a symmetrical (in-phase) pattern. The first pattern was stable, and at a critical frequency, this changed abruptly to a different pattern, which was also stable. This so-called phase transition, reported by Kelso in 1981 (in Haken et al. 1985), has been replicated many times since, demonstrating the same phenomenon in different scenarios, including quadrupedal gait (Schöner et al. 1991). These experiments demonstrate that individual body segments can be coupled together and behave as coupled oscillators in a stable coordination pattern.

parameter may not be mirrored in a similar change in the order parameter, but that sudden changes may occur in the entire coordination pattern of an organism.

What is the role of non-linearity in motor control? Haken et al. (1985, Haken and Wunderlin 1990) argued that non-linearity enables reproducible behaviour, i.e. stable coordination patterns (so-called *attractor states*) while control parameters (e.g. movement frequency) may vary considerably. It is only at a critical value of the control parameter that the stable coordination pattern becomes unstable – while nonlinearity also enables the system to switch between different stable patterns.

How does the dynamical systems approach solve the ubiquitous degrees-of-freedom problem? According to Haken et al. (1985), describing coordination in terms of order parameters reduces the degree-of-freedom problem, as it is no longer burdened with specifying the movements of individual body segments. Furthermore, it has been proposed that movement control emerges from different subsystems working together (e.g. vision, proprioception and the musculoskeletal system), with fine-tuning of the movement being undertaken by relatively autonomous subsystems (e.g. reflex mechanisms, discussed in Chapter 6). Actual movement is produced by so-called **coordinative structures (or synergies)**, which are functional linkages of muscle groups that work together in achieving certain tasks (Bernstein 1984/1935, Turvey 1990, Latash 2008). The term synergy has been described in many different ways, but in principle it refers to a *'correlated output of muscles/joints/effectors in voluntary multi-joint movements'* (Latash 2008, p. 39). Taking a cup to your mouth may be undertaken using different synergies, but trunk lateral flexion and shoulder elevation are normally not part of these. In people with stroke, however, such abnormal synergies are common coordination patterns (Archambault et al. 1999, Cirstea and Levin 2000).

Taken together, the dynamical systems approach provides an entirely paradigm for the study of movement compared to the motor programming approach introduced earlier. Drawing on an understanding of complex systems in physics, this approach is particularly well equipped to explain important non-linear phenomena that none of the other theories discussed earlier has managed to explain satisfactorily, e.g. transitions of movement patterns.

An interesting clinical application of this approach is the use of bilateral simultaneous task training in people with stroke. In this type of intervention, the patient performs the same movement with each arm simultaneously – but independently, e.g. moving the two hands at the same time, each placing a peg in a hole. There are a number of theoretical foundations for this intervention, one of which is the dynamical systems approach. Based on this theory, the two upper limbs can be seen as coupled oscillators. The hypothesis is that the more affected arm is coupled to the less affected arm, being 'entrained' by it to perform in the same way. Early studies (Mudie and Matyas 1996) were promising, although a recent Cochrane systematic review concluded that there was no additional benefit of this type of training compared to other forms of upper limb therapy or 'usual care' (Coupar et al. 2010). As bilateral task training is an umbrella term for a diverse range of stimuli (from highly constrained movements executed with the aid of a mechanical device to functional tasks undertaken more freely), further research is required to unravel the perceptuo-motor control processes involved in different forms of bilateral simultaneous task training.

Another clinical application of dynamical systems theory in PD is shown in Research box 7.5.

Motor control in context

Reflecting on the different theories that endeavour to explain motor control, it will hopefully have become apparent that there is more to motor control than just the 'motor'. As the eminent Nikolai Bernstein said (1984/1935, p. 359):

> *'Every intelligent purposeful movement is made as an answer to a motor problem and is determined – directly or indirectly - by the situation as a whole.'*

In order words, we don't just produce shoulder flexion with elbow and finger extension; we reach, and we reach *for something* – and in a *specific environment*.

There are two key points in Bernstein's statement that are worth elaborating: firstly, the notion that purposeful movement represents an answer to a motor problem. Restoring purposeful movement is of considerable interest to patients and health-care professionals; activities of daily living such as dressing, going up and down stairs, and communicating with others are just a few examples. Undertaking purposeful movement implies that the individual is solving a problem – through action. Reaching for your cup of coffee is a problem – even if you are not consciously aware of this, your motor control system has to work out how to do it. Initial conditions are picked up prospectively and through a process of working backward – known as inverse modelling – (Berthoz 2000) the system works out how to reach its desired state. The notion of the patient as a problem solver has important implications for the role of the health-care professional in the rehabilitation process, as we shall see in the next chapter.

The second aspect of Bernstein's quotation that is worth highlighting is the notion that purposeful movement is 'determined...by the situation as a whole'. What does this mean? Studying motor control from the perspective of the individual provides us with important information, e.g. about the *individual's* nervous, musculoskeletal, cardiopulmonary systems and any impairments there may be. This information is necessary, but not sufficient. For example, reaching for that cup of coffee again, you may be able to undertake this without much conscious attention if the cup is only half full. However, your control will need to be adapted if the cup is full to the brim; in order to reduce the chance of spilling you will need to minimise accelerations and decelerations. This is an example where the specific *task* requirements influence motor control. Finally, you may be able to pick up this cup competently in an environment with a stable base of support, but the same task on a train may cause some unexpected complications for your perceptuo-motor control system. This is an example where the *environment* plays an important role in the control of the action.

Research box 7.5

The relation between clinical signs and symptoms and coordination in PD: a dynamical systems approach

Winogrodzka and colleagues (2005) were interested in coordination problems in Parkinson's disease (PD) and examined the impact of bradykinesia, rigidity and the extent of dopaminergic degeneration on interlimb coordination during walking in a group of 29 early PD patients, who were not receiving medication.

Based on a dynamical systems approach, previous work by Wagenaar and van Emmerik (1994) had shown that in healthy controls, changing walking speed (the control parameter) resulted in a phase change between arm and leg swing (the order parameter).

You can try this experiment for yourself: start walking at a very low speed, and you will find that your arms move in phase and at a frequency twice that of your legs. As you increase your walking speed, your arms will start to move in an out-of-phase mode and at the same frequency as the legs (the changes in frequency had been reported by Craik et al. in 1976). Studies with people with PD had shown that these phase transitions did occur but were less pronounced than in healthy controls (van Emmerik and Wagenaar 1996, van Emmerik et al. 1999). These findings match the clinical notion of rigidity in PD, including reduced arm and leg swing. However, what had not been investigated was the association between the phase changes during walking, the severity of typical clinical symptoms of PD (i.e. bradykinesia and rigidity) and the severity of the dopaminergic degeneration.

The main hypothesis in this study was that the severity of rigidity, bradykinesia and extent of dopaminergic degeneration would be correlated with the magnitude of the phase changes between arm and leg swing during walking, such that a greater severity would be associated with reduced phase changes.

To manipulate walking speed, the researchers used a treadmill so they could incrementally vary walking speed from 0.6 km/h to 5.4 km/h while they measured changes in the relative phase between arm and leg swing, using accelerometers.

The findings demonstrated that phase changes between arm and leg swing did occur with changes in walking speed, but that there was marked variation between different patients. Overall, the more severe the rigidity and bradykinesia, the smaller the phase changes as well as the maximum phase between arm and leg swing that could be achieved. There was no correlation, however, between the extent of dopaminergic depletion and the coordination measures – although there was a correspondence between the side of the body with the more severe coordination deficits and the side of the brain showing more severe dopaminergic depletion.

In conclusion, although the relationship between the reduction in dopaminergic integrity and coordination needs to be more fully explored, this study with early PD patients who were not on medication, suggests that the severity of a number of cardinal signs and symptoms of PD is associated with a pathologically increased stability (or diminished adaptability) of the coordination between arm and leg swing. Thus, this study has demonstrated that patients with PD show reduced phase changes, and the dynamical systems approach has provided a useful way to examine complex coordination of movement in these patients.

Shumway–Cook and Woollacott (2007) illustrate the interaction between the individual, the task and the environment in terms of motor control very effectively (Fig. 7.4). The implication for health-care professionals is that, in their assessment of a patient's movement problems, they need to consider not just the individual and their impairments, but also the ways in which different tasks and environments influence their motor control difficulties. As we have seen in the case of PD, changing the environment by adding cues considerably improved walking ability.

Summary

This chapter has provided an introduction to the concept of motor control and explained how this is aimed at reducing the numerous degrees of freedom involved in human movement and render movement both effective and efficient. Different theories propose different solutions to the degree of freedom problem. Schmidt's model, as a proponent of the 'motor theories', proposes that movement is controlled through a generalised motor programme (GMP) that stores the blueprint for a particular class of action, which is then fine-tuned to the specific requirements of the task within the environment in which it is taking place. However, those representing the 'action theories' propose different solutions: direct perception theory suggests that movement is specified by invariants in the environment, while dynamical systems theory proposes that coordination involves order parameters instead of individual degrees of freedom, and that movements emerge from coordinative structures or synergies.

"Motor control emerges from an interaction between the individual, the task and the environment"

SHUMWAY-COOK & WOOLLACOTT (1995)

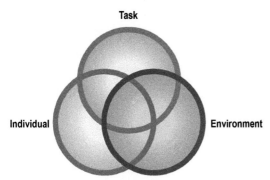

Task

Individual

Environment

Fig. 7.4 • Adapted from Shumway–Cook and Woollacott (2007), with permission from Wolters Kluwer Health.

We have seen that motor and action theories offer different interpretations of motor problems. There is no such thing as 'the correct' theory – the question is whether the theory matches the type of question you wish to answer.

But whichever theoretical approach you take, purposeful movement has been proposed as a **problem-solving activity**, which needs to take account of the specific task requirements, as well as environmental conditions. In the next chapter, we shall explore how movements and skills are acquired, and what this means for the role of the health-care professional, involved in improving movement and activity.

SELF-ASSESSMENT QUESTIONS

Following this chapter, can you:

1. Define motor control and co-ordination
2. Describe, in your own words, the 'degrees of freedom' problem and explain its importance for understanding perceptuo-motor control
3. Explain, in general terms, how perceptuo-motor control strategies are dependent on the following three factors: the individual, the task and the environment
4. Explain the main roles of sensory information in the control of movement
5. Describe and explain Schmidt's hierarchical model of motor control
6. Within Schmidt's model, compare and contrast closed loop and open loop modes of motor control
7. Define the term generalised motor programme (GMP) and explain how this is purported to work; in general terms as well as for a specific activity:
   - Discuss the strengths and limitations of Schmidt's hierarchical model of motor control.
   - Explore how Schmidt's model may inform rehabilitation practice.
8. Compare and contrast Schmidt's motor programming theory with the direct perception approach and dynamical systems approach in terms of:
   - the perspective each takes on describing human movement
   - the role of cognition in motor control
   - the nature of perception-action coupling
   - the solution to the degrees of freedom problem
   - how each theory may be applied to rehabilitation.

Further reading

Altenmüller, E., Wiesendanger, M., Kesselring, J., 2006. Music, Motor Control and the Brain. Oxford University Press, Oxford.

Bernstein, N., 1967. The Coordination and Regulation of Movements. Pergamon Press, New York.

Freund, H.J., Jeannerod, M., Hallett, M., et al., 2005. Higher Order Motor Disorders. From neuroanatomy and neurobiology to clinical neurology. Oxford University Press, Oxford.

Kugler, P.N., Turvey, M.T., 1987. Information, Natural Law and the

Self-assembly of Rhythmic Movement. Lawrence Erlbaum Associates, Hillsdale, NJ.

Thaut, M.H., 2008. Rhythm, Music and the Brain. Scientific foundations and clinical applications. Routledge, New York.

References

Adams, J.A., 1971. A closed-loop theory of motor learning. J. Mot. Behav. 3, 111–149.

Archambault, P., Pigeon, P., Feldman, A. G., et al., 1999. Recruitment and sequencing of different degrees of freedom during pointing movements involving the trunk in healthy and

hemiparetic subjects. Exp. Brain Res. 126, 55–67.

Azulay, J.P., Mesure, S., Amblard, B., et al., 1999. Visual control of locomotion in Parkinson's disease. Brain 122, 111–120.

Bernstein, N.A., 1984/1935. Some emergent problems of the regulation

of motor acts. In: Whiting, H.T.A. (Ed.), Human motor actions: Bernstein re-assessed. North Holland, Amsterdam.

Berthoz, A., 2000. The brain's sense of movement. In: Kosslynn, S.M. (Ed.), Perspectives in Cognitive Neuroscience. Harvard University Press, Cambridge Massachusetts.

Bloem, B.R., van Vugt, J.P., Beckely, D.J., 2001. Postural instability and falls in Parkinson's disease. Adv. Neurol. 87, 209–223.

Bobath, B., 1990. Adult Hemiplegia Evaluation and Treatment, third ed. Heinemann Medical Books, Oxford.

Bongaardt, R., 2001. How Bernstein conquered movement. In: Latash, L.M., Zatsiorsky, V.M. (Eds.), Classics in Movement Science. Human Kinetics, Champaign, Illinois, pp. 59–84.

Butler, P.B., 1998. A preliminary report of the effectiveness of trunk targeting in achieving independent sitting balance in children with cerebral palsy. Clin. Rehabil. 12, 281–293.

Cirstea, M.C., Levin, M.F., 2000. Compensatory strategies for reaching in stroke. Brain 123, 940–953.

Coupar, F., Pollock, A., van Wijck, F., et al., 2010. Simultaneous bilateral training for improving arm function after stroke. Cochrane Database Syst. Rev. 4, CD006432. doi: 10.1002/14651858.

Craig, G.M., Grealy, M.A., Lee, D.N., 2000. Detecting motor abnormalities in preterm infants. Exp. Brain Res. 131, 359–365.

Craik, R., Herman, R., Finley, F.R., 1976. Human solutions for locomotion. Interlimb coordination. In: Herman, R. M., Grillner, S., Stein, P.S.G. (Eds.), Neural Control of Locomotion. Plemum Press, New York, pp. 51–63.

Dennett, D.C., 1997. Brainstorms: Philosophical essays on mind and psychology. Penguin, London.

Farmer, S.E., Butler, P.B., Major, R.E., 1999. Targeted training for crouch posture in cerebral palsy. Physiotherapy 85, 242–247.

Gibson, J.J., 1958. Visually controlled locomotion and visual orientation in animals. Br. J. Psychol. 49, 182–194.

Gibson, J.J., 1963. The useful dimensions of sensitivity. Am. Psychol. 18, 1–15.

Gibson, J.J., 1977. The theory of affordances. In: Shaw, R.E., Bransford, J. (Eds.), Perceiving, acting and knowing: toward an ecological psychology. Erlbaum, Hillsdale NJ.

Gibson, J.J., 1979. The Ecological Approach to Visual Perception. Houghton Mifflin, Boston.

Goodale, M.A., Milner, A.D., 1992. Separate visual pathways for perception and action. Trends Neurosci. 15, 20–25.

Gordon, J., 2000. Assumptions underlying physical therapy intervention: theoretical and historical perspectives. In: Carr, J., Shepherd, R. (Eds.), Movement Science. Foundations for physical therapy rehabilitation, second ed. Aspen Publishers, Gaithersburg, Maryland, pp. 1–32.

Haken, H., Wunderlin, A., 1990. Synergetics and its paradigm of self-organisation in biological systems. In: Whiting, H.T.A., Meijer, O.G., van Wieringen, P.C.W. (Eds.), The Natural-physical Approach to Movement Control. VU University Press, Amsterdam, pp. 1–36.

Haken, H., Kelso, J.A.S., Bunz, H., 1985. A theoretical model of phase transitions in human hand movements. Biol. Cybern. 51, 347–356.

Hoff, B., Arbib, M.A., 1993. Models of trajectory formation and temporal interaction of reach and grasp. J. Mot. Behav. 25, 175–192.

Jeannerod, M., 1984. The timing of natural prehension movements. J. Mot. Behav. 26, 235–254.

Jeannerod, M., 1988. The Neural and Behavioural Organisation of Goal Directed Movements, vol. 15. Clarendon Press, Oxford.

Kamm, K., Thelen, E., Jensen, J.L., 1990. A dynamical systems approach to motor development. Phys. Ther. 70, 763–775.

Kolb, B., Whishaw, I.Q., 2009. Fundamentals of human neuropsychology, sixth ed. Worth Publishers, New York.

Latash, M., 2008. Synergy. Oxford University Press, Oxford.

Latash, L.M., Zatsiorsky, V.M., 2001. Classics in Movement Science. Human Kinetics, Champaign, Illinois.

Lee, D.N., 1976. A theory of visual control of braking based on information about time-to-collision. Perception 5, 437–459.

Lee, D.N., 1998. Guiding movement by coupling taus. Ecol. Psychol. 10, 221–250.

Lee, D.N., 2009. General Tau Theory: evolution to date. Perception 38, 837–850.

Lee, D.N., Aronson, E., 1974. Visual proprioceptive control of standing in infants. Percept. Psychophys. 15, 529–532.

Lee, D.N., Young, D.S., 1986. Gearing action to the environment. In: Experimental Brain Research Series 15. Springer-Verlag, Berlin-Heidelberg, pp. 217–230.

Lee, D.N., Young, D.S., 1986. Gearing action to the environment. In: Experimental Brain Research Series 15, Springer-Verlag, Berlin-Heidelberg, pp. 217–230.

Lee, D.N., 2009. General Tau Theory: evolution to date. Perception 38, 837–850.

Lim, I., van Wegen, E., de Goede, C., et al., 2005. Effects of external rhythmical cueing on gait in patients with Parkinson's disease: a systematic review. Clin. Rehabil. 19, 695–713.

Major, R.E., Johnson, G.R., Butler, P.M., 2001. Learning motor control in the upright position: a mechanical engineering approach. Proceedings of the Institute of Mechanical Engineers 215 H, 315–323.

Marteniuk, G., MacKenzie, C.L., Jeannerod, M., et al., 1987. Constraints of human arm trajectories. Can. J. Psychol. 41, 365–378.

Meijer, O.G., 2001. Making things happen: an introduction to the history of movement science. In: Latash, L.M., Zatsiorsky, V.M. (Eds.), Classics in Movement Science. Human Kinetics, Champaign, Illinois, pp. 1–58.

Meijer, O.G., Roth, K. (Eds.), 1988. Complex Movement Behaviour: 'The' motor-action controversy. North Holland, Amsterdam.

Mudie, M.H., Matyas, T.A., 1996. Upper extremity retraining following stroke: effects of bilateral practice. J. Neurol. Rehabil. 10, 167–184.

Nagasaki, H., 1989. Asymmetric velocity and acceleration profiles of human arm movements. Exp. Brain Res. 74, 319–326.

Nieuwboer, A., Kwakkel, G., Rochester, L., et al., 2007. Cueing training in the home improves gait-related mobility in Parkinson's disease: the RESCUE trial. J. Neurol. Neurosurg. Psychiatry 78, 134–140.

Purdon Martin, J., 1967. The Basal Ganglia and Posture. Lippincott McIntosh GC, Brown, Philadelphia.

Raine, S., 2009. The Bobath Concept: developments and current theoretical underpinning. In: Raine, S., Meadows, L., Lynch-Ellerton, M. (Eds.), Bobath Concept: theory and clinical practice in neurological rehabilitation. Wiley-Blackwell, Oxford, pp. 1–22.

Raibert, M.H., 1977. Motor Control and Learning by the State-space Model. Massachusetts Institute of Technology, Artificial Intelligence Laboratory, Cambridge.

Rand, M.K., Squire, L.M., Stelmach, G. E., 2006. Effect of speed manipulation on the control of aperture closure during reach to grasp movements. Exp. Brain Res. 174, 74–85.

Rochester, L., Baker, K., Hetherington, V., et al., 2010. Evidence for motor learning in Parkinson's disease: acquisition, automaticity and retention of cued gait performance after training with external rhythmical cues. Brain Res. 1319, 103–111.

Rushton, S.K., Wann, J.P., 1999. Weighted combination of size and disparity: a computational model for timing a ball catch. Nat. Neurosci. 2, 186–190.

Schmidt, R.A., 1975. A schema theory of discrete motor skill learning. Psychol. Rev. 82, 225–260.

Schmidt, R.A., 1988. Motor Control and Learning. A behavioural emphasis, second ed. Human Kinetics, Champaign Illinois.

Schmidt, R.A., Wrisberg, C.A., 2008. Motor learning and performance. A situation-based learning approach. Human Kinetics, Champaign Illinois.

Schöner, G., Jiang, W.Y., Kelso, J.A.S., 1991. A synergetic theory of quadrupedal gaits and gait transitions. J. Theor. Biol. 142, 359–391.

Schwarz, C., 1990. Chambers English Dictionary (7th edition). University of Michigan, Ann Arbor, USA, Chambers.

Shumway-Cook, A., Woollacott, M.H., 2007. Motor control. Translating research into clinical practice, third ed. Lippincott Williams & Wilkins, Baltimore.

Summers, J., 2004. Historical perspective on skill acquisition. In: Williams, A.M., Hodges, N.J. (Eds.), Skill Acquisition in Sport. Research, theory and practice. Routledge, London, pp. 1–26.

Thelen, E., Fisher, D.M., Ridley-Johnson, R., 1984. The relationship between physical growth and a newborn reflex. Infant Behav. Dev. 7, 479–493.

Turvey, M.T., 1990. Coordination. Am. Psychol. 45, 938–953.

Ungerleider, L.G., Mishkin, M., 1982. Two cortical visual systems. In: Ingle, D.J., Goodale, M.A., Mansfield, R.J.W. (Eds.), Analysis of Visual Behaviour. MIT Press, Cambridge, Massachusetts, pp. 549–586.

van Emmerik, R.E., Wagenaar, R.C., 1996. Dynamics of movement coordination and tremor during gait in Parkinson's disease. Hum. Mov. Sci. 15, 203–235.

van Emmerik, R.E., Wagenaar, R.C., Winogrodzka, A., et al., 1999. Identification of axial rigidity during locomotion in Parkinson disease. Arch. Phys. Med. Rehabil. 80, 186–191.

van Wieringen, P.C.W., 1989. Compendium van de Psychologie. Deel 2/1 Waarneming. Dick Coutinho, Muiderberg, The Netherlands.

Wagenaar, R.C., van Emmerik, R.E., 1994. Dynamics of pathological gait. Hum. Mov. Sci. 13, 441–471.

Warren Jr., W.H., 1984. Perceiving affordances: visual guidance of stair climbing. J. Exp. Psychol. Hum. Percept. Perform. 10, 683–703.

Warren Jr., W.H., 1988. Action modes and laws of control for the visual guidance of action. Complex movement behaviour. In: Meijer, O. G., Roth, K. (Eds.), The Motor-action Controversy. Elsevier Science publishers, North Holland, pp. 339–380.

Wing, A.M., Turton, A., Fraser, C., 1986. Grasp size and accuracy of approach in reaching. J. Mot. Behav. 18, 245–260.

Winogrodzka, A., Wagenaar, R.C., Booij, J., et al., 2005. Rigidity and bradykinesia reduce interlimb coordination in Parkinsonian gait. Arch. Phys. Med. Rehabil. 86, 183–189.

Perceptuo-motor learning

8

CHAPTER CONTENTS

LEARNING OUTCOMES

At the end of this chapter, you should be able to:

- describe the concept of perceptuo-motor learning and differentiate this from motor performance
- apply an information-processing (or motor programming) model to the process of perceptuo-motor learning
- distinguish between three main stages of motor learning and compare and contrast the needs of the patient (or learner) in each of these stages
- explain how perceptuo-motor learning may be facilitated through motivation, practice and feedback
- discuss how this information may be applied to rehabilitation practice.

Introduction

'Practice makes perfect' is a well-known adage used in a range of scenarios to encourage learning, from learning to play a musical instrument or a sport for the first time, to re-learning functional skills in the context of rehabilitation. Consider the case study below (Case study 8.1).

Following on from the chapter on perceptuo-motor control, this chapter will begin by introducing a number of key concepts and present an overview of the main stages of the perceptuo-motor learning process. We will build on the **information processing approach** to perceptuo-motor control, introduced in Chapter 7, for reasons explained there. A more detailed discussion will follow about key factors that impact on the process of skill acquisition, and what the implications for health care professionals involved in rehabilitation may be. But first, we need to go back in time and discuss how 'learning' has been studied in the past in order to avoid some pitfalls. For a more comprehensive overview of the history of motor learning research, the reader is referred to Summers (in Williams and Hodges 2004).

Case study 8.1

Re-learning functional skills following traumatic brain injury

Mrs S. is a 34-year-old mother of two, who has been referred for rehabilitation following a road traffic accident. She has sustained multiple injuries, including a traumatic brain injury (TBI) with diffuse axonal tearing as well as frontal lobe damage, and requires extensive rehabilitation. Following a 3-month period in hospital, Mrs S's musculoskeletal injuries have recovered sufficiently for her to be transferred to a neurological rehabilitation centre for further specialist care.

The neurorehabilitation programme comprises input from a multidisciplinary team, involving physiotherapy, occupational therapy, and speech and language therapy.

The overall aim is to improve a range of skills, including transfers and mobility, arm function, activities of daily living, feeding and communication, all to a level to enable Mrs S. to be discharged home in 3 months' time. This will involve a process of re-learning skills that the patient previously mastered but needs to re-acquire, as well as learning new skills (e.g. wheelchair transfers).

Clearly there are a considerable number of activities to be covered in the rehabilitation programme. In this context, what does 'practice' involve and how may this improve performance? What is the role of health care professionals in facilitating the (re-) learning process?

The learning curve: performance versus learning

How do we know whether patients have learned anything from what they practised? A 'learning curve' is a graphical representation of performance over time. Typically, performance on an outcome measure (Y-axis) is plotted at specific points in time (X-axis). Figure 8.1 presents a learning curve from a classic study by Stelmach in 1969, where performance was measured as the number of rungs climbed on the Bachman ladder (a novel ladder with unequally distributed rungs on either side of a vertical beam in the middle of the ladder). The purpose of the experiment was to compare the effectiveness of two

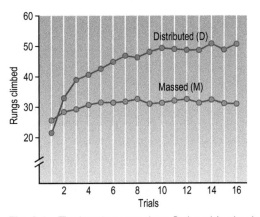

Fig. 8.1 • The learning curve from Stelmach's classic experiment on learning the Bachman ladder task (1969), with permission from the American Alliance for Health, Physical Education, Recreation and Dance.

different training regimes; 'distributed practice' (i.e. practice interspersed with rest, with more rest than practice) and 'massed' (i.e. more practice than rest).

Looking at figure 8.1, which schedule was more effective? Clearly, the distributed practice schedule resulted in a higher number of rungs climbed, compared to the massed practice schedule. Thus, motor performance appeared to be better following distributed practice.

In order to assess the effect of practice on learning, performance is usually tested again after a delay, with either a '**retention test**' or a '**transfer test**'. A retention test occurs some time (minutes, days or weeks) after the practice has been completed, with the aim to determine how much the individual has retained. In the retention test, the task that has been practised is the same as the one that is assessed. A transfer test is different, in that the task that is assessed is similar but not identical to the task that has been practised. The purpose of a transfer test is to determine to what extent the person can transfer (carry over) what they have learned to a problem that is slightly different.

In Stelmach's study, a retention test was used, following a short delay (4 minutes only). It is interesting to note that at the retention test, there is now hardly any difference between the two practice schedules (Fig. 8.2). What happened in that short period of time? Imagine yourself undertaking the Bachman ladder task under the massed practice schedule: stepping up and down as fast as you can, again and again. It is likely that fatigue would set in and impair your performance: your leg extensors would fatigue quickly with the fast concentric and eccentric contractions. However, after a short break the increased muscle tension reduces,

Fig. 8.2 • The learning curve from the same experiment as Fig. 8.1 (Stelmach1969), with permission from the American Alliance for Health, Physical Education, Recreation and Dance.

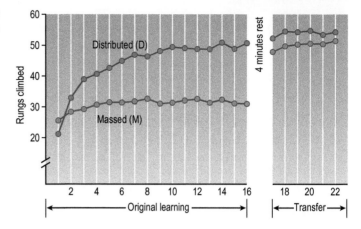

circulation improves, your attention may also become more focused, and altogether you are able to deliver a much better performance.

Based on this classic, and similar experiments, it became clear that a distinction had to be made between 'performance' and 'learning'. **Motor performance** is defined as:

'the behavioural act of performing a skill at a specific time and in a specific situation.'

(Magill (2007), p. 440)

In contrast, **motor learning** can be defined as:

'a set of processes associated with practice/ experience leading to relatively permanent changes in the capability for producing skilled action.'

(Schmidt, 1988, p. 346)

Three points are worth noting in the motor learning definition:

1. *Practice or experience* is required, i.e. an initial successful attempt would not be defined as a learned action stored in memory
2. Changes in performance are *relatively permanent*
3. Motor learning is concerned with *skilled action*, i.e. goal-oriented behaviour, but not reflex-like behaviour, which is largely automatic.

What is the moral of the study by Stelmach? The important point to take away is that one should not jump to conclusions about the effectiveness of a specific training schedule, if performance has only been tested immediately at the end of the training. The clinical equivalent would be to use an outcome measure at the start and immediately after practising a specific activity, and base conclusions about the effectiveness of the intervention on just this outcome.

In this case, the clinician will only have tested the patient's performance. Patients may appear to perform well following the end of an intervention, but effects may not be sustained without further practice. The need to include a follow-up after the end of an intervention is illustrated in Research box 8.1 below on cueing in patients with Parkinson's disease (PD).

We mentioned earlier that some factors may mask learning. For example, in neurological rehabilitation, pain and fatigue are common (Chapter 14). Physical practice may exacerbate pain and fatigue, which in turn may have a detrimental effect on concentration. Patients may even get bored with an activity! All these factors may affect performance. So how may a therapist obtain a more accurate picture of what a patient has actually learned? The evidence from experiments such as that by Stelmach (1969) shows that it is essential to:

1. undertake a **retention test** sometime after the end of the intervention. This will help reduce any practice-related effects on pain, attention and fatigue and show how much has actually been retained in memory. Assessing performance immediately after an intervention will merely show performance effects.

2. utilise a **transfer test**, i.e. a slight variation from the task that has been practised. This will reveal to what extent the patient is able to adapt what has been learned. This means that the outcome measure must be related but not identical to the tasks that were practised in the intervention.

One point worth making here is that it is not advisable to change established, standardised outcome measures for the sake of a transfer test, as this would invalidate the measure. However, if one was using a simple measure such as time taken to stand up, the standing up movement could be done slightly

Research box 8.1

Short- and longer-term effects of cueing on the coordination of gait in Parkinson's disease

The Rehabilitation in Parkinson's Disease: Strategies for Cueing (ResCUE) trial, the first large scale randomised trial on cueing in Parkinson's disease (PD), was designed to examine the effects of a home-based cueing programme on gait parameters, gait-related activity and health-related quality of life in people with PD (Nieuwboer et al. 2007). In this randomised cross-over trial, a total of 153 people with PD participated in a cueing intervention, which comprised a 3-week programme with nine treatment sessions of 30 minutes each. In the first week, patients tried auditory, visual as well as somatosensory cueing modalities, i.e. beeps administered via an earpiece, flashes from an LED mounted on a pair of glasses, and pulsed vibrations applied via a wristband-mounted device. Having tried each of these modalities, patients then continued training with the one they preferred. Most patients (67%) selected the auditory, while the remainder chose the somatosensory modality. While being instructed to time their heel strike according to the rhythm provided and to continue stepping through turning and other transitions, patients undertook a variety of tasks. These included starting and stopping walking, sideways and backward stepping, walking while doing another task (i.e. dual tasking), and walking outside over different surfaces. More information about the specific cueing intervention and the underlying evidence is detailed on the ReSCUE project CD-ROM (2002/3, http://www.rescueproject.org/). Depending on group allocation, this intervention was either preceded or followed by a 3-week period without any training, after which a 6-week follow-up period ensued.

The primary outcome measure was a composite score of five items on the Unified Parkinson's Disease Rating Scale, reflecting gait and balance. Secondary outcomes included measures of gait and balance, functional activity, falls-related self-efficacy, participation and carer strain. All outcome measures were assessed – without patient using the cueing device – by a blinded assessor in weeks 3, 6 and 12.

Straight after the intervention, the results demonstrated significant improvements in the primary outcome measure of 4.2%, while median gait speed improved by 5 cm/s and median step length improved by 4 cm. Significant improvements were also found in balance tests, while self-reported confidence in gait-related activities had increased. A significant reduction of freezing episodes was found in so-called 'freezers' only. There were no significant changes in any of the other outcomes. However, at the *12-week follow-up assessment*, most outcomes had deteriorated significantly compared to those after the intervention at week 6.

What do these findings mean for clinical practice? The results from this trial demonstrated that a 3-week programme of nine cueing sessions can result in significant – albeit small – improvements in specific aspects of gait and balance in people with mild to moderate PD. Interestingly, the effects were noted *without* patients wearing their cueing device, which indicates that some carry-over had taken place. However, although these effects were seen immediately after the intervention, they were not retained at follow-up. This suggests that the effects of cueing were more due to performance than learning, with the clinical implication that continuing use of cueing may be required to sustain its effects.

differently on the transfer test, e.g. by using a different chair, placed on a different surface.

The transfer test (or task) is a crucial concept in clinical practice, as rehabilitation programmes – which can't possibly incorporate all potential problems a patient may encounter after discharge – are designed on the assumption that what patients learn during treatment will carry over to their own activities of daily living in their own environment. This is more of a challenge than we may appreciate, and this topic will be further discussed below.

Perceptuo-motor learning: what do we learn?

What is actually stored in long-term memory during the skill acquisition process? Based on Schmidt's motor control model (Schmidt and Wrisberg 2008, see Chapter 7), the following elements of information are stored:

1. The initial conditions. E.g. if you were to reach for an object, this would involve information about the object, its location in relation to you and any other environmental conditions (e.g. predictability) that need to be incorporated in programming the action.
2. The parameters assigned to the generalised motor programme (GMP):
   ○ specific muscles
   ○ absolute force
   ○ absolute duration of muscle activation.
3. Feedback: both intrinsic and extrinsic.

In other words, motor learning is the process of working through the motor control process, time and time again, utilising any feedback available to improve performance. Through extensive repetition and trial and error, an increasingly reliable relationship is established between sensory input and motor output that is stored in long term memory – hence the term 'perceptuo-motor' learning.

In summary, this section has highlighted the difference between motor performance and learning and recommended that health care practitioners consider a delay between practice and outcome assessment, and utilise a transfer task to examine carry-over of what has been learned. From an information processing perspective, motor learning reflects the extent to which a GMP has been stored in long-term memory.

How do we learn? Stages of learning

Learning a new skill requires practice, and resultant changes in performance emerge over time. An understanding of this process, which can be described in stages, is important to therapists, as patients require different forms of guidance as they progress. The key stages, which were originally proposed by Fitts and Posner (1967), and later updated by Schmidt and Wrisberg (2008), are described below.

Verbal-cognitive stage

This is the first stage of skill acquisition, where the patient needs to get 'the idea' of the activity to be learned (e.g. walking with crutches for the first time). This stage is labelled verbal- cognitive as there is often a considerable amount of self-talk going on, with the patient guiding themselves through the solution (e.g. 'left foot - right crutch. . .'). Information processing at this stage is predominantly conscious and deliberate; hence the term 'cognitive': this stage involves thinking through the activity and working out how to do it. Performance improves quickly but is often variable, as the patient tries different strategies to solve the problem.

What do you think is the main role of the therapist in this stage? Obviously, giving a clear explanation is crucial. Demonstration, either 'live' or on video, can be very useful to convey a clear image of the activity, without the need to use complex verbal descriptions. Manual guidance can also be effective in providing the patient with the necessary sensory information. Feedback on performance is also very important for

this and the following stages and is discussed in detail later in this chapter.

Is there anything that therapists should try and avoid at this stage? It is easy to overload the patient with detailed information, or to talk, manually guide and demonstrate all at the same time, but this may well lead to *information overload* – causing the patient to get 'lost'. Short-term memory has only limited capacity, restricted to around an average of 7 ± 2 chunks of information in healthy people, while it can only retain information for around 20 s. Short-term memory is vulnerable to interference, mainly caused by an overload of information.

Given the limitations of short-term memory, which are often even further compromised in people with a condition affecting the CNS (Chapter 9), it is essential that therapists select key information, e.g. where to look during a balance task (rather than prescribing the optimal position of individual joints). It is important for therapists to consider the patient's capacity to process information. For example, physiotherapy gyms or occupational therapy kitchens are often lively environments, where music may be used to create an enjoyable atmosphere. While not denying the importance of this, therapists need to consider whether this environment actually enables the patient to focus their attention on the task in hand. As Chapter 9 will explain, information that is not attended to will be poorly remembered.

Motor stage or associative stage

Now that the patient has a clear idea of what to do and some idea of how best to do it, the process of putting this knowledge into practice and fine-tuning performance can begin. At this stage, improvements tend to be smaller, but performance becomes more consistent.

What is the main role of the therapist at this stage? Providing safe opportunities for practice (including trial and error where appropriate), allowing the patient to become proficient at the skill and solve more complex variations of the task. This could be done by adding 'noise' to the system, e.g. when practising walking, therapist could start talking at the same time (dual tasking), walking outside where the terrain is more variable (variable practice), interspersing walking with another task (random practice), all of which are examples of **contextual interference** – a concept we will discuss under random practice below.

With the patient gaining proficiency, the therapist should prepare for handing over control to the patient and gradually withdraw their input – eventually, the patient needs to be become as autonomous as possible.

Autonomous stage

This is where the patient masters the activity automatically and performance becomes more stable; little conscious attention is required. The patient may be able to dual task (e.g. walk with crutches and talk at the same time without this affecting their performance) and learns to adapt their performance to suit different situations. The main role of the therapist at this stage is to provide practice situations in which the patient can consolidate their performance and have the opportunity to problem-solve how the movement should be adapted to meet changing environmental conditions. At this stage, the therapist is usually no longer needed to provide detailed task instructions.

In summary, the process of skill acquisition progresses through stages. Different authors have proposed more or fewer stages (e.g. see Gentile 2000), and may have used slightly different terminology. However, it is important to bear in mind that the boundaries between the stages are rather blurred. Therefore, it is sufficient to have a broad understanding of these main stages of motor learning – and the key role of the therapist in each stage.

Facilitating skill acquisition

Having briefly introduced the role of the therapist in each of the stages of skill acquisition, it is now time to look in more detail at how this process can be facilitated. Several key factors impact on this process:

- Motivation
- Practice: amount, type and scheduling of practice,
- Feedback: type and content of feedback, attentional focus, feedback scheduling.

We will now discuss each of these points in more depth.

Motivation

Motivation is a key factor in any learning process; highly motivated patients are more likely to practise more and may require less therapist input than those who have low motivation. Although an in-depth discussion of the topic of motivation is beyond the scope of this text, it is important for therapists to have a good working understanding of motivation and how this may be enhanced.

Firstly, it may be helpful to differentiate between intrinsic motivation, which is directed at achieving internal satisfaction (e.g. enjoyment, having a sense of autonomy), and extrinsic motivation, which is aimed at external rewards, (e.g. recognition or positive feedback from the therapist). In order to nurture intrinsic motivation, it is important that the patient feels that what they are trying to achieve is meaningful and relevant to their own life and aspirations. E.g. patients may not automatically feel motivated to undertake straight leg raise exercises to improve quadriceps strength. However, the same exercise formulated as a short term goal to achieve the more functional goal of being able to go up and down stairs independently is more likely to be seen as relevant, and encourage a patient to practise.

A technique to enhance motivation and engagement is **goal setting**, which is widely recognised in rehabilitation settings as a useful tool, even though there is a lack of robust evidence on its effectiveness in clinical populations (Levack et al. 2006) as well as debate on how best to conduct the process (Playford et al. 2009). Despite these uncertainties, goal setting is recommended in a number of UK clinical guidelines (RCP 2008, SIGN 2010) and there is broad consensus that the characteristics of successful goals should follow the SMARTER acronym, i.e. they should be:

Specific: goals need to be specific in order to focus one's effort. Goals such as 'I want to be normal again' lack precision about the aim, and about how progress can be ascertained. A more specific goal could be: 'I want to be able to ascend and descend one flight of stairs without assistance'.

Measurable: as indicated above, it is necessary to be able to assess to what extent a goal has been achieved. For example, 'I want to be able to ascend one flight of stairs in 2 minutes without assistance'. Outcome measures comprising timed tests (e.g. the Timed Up and Go test) may be useful to provide detailed information on progress in function and activity.

Agreed: it is important that a goal is agreed between the patient and the therapist, since ownership of the goal is key to intrinsic motivation. Other authors recommend that the 'A' stands for 'achievable', while others argue this should stand for 'ambitious'.

Relevant: as indicated above, goals need to be seen to be relevant by the patient. However, it is not always possible to formulate goals that meet this criterion. E.g. for a patient with traumatic brain injury, who has to have a plaster applied to his leg to prevent contracture of the ankle plantar flexors, the goal to increase range of movement in the ankle may not seem to be immediately relevant. However, having sufficient ankle movement to achieve 90 degrees of dorsiflexion is an essential requirement for weight bearing, which in turn is necessary to reach the longer term goal of being able to walk. Therapists often need to translate short-term, impairment-based goals into goals that are perceived to be relevant in the eyes of the patient.

Time-based: goals need a timeline, otherwise interventions could be endless. Setting deadlines is one of the most difficult aspects of goal setting in clinical practice however, due to the problems with predicting outcomes. For example, 'In 1 week from now I want to be able to ascend one flight of stairs in 2 minutes without assistance'.

E: engaging: health care professionals may forget that therapeutic activities – however beneficial for the patient - can sometimes be tedious. Devising activities that are engaging and enjoyable is key to stimulating intrinsic motivation – the stepping stone to successful self-management after discharge. The rapidly growing field of 'games for health', using technology such as the Nintendo Wii and Microsoft Kinect, is an interesting development in this respect.

R: reviewed. In order to keep on track, or identify what holds patients back, goals need to be regularly reviewed.

In summary, motivation is key to engaging the patient in their rehabilitation process. Goal setting, based on the SMARTER acronym, is a technique for enhancing motivation. Finding out what motivates patients, integrating this with goal setting, designing targeted interventions and seeing patients achieve their own goals is probably one of the most rewarding aspects of clinical practice.

Practice: amount, types and schedules of practice

How much practice do patients need? Referring back to our case study at the start of this chapter, is there an optimum way to organise therapy sessions when a range of tasks need to be practised, e.g. should it be drill-like, or more variable? Are there any alternatives for practice when a patient is limited in their capacity to practice, e.g. because of pain, fear or fatigue?

Amount of practice

To master a skill, one needs to physically practise it, but how many times? It is clear that there is a lack of clarity on this issue. Ideally, several thousands of repetitions may be required to build and refine the required motor program and for this to be mastered at an automatic level, but this depends on the individual, their baseline performance, and the nature of the skill. For example, a group of people with stroke improved upper limb function significantly by practising an average of 322 repetitions per session (3 sessions a week for 6 weeks). (Birkenmeier et al. 2010). The consensus in the skill acquisition literature is, ideally, that '**overlearning**' is required, i.e.continuing to practice beyond proficiency. Overlearning involves using the neural network required for the execution of a task over and over again, increasing efficiency and processing speed.

In reality, do patients get an opportunity to overlearn in the clinical setting? A study by de Wit et al. (2005) showed that, in the UK, stroke patients on stroke units (the accepted gold standard for hospital care after stroke) spent on average just 10% of their waking hours in therapy. Lang et al. (2009) showed that the average number of repetitions of task-specific training for people with stroke in a number of rehabilitation units in the USA was only 32 per therapy session. It is essential that therapists make the most of the very limited time available to increase opportunities for patients to practise the skills they need to be ready for discharge. One way to do so is to extend what we mean by 'practice'.

Mental practice and observational learning

Traditionally, what we think of as practice is 'doing', i.e. physically performing an activity, over and over again. This is known as **overt practice**; the behaviour can be observed. However, ask professional dancers, athletes and musicians how they attain and maintain their level of proficiency and they are likely to reply that they use observation and going through an activity 'in their mind' as additional strategies. Below, we will briefly address each of these forms of **covert practice** and explain how they may be effective.

Observational learning can be defined as:

'Learning a skill by observing a person performing the skill.'

(Magill 2007, p. 439)

Since the pioneering work by Bandura (1986), we have known that observation can be a powerful tool in learning. Social situations offer opportunities for role-modelling; a principle that is widely used in education in general and the field of skill acquisition in particular. However, it was not until relatively recently that a *neural explanation* for the phenomenon of observational learning emerged. Pioneers in observational learning, Di Pellegrino and his group, made their discovery in 1992 purely by serendipity. They observed monkeys interacting with objects, using single cell recordings of neurones in the monkeys' cerebral cortex. To cut a long and fascinating story short, they discovered that the same network of neurones was activated when the monkey was looking at an experimenter interacting with an object, as when the monkey itself was interacting with the object (Rizzolatti and Fadiga 2005). This discovery led to the '**direct matching hypothesis**', which postulates that by observing an actor interacting with an object, the visual representation of that activity is mapped onto the motor representation of the same activity (quite literally, a case of 'monkey see, monkey do'). In other words, the visual map of the activity is reflected onto the motor map of the same activity. The neural network involved in this process of 'reflection' was aptly named the '**mirror neurone system**'. Much more work has been done since on the roles of the mirror neurone system including on humans, where a similar system has been confirmed. This discovery is so exciting, as it not only confirms earlier findings that observational learning can be effective, but it provides us with a much deeper understanding of how this process is thought to work.

Another type of covert practice is **mental practice**. This has been defined as follows:

'The cognitive rehearsal of a physical skill in the absence of overt physical movements; it can take the form of thinking

about the cognitive or procedural aspects of a motor skill, or of engaging in visual or kinaesthetic imagery of the performance of a skill or part of a skill.'

(Magill 2007, p. 423)

The literature on this topic uses a number of different terms (e.g. mental imagery, or imagery) and a range of definitions and interpretations. Some forms of mental imagery may be used to achieve a state of relaxation, or increase confidence. Within this chapter however, we will interpret mental practice as practising a specific skill in the mind. How does that work? Some of you may engage in mental practice without realising it; others may use it purposefully in athletics, dance or playing music. Here is an example: imagine walking over a tightrope; you visualise the rope in front of you and fix your eyes on the imaginary horizon. You may also 'feel' imaginary balance reactions and the contact between your feet and the rope, as you walk forward.

Mental practice is a skill that can be acquired, just like any other skill. Some patients may find it difficult (if not unusual!) to begin with but with guidance and practice, their imagery may become more and more vivid.

Thus, learning a new skill can be undertaken using overt as well as covert techniques (i.e. observational learning and mental practice). According to Jeannerod (2005, p. 173), these forms of skill acquisition can be placed on a continuum:

'Covert and overt stages represent a continuum, such that every overtly executed action implies the existence of a covert stage, whereas a covert action does not necessarily become an overt action.'

How may Schmidt's model of motor control help to explain the notion of a continuum from covert to overt action? The covert stage of any skilled action involves the response selection and programming components, which will be undertaken in all types of practice (i.e. physical and mental practice, as well as observational learning). One important difference in the case of mental practice is that the process of actually sending action potentials down the spinal cord and to the motor endplates does not occur. What are the differences between observational learning and mental practice? Again, the response selection and programming components are the same, but during observational learning, actual visual stimuli are provided whereas during the mental practice, they have to be retrieved from memory.

So if overt and covert strategies can all be used to enhance motor learning, how do they compare in terms of their effectiveness? This question has been subject to much research. In a classic review, Feltz and Landers (1983) compared overt practice with mental practice and no practice in a healthy population. Their findings indicated that overt practice is more effective than mental practice, which in turn is more effective than no practice. Why would overt practice be more effective than mental practice? Refer back to Schmidt's model – the difference lies in the feedback. At some point, the learner does need feedback to verify that what they are mentally practising actually works. Further research has suggested that overt practice should precede mental practice, as the learner requires the *experience* of the activity in order to have a basis for mental practice (Jeannerod 2006). Research box 8.2 presents findings from a clinical trial using mental practice to improve arm function in people with stroke.

How may this information guide clinical practice? We opened this section by stating that, for patients to gain the necessary level of proficiency, over-learning needs to take place. Within the health-care system, however, there tends to be a dearth of opportunity for patients to achieve this. We have now seen that, in addition to the overt method of practice, observational learning and mental practice can be included.

This may be especially useful in cases where fatigue or other factors (e.g. immobilisation, increased risk of falls) constrain the amount of overt practice that can be undertaken. Video feedback of the patient themselves, as well as peer observation (provided the required consent has been obtained) could be used, as a form of observational learning.

Research on mental practice in neurological rehabilitation has taken off rapidly in the last few decades, accelerated by information provided by neuroimaging technology. This has increased our understanding of what happens in the brain as a result of an activity (or even thinking about it), which has demonstrated considerable overlap in brain areas involved in overt and covert rehearsal of the same task (Jeannerod, 2005). It is now even possible to harness EEG and other brain activity signals in brain-computer interfaces to actuate remote controls. Examples are communication devices, actuated through EEG by a tetraplegic person with muscular dystrophy (Hashimoto et al. 2010) or robotic navigation and communication devices for a person with Amyotrophic Lateral Sclerosis (or ALS, Escolano et al. 2010). Many of these initiatives are still in the proof-of-concept stage and involve only small numbers of patients, but this area is of enormous interest and promise for rehabilitation, especially for people with intact cognition and very severe motor impairments.

Research box 8.2

Using mental practice to improve arm function after stroke

In a single-blind RCT, Page and colleagues (2007) examined the effects of mental practice on arm function in people in the chronic stage after stroke. A total of 32 patients (mean time post stroke 42, range 12–174 months) were randomised into either a mental practice with physical practice (MP+PP) group, or relaxation with physical practice (R+PP) group. All participants practised bimanual, functional upper limb tasks (i.e. reaching and grasping objects, turning a page in a book and using a writing utensil) in 30-minute sessions, twice per week, for 6 weeks. Outcome measures were the Fugl-Meyer Assessment of Motor Recovery after Stroke and the Action Research Arm test, which assess upper limb coordination and function, respectively. Those in the MP+PP group additionally engaged in a 30-minute MP session after each PP session. They listened to a tape that, following a short episode to encourage relaxation, provided instructions on how to mentally rehearse the activities that had been undertaken during the physical practice. Those in the R+PP group also spent 30 minutes listening to a tape, which provided a progressive relaxation programme, in

order to control for attention effects, but which did not focus on the activities undertaken in the physical practice sessions.

One week after the intervention had finished, participants returned for their assessments. Two baseline assessments had demonstrated that motor performance was stable across all participants, and that there were no significant differences in key variables (such as time post stroke) between the two groups. Compared to baseline, changes in both outcome measures were negligible in the R+PP group. In contrast, those in the MP+PP group demonstrated changes that were both statistically and clinically significant.

A retention test, undertaken longer after treatment finished, would have been useful to gauge how long treatment effects persisted, or whether continued mental and physical practice would be required.

However, these findings show that, even in the chronic stage after stroke, considerable improvement in functional activity may be achieved through a *combination* of task-specific mental and physical practice.

Practice schedules

To progress physical practice along the stages of learning, therapists have a number of different options, related to the scheduling or structure of practice. We will begin with briefly describing each of the different practice schedules, after which we will discuss in more detail how these could be progressed along the stages of learning.

The structure of practice can be described according to the following categories (Schmidt and Wrisberg, 2008):

- Constant and variable practice: this distinction refers to the situation where a patient practises a single class of activities (e.g. rising from sit to stand):
  - Constant practice means that exactly the same task is practised (e.g. the same chair in the same location, moving at the same speed)
  - Variable practice means that different 'variations to the theme' are practised, remaining within the same class of activity (e.g. different chairs with/ without arm rests, in different locations, moving at different speeds).
- Blocked and random practice: this distinction refers to a situation where a patient practises different classes of activity within the same session (e.g. sit to stand, walking and reaching):
  - Blocked practice: the same class of activity is practised for a number of repetitions before moving onto a different class of activity (e.g. a block of repetitions of reaching are undertaken, followed by a block of repetitions of sit-to-stand)
  - Random practice: the order in which different classes of activity are practised is randomised (e.g. a reaching activity may be followed by sit-to-stand, which is followed by walking, etc.).
- Whole task – part task: this distinction refers to a situation where a task is practised in its entirety, or split up into components:
  - Whole task practice refers to a situation where the entire task is practised, e.g. a complete dressing routine
  - Part task practice means that a component of a task is practised, e.g. doing buttons as part of a dressing routine
- Massed – distributed practice:
  - Massed practice refers to a practice schedule where the amount of practice exceeds the amount of rest in any given training session
  - Distributed practice indicates a practice schedule where the amount of rest exceeds the amount of practice.

How do you think practice should be structured to facilitate progress through the stages of motor learning?

Verbal – cognitive stage of learning

Remember that in this stage, the patient tries to form a clear image of the task. It is also important that the patient achieves success at this early stage, in order to enhance motivation and encourage further (self) practice. How could you achieve these aims through structuring practice?

Constant vs. variable practice: Constant practice, where the same task is practised each time, will help the patient to develop a clear and stable image of the task. In contrast, variable practice at this stage might confuse the learner and impact negatively on performance.

Random vs. blocked practice: A similar rationale applies to blocked and random practice: repeating the same task over and over again, as in blocked practice, is likely to help the patient to develop their GMP and, from a neural perspective, activate the same neural networks over and over again. However, random practice would likely result in chaos and confusion and dishearten the patient, as it is difficult to obtain any clarity and consistency on how to complete a task.

Part vs. whole practice: Practising a whole task in its entirety (e.g. a full dressing routine) may present too much of a challenge at this stage. Provided that the task lends itself to being compartmentalised into discrete units, it may be better to focus on a specific component. However, it is important to remember that the patient needs to develop a clear and coherent image of the activity as a whole. It may therefore be advisable to proceed from whole to part to whole.

Massed vs. distributed practice: In healthy populations, research has shown that distributed practice generally yields better results than massed practice when learning a new skill, but this depends to some extent on the type of task and the amount of time between repetitions (Donovan and Radosevich 1999). For motor tasks that require considerable physical skill but involve little cognitive complexity (e.g. tossing a ball), distributed practice was clearly superior. For tasks involving both physical and cognitive complexity (e.g. balancing, playing music), the difference between massed and distributed practice was less pronounced.

For continuous tasks, distributed practice is recommended, as massed practice leads to fatigue (Lee and Genovese 1988). In the reality of clinical practice however, it is more the patient's tolerance to practice that informs the therapist about the amount of practice that can be undertaken. Reduced physical fitness is a common problem in patients with neurological conditions such as stroke (Brazzelli et al. 2011), which means that patients may only tolerate a limited number of repetitions. Where fatigue affects safety (e.g. in balance and transfer tasks) therapists need to closely monitor patients and adjust the amount of rest accordingly.

Associative stage of learning

As you remember, this is where the GMP for a class of activity is fine-tuned, perfected and extended to apply to a range of variations within the theme. Would the same strategies that boosted performance in the previous stage be as effective here?

Constant vs. variable practice: at this stage, the question is whether the patient is still problem solving, or merely running off a pre-prepared motor program. Practising the same task without any variation is now likely to result in a drop in attention; patients may get bored, and not learn anything new. In contrast, variable practice is more likely to keep the patient interested and attentive. Variable practice extends the GMP to related, but slightly different situations where the initial conditions of the task vary, and where the parameters need to be fine-tuned. This is where more flexible learning takes place: time and time again, the patient needs to work through the motor programming process, taking error signals into account to improve the next attempt. Moreover, variable practice is essential if we want patients to be prepared for an independent life beyond rehabilitation, where probably no two activities are identical! Thus, variable practice continues well into the 'autonomous stage'.

Random vs. blocked practice: This is where science and common sense seem to have come into conflict with one another. Let us refer to the classic study by Shea and Morgan (1979, Research box 8.3).

The superiority of random over blocked practice can be explained on the basis of the concept of **contextual interference**. This concept, introduced by Battig in the 1970s, refers to interference associated with varying intrinsic factors (variations to the task itself), or extrinsic factors (e.g. environmental variations) in the task being learned (Battig 1979). Dual tasking, where two tasks need to be carried out simultaneously (e.g. walking and talking) can also be seen as form of contextual interference.

In the case of the Shea and Morgan experiment, intrinsic interference was introduced in the random practice group by constantly switching between different sequences. This meant that participants were prevented from carrying out the task automatically; unable to re-use the solution for the previous task, they had to develop more elaborate problem solving strategies to learn the task, compared to those in the blocked practice group. In terms of Schmidt's model of motor control, once a task is understood and the GMP has been programmed, blocked practice requires little further problem solving, allowing the learner to 'switch off'. In contrast, random practice requires the learner to select different GMPs each time. Although random practice impairs performance initially, in the longer term it produces better outcomes. The latter is particularly interesting for clinical practice, where therapy is designed not just to improve performance on activities that have been trained, but also to enhance carry-over into related – but slightly different – activities.

How may the findings from Shea and Morgan's experiment apply to clinical practice, especially to neurological rehabilitation? Although there is a substantial body of evidence on this topic with non-impaired participants, only very few studies have actually been replicated in neurological rehabilitation contexts. Research boxes 8.4 and 8.5 present some contradictory findings.

The findings from the study by Dick et al. (2000), which were supported by findings from a later study by Kessels and Olde Henskens (2009) in people with dementia, indicate that for learning to succeed in people with memory impairments, contextual interference needs to be minimised.

This brings us to the concept of **errorless learning**, introduced by Baddely and Wilson (1994). Errorless learning has been tested in numerous areas of neuropsychological rehabilitation, and found to be superior for retaining information in patients with amnesia (Kessels and de Haan 2003). Errorless learning avoids learning through trial-and-error experiences. One hypothesis is that people with amnesia have difficulty eliminating errors and therefore trial-and-error learning may lead to retaining erroneous solutions.

Research on the effectiveness of errorless compared with trial-and-error learning for acquiring 'real-life' skills however, is less well developed. An innovative study by Mount et al. (2007) compared errorless with trial-and-error learning of a wheelchair transfer task

Research box 8.3

Testing the effects of random versus blocked practice on learning a new task

Shea and Morgan (1979) undertook a novel experiment with 72 healthy participants to compare the effects of random with blocked practice. Holding a tennis ball in their right (dominant) hand, participants had to knock down a selection of six barriers, mounted on a table top, in a pre-specified sequence and as fast as possible. During the acquisition phase, a total of 54 trials were practised in three different sequences. The same sequences were also examined during the retention test. At the end of the training, two transfer tasks (one easier, one more difficult) were undertaken using a new sequence.

Participants were divided into two groups: one group trained the tasks under blocked conditions and the second group trained the same tasks under random conditions. In the retention test, each group undertook a total of 18 trials: 9 trials in a blocked, and 9 trials in a random order, thus creating four comparisons (i.e. blocked->blocked, blocked->random, random-> blocked and random->random, see Fig. 8.3). There was a retention test after a delay of 10 minutes and one after 10 days. Immediately following the retention trials, all participants undertook both transfer tests. The primary outcome measure was time taken to complete the task.

Figure 8.3 shows that in the acquisition (or verbal-cognitive) stage, participants who practised in a blocked schedule quickly improved their performance, which then remained fairly constant. In comparison, those in the random practice group were much slower at the start and continued to perform worse than those in the blocked practice group. However, at the end of the acquisition stage, there was little difference between the two groups.

Now let's look at the data from the retention test. Those who learned the task on a *random* schedule and were tested on a blocked retention test came out best, both at 10 minutes and at 10 days. In contrast, those learning the task on a blocked schedule and tested on a random retention test had the poorest performance at both time points. Apparently, this group improved their motor performance in the acquisition phase, but were probably learning very little. Despite a considerable amount of practice, the data show that their final performance was worse than when they started!

In terms of transfer, the random practice group also outperformed the blocked practice group, especially on the more complex transfer task.

These results shook the commonly held belief at the time that blocked (or drill-like) practice was the optimum method for improving motor performance. How can these results be explained?

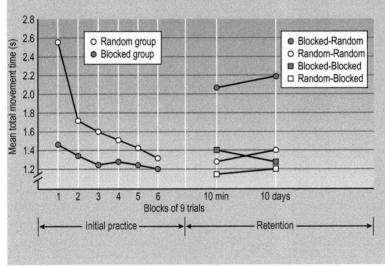

Fig. 8.3 • Results from the classic experiment by Shea and Morgan (1979). Reprinted with permission from Shea and Morgan

and a sock-donning task in people with acute stroke, who had either intact or impaired explicit memory (i.e. conscious memory for events, facts and figures, see Chapter 9). They were primarily interested in carry-over, using variations of each of the two tasks during retention testing. The findings showed that there were no significant differences between the errorless and trial-and-error conditions in terms of time required to learn the tasks. However, carry-over was significantly better following trial-and-error compared with error-less learning of the sock-donning task, regardless of memory function. No significant difference could be detected with respect to the wheelchair task, though, when the two learning strategies were compared.

Research box 8.4

Testing the effects of random versus blocked practice in patients with stroke

Hanlon (1996) reported the first trial with 24 participants at least 6 months after stroke, in which blocked practice was compared with random practice involving functional tasks with the hemiparetic upper limb. The experimental task simulated a 5-step sequence of opening the door of a cupboard, picking up a coffee cup, placing it on a counter, and releasing the cup. The blocked practice group practised this sequence only, while the random practice group practised the same sequence, with the difference that each trial was interspersed with three different upper limb tasks, i.e. pointing, touching specific objects and touching specific locations on a horizontal surface, all with the affected hand. There was also a control group of six participants who did not undertake any practice at all.

The experimental task was practised 10 times per day until the criterion of being able to complete the task 3 times in a row had been achieved. The outcome measures were achievement of performance criteria, judged by an observer, on each of the two retention trials at 2 and 7 days after training, and the number of practice trials required to achieve the criterion.

The results indicated that performance accuracy in the random group was significantly better than in the other two groups at both retention tests, but there was no difference between the random and blocked practice group in terms of the number of trials required to achieve the criterion. Interestingly, random practice did not seem to have affected the rate of acquisition, as had been observed in the Shea and Morgan (1979) experiment. In Hanlon's study, participants in the random practice group did indicate however that they found it difficult to perform the task correctly, which ties in with the hypothesis, mentioned earlier, that in random practice one requires to select the GMP each time the task changes.

Although the findings from Hanlon's study were promising, there were several limitations; the sample size was relatively small and it was not entirely clear how performance accuracy – an important outcome measure – had been measured. Additionally, there was a potentially confounding variable in that the random practice group included the additional three tasks and hence the increased dose of practice may have biased the results.

Research box 8.5

Testing the effects of random versus blocked practice in patients with Alzheimer's disease

Interestingly, a study by Dick et al. (2000) with patients with Alzheimers disease (AD) found contrasting results to those reported by Hanlon (1996). This study compared performance of a tossing task, learned under random, blocked, constant or no practice (control) conditions in 58 patients with AD and 58 healthy controls, matched for age and level of education. The training task involved tossing a bean bag onto a vertical target board. Participants in the experimental groups practised the training task 32 times per session, 2 sessions per week, for a total of 10 weeks. In the constant practice group, the distance to the target was kept the same throughout. In the blocked and random practice groups, participants practised the task at four different distances. Interestingly, in a preceding pilot study with the AD group, the researchers had been unable to change the distance for each trial as this had been too confusing for the participants. Therefore, in this study, the distance was only changed on every fourth trial.

A total of eight post-tests were undertaken over a period of around 1 month, including a retention test (using the same tasks that had been practised before), a 'near transfer task' (the same as the training task, but with heavier bean bags) and an 'intermediate transfer task' (which involved tossing a horse shoe onto a horizontal target mat) at the very end of the study period.

The main findings showed that both the AD and healthy groups managed to learn the task to the same extent, as there was no significant difference between the groups in terms of changes in performance between pre-test and retention test. However, when comparing the effects of different training methods, the results showed that constant practice was the only condition that facilitated learning on all post tests in participants with AD. Random practice was not effective in the AD group. In fact, those in the AD group who had trained on a random schedule appeared to perform worse than the control group who had had no practice at all. This was in contrast to the healthy older participants, who achieved as much through either random, blocked or constant practice.

How can these findings be explained? The authors postulated that random practice requires patients to compare recent experiences that are different from each other. This function is known to involve the hippocampus – a structure that is often affected in AD. The findings from this study emphasise that caution should be exercised in generalising findings from motor learning research – which to date has predominantly involved cognitively intact people – to neurological populations.

The authors suggested that different learning strategies may be more effective for different tasks and recommended further research.

In summary, once a patient has passed the verbal-cognitive stage of learning, contextual interference should be introduced where possible, either through variable or random practice, and/or dual tasking. However, this may not be suitable for all patients, especially for those with memory impairment. The disadvantage of contextual interference is that it renders practice more demanding. It requires more attention, it may be more confusing, fatiguing or frustrating to some patients. Performance gains may not be visible, especially early on in the learning process. It is therefore important that the therapist, if deciding to introduce contextual interference, explains to the patient why making learning more effortful in the short term may yield better outcomes in the longer term. The rationale could include the need to prepare the patient for independent problem solving prior to discharge, when they need to be able to cope with the unpredictable and complex nature of daily living.

Part vs. whole practice: With regard to part or whole task practice, we need to clarify what we mean by 'part'. If a 'part' is a discrete unit within a serial task (e.g. pouring water into a cup as part of making a cup of tea), practice of this part may be efficient if the other parts do not require as much practice. This enables the patient and therapist to focus their efforts on the part(s) of the task that require most practice. It is important to finish with practising the task as a whole however, to ensure that the patient is able to link the isolated part with the neighbouring parts.

In contrast, if a part is not a discrete unit of a task (e.g. extending one's leg backwards to kick a ball), breaking up the task may disrupt the kinematics. Moreover, practising a part in a way that is dissimilar to how it is performed in the whole task may not transfer to the task as a whole. A study by Winstein et al. (1989) is an interesting example. The aim was to explore the effects of balance retraining on standing balance and gait in people with stroke. After stroke, weight bearing on the affected side during standing and walking is typically reduced, leading to asymmetry. This means that patients often lean towards the less-affected side of the body, putting less weight on the affected side. The rationale was that practising a more even weight distribution over both feet during standing would improve weight-bearing

on the affected side during standing and walking, thereby reducing the asymmetry. The results showed that the group that had practised standing balance had indeed improved weight bearing symmetry during standing. Interestingly, however, this did not carry over into walking; the gait asymmetry in the standing balance group was no different from that in the control group. Why would standing balance not have transferred into more symmetrical walking? Think of the dynamics of gait – is there ever a movement where you actually stand still on one leg? An inherent feature of walking is transferring one's body through space and therefore static balance is not actually a component of gait. In terms of Schmidt's model of motor control, the order of the movement, relative timing and relative forces of walking are different from those during standing, indicating that a different GMP is at work. Perhaps it is not surprising then, that practising this particular 'component' does not carry over to a dynamic task like gait. This study is a good example of the specificity of learning principle, which will be explained later.

Taken together, the body of research discussed above characterised practice in the context of skill acquisition as **'problem solving'**. In the verbal-cognitive stage, the learner needs to form a clear image of the problem and an initial idea about how to solve it. Constant, blocked and errorless practice is useful to achieve this goal – and gain quick performance gains, thus boosting motivation and self-efficacy. However, where possible the associative stage needs to provide opportunities for a deeper level of problem solving by including variable and random practice.

Going back to our case study, one would expect Mrs S.'s TBI to affect her ability to focus her attention, problem solve and govern her behaviour. Chapters 9 on attention and 12 on executive functions will explain these difficulties in more detail, but it would be plausible that Mrs S would have more difficulty with concentration, adjusting to the changes involved in random practice, and that the lack of progress would cause considerable frustration and even emotional outbursts. As a clinician, how do you select the optimum practice schedule for an individual? It is important to acknowledge that there is no single solution; evidence provides the necessary starting point but practitioners should also use their clinical judgement – and be willing to adjust their treatment plan if necessary. In the case of Mrs. S, you may need to minimise contextual interference, especially in the verbal-cognitive stage of learning. Variable and random practice may need to be introduced later and more gradually – depending on the patient's response.

Feedback: type and content, attentional focus, scheduling

Type and content

Feedback is the general term for any type of information that is generated by an action. This information can be relayed through a range of sensory systems, including:

- Visual
- Vestibular
- Proprioceptive
- Olfactory
- Gustatory
- Tactile
- Acoustic systems.

For example, a patient moving from sit to stand will see a change in the position of the horizon in relation to their own position, feel the acceleration when rising to stand, sense the contraction in their leg muscles, feel the pressure changes under their feet and hear the chair moving over the floor as they push off.

Movement-related feedback can be divided into **intrinsic feedback** (i.e. information arising from sensory systems of the person who is moving, such as how the movement feels) or **extrinsic feedback** (or augmented feedback, i.e. additional sensory information provided by an external source, such as a therapist providing commentary on a patient's movements, or a video replaying a movement). In this section, we will focus on augmented feedback.

Augmented feedback pertains either to the pattern or the outcome of the movement (Magill 2007):

- Feedback about the movement pattern is known as **Knowledge of Performance** (KP). An example is stating to a patient that they had insufficient hip and knee extension during stance phase of walking, or insufficient elbow extension in an aiming task.
- Feedback about the movement outcome is known as **Knowledge of Results** (KR). Examples include stating to a patient how long it took them to walk 10 m., or what their accuracy was in an aiming task.

In addition, therapists often use feedback to enhance *motivation* to reinforce a particular behaviour. Based on Thorndike's 1905 Law of Effect (cited in Sternberg 2003), increasing the likelihood that a person will demonstrate a particular behaviour can be achieved through positive reinforcement (a pleasant event following the behaviour) or through negative reinforcement (the removal of an unpleasant event following the behaviour). Let's take an example where the goal of occupational therapy is for a patient to dress independently. Positive reinforcement would be praise from the therapist when the patient manages to dress with fewer prompts. An example of negative reinforcement would be the patient experiencing reduced fatigue. A wealth of research indicates that positive reinforcement is more effective than negative reinforcement for encouraging behaviour. *Shaping* techniques, which work towards the target behaviour in a step by step manner, could use goal setting as described above, if the long-term goal is too far removed from current behaviour.

Although *motivational* feedback (e.g. 'well done') plays an important role in encouraging the learning process, it is worthwhile to note that it does not actually provide the patient with any *information* on how to improve their performance. Research box 8.6 provides some information on how much therapists tend to use motivational as opposed to feedback with informational content.

Attentional focus of feedback

Feedback can induce an *internal focus* of attention in the learner (about the body and body parts) or an *external focus* of attention (about effects of the movement on the environment). This distinction is relevant, as a considerable body of evidence suggests that external focus feedback is more effective for the acquisition of a range of skills compared to internal focus feedback in healthy people (Wulf et al. 1999, McNevin et al. 2003, Wulf et al. 2002, Wulf and Prinz 2001). For example, to encourage greater extension of the elbow in a reach-to-grasp movement, saying 'next time, move closer to the cup' (external focus) could be more effective than 'next time, straighten your elbow more' (internal focus). The predominant explanation for this finding is that feedback with an internal focus may interfere with automatic motor control processes (van Vliet and Wulf 2006); most people may be entirely unaware of the kinematics of their various degrees of freedom, and explaining this to them may well lead to some interference! Focusing on kinematics (e.g. avoiding shoulder elevation when reaching for a cup by a person with a

Research box 8.6

Exploring the use of feedback in stroke rehabilitation

Durham et al. (2009) observed the use of feedback by physiotherapists during treatment sessions for the upper limb after stroke. Eight physiotherapists and eight patients with stroke from two hospitals participated. Data were collected by video recordings of treatment, followed by interviews with therapists and patients and questionnaires with the therapists. Information feedback, instructions and motivational statements were identified from transcripts of the video recordings. Examples of motivational statements were 'keep going' and 'well done', to encourage or act as reinforcement to facilitate the motor performance, whereas information feedback provided information that could be used to improve the movement such as 'your arm did not lift high enough'.

The results showed that two hundred and forty-six (13%) of the total 1914 statements identified in the videos were feedback, the rest comprising 1024 instructions (54%) and 641 statements of motivation (33%).

The finding that instruction was the predominant choice of communication by the therapists is similar to that in a study by Talvitie, U. and Reunanen (2002). Therapists in the study by Durham et al. felt satisfied that the amount of feedback they had given was sufficient. It could be that the therapists preferred to deliver corrective information indirectly by further instruction thus avoiding any negative feedback. However, a lack of information feedback may be detrimental to motor learning. Evidence from the stroke population (van Vliet and Wulf 2006) has shown that informational feedback can be beneficial to improve motor performance.

stroke) may also change the goal of the original task (i.e. reaching for the cup without knocking it over).

Implementing this body of evidence in clinical practice is not straightforward, especially in cases where patients do achieve an acceptable result in terms of outcome (e.g. reaching speed), but at the expense of the movement pattern (e.g. using compensatory techniques that may increase the risk of knocking an object over). Clearly, patients need to be provided with some essential internal focus information in order to avoid movement patterns that are potentially detrimental, but the evidence suggests that the effects of relying on this alone are limited and that feedback on the effects of the action on the environment may be more productive.

Studies of attentional focus in patient groups to date tend towards evaluation of instructions rather than feedback. Laufer et al. (2007) compared the effect of instruction inducing either an internal or external focus of attention in patients who had sustained an ankle sprain. Pre-test balance stability was measured followed by 3 days of balance training with one group receiving internal focus instructions and the other group receiving external focus instructions. After training, the group where an external focus was induced showed significantly improved balance compared to the internal focus group, which was maintained in a retention test 48 hours later where no attentional focus instructions were given. An advantage for external focus instructions has also been found in patients with Parkinson's disease who were learning balance tasks (Wulf et al. 2009) and people with stroke learning reaching tasks (Fasoli

et al. 2002). More research needs to be done but one could hypothesise that if external focus instructions are more effective, then the same could apply to feedback.

Scheduling feedback

How much augmented feedback should ideally be provided – and when? Intuitively, therapists may believe that 'more is better'; after all, providing expert feedback is perceived to be an important part of their role as health care professionals. But is there any evidence to show that augmented feedback may not necessarily add to the learning process – or even be counterproductive?

First of all, it is useful to consider that some augmented feedback may be *redundant* – this is often the case in situations where the patient is able to glean the same information through their own (i.e. intrinsic) feedback. For example, it is probably not useful to inform a patient that they have knocked over a cup during a reaching exercise! Furthermore, too much augmented feedback may create a *dependency*, whereby the patient learns to rely on the therapist's feedback and fails to develop their own error-detection capabilities. This is evident in scenarios where a patient immediately asks for the therapist's comments after having completed a task – without having evaluated it for themselves. This situation is understandable in the beginning of a rehabilitation programme, but is not productive in the longer term, as at the time of discharge, the patient should be able to rely on their own intrinsic feedback. Thus, augmented feedback may be redundant – and it may be counterproductive.

The need for augmented feedback relies on:

1. whether the patient can obtain the same information through intrinsic feedback
2. to what extent the patient understands the task requirements and is experienced at the task
3. the complexity of the task.

Amount of feedback: Care must be taken not to overload patients with information. Especially in the verbal-cognitive stage of learning, the enthusiastic therapist may provide the patient with verbal instructions (acoustic information) together with 'hands-on' guidance (tactile and/ or proprioceptive information) – perhaps even in front of a mirror (visual information). Patients with reduced attentional capacity (e.g. dementia) may especially become overloaded. Carefully selecting key points for the beginner and gradually adding other information as learning progresses is a key teaching skill in clinical practice.

Frequency of feedback: Research involving people with traumatic brain injury (Croce et al. 1996) and Parkinson's disease (Adams et al. 2002) has shown that providing feedback on 50% of the attempts at a task is often more effective than providing feedback on 100% of the attempts (i.e. every time). Initially, this may seem counterproductive; as therapists we may feel that, surely, more feedback is better! However, these findings may be explained by the notion of *problem solving*. By evaluating the movement for themselves, the patient uses their intrinsic feedback to build an internal representation of the correct task. If they receive feedback 100% of the time, they may become dependent on the therapist and do not develop this problem-solving ability.

There are several ways to reduce the *amount* of feedback throughout the stages of learning:

- **Summary feedback** is a schedule where feedback provided about each attempt, but only after a certain number have been completed. One way of doing this could be by keeping a log or making a diagram of subsequent attempts at a task, e.g. the amount of grip force produced at each attempt, before feeding this back to the patient. Schmidt et al. (1990) found that a summary of five attempts yielded superior results compared to summaries of 1, 10 or 15 attempts. However, this was a laboratory-based task. In clinical practice, the optimal number of attempts per summary probably depends on the complexity of the task, the patient's level of experience and their capacity to remember relevant information.

- **Average feedback** is a schedule where performance is averaged over subsequent attempts. In addition to the average, a measure of the variation could also be provided (e.g. the average and range of 5 repetitions of trying to pronounce a word).

- **Bandwidth feedback** is a schedule where feedback is given only when performance falls outside specified criteria. For example, a person with stroke may move the foot of their stronger leg back at the beginning of standing up, in order to take more weight on it. The therapist may want to discourage this, so that the patient puts weight on the affected leg to strengthen the muscles on the hemiparetic side. By placing an object to block the movement of the stronger leg, the patient will realise their mistake when their foot touches the object. Note that they only receive this feedback if they do something wrong, otherwise practice continues with the patient knowing their performance is correct. This type of bandwidth feedback promotes consistency of performance.

The *timing* of delivering feedback can also exert a powerful influence over motor learning:

- **Instantaneous vs. delayed** feedback. A classic study by Swinnen et al. (1990) compared instantaneous KR (i.e. delivered immediately after the completion of the task) with delayed KR, and with the participant's estimate of their performance. Interestingly, the results showed that instantaneous KR was not effective, as performance after a 2-day retention period was comparable to that at baseline. Performance under delayed KR conditions was better than under instantaneous KR, but the best performance was seen in the condition where the participants had to estimate their own performance. Subsequent work has confirmed that delayed augmented feedback is more effective for skill acquisition than instantaneous feedback. How can this finding – which seems counter-intuitive – be explained? The opportunity for participants to process their own intrinsic feedback and learn from their own performance, again appears to be the key factor in motor learning.

- Giving patients the opportunity to decide when they need feedback may also influence outcomes. One study (Chiviacowsky and Wulf

2005) gave healthy individuals who were learning a sequential timing task a choice as to when to request feedback; one group had to make this decision before each attempt, while the other group made this decision after each attempt. On the transfer tests, participants in the 'after' group improved more with regard to overall timing and accuracy than participants in the 'before' group. How may this be explained? The authors postulated that being able to request feedback after an attempt enables the learner to estimate their own errors – similar to the findings by Swinnen et al. (1990) mentioned above.

In summary, augmented feedback plays an important role in skill acquisition. It has the potential to motivate the patient, encourage persistence to master a skill, increase skill level, speed up learning and enhance self-efficacy. However, an overload of augmented feedback may create a dependency that impairs this process. Thus, therapists need to select key information and tailor this to the complexity of the task, the patient's level of experience, their attentional capacity and their level of motivation and confidence. As the learning process progresses from the verbal-cognitive stage to the associative stage, and henceforth to the autonomous stage, augmented feedback should be faded in order to enable the patient to problem solve more independently.

Transfer and the specificity of training hypothesis

As stated before, resource limitations within clinical practice place constraints on the amount of time available for supervised therapy and the opportunity for practice. This means that therapists need to prioritise which skills need to be practised. There are often implicit assumptions that practising one skill will carry over onto another skill. For example, one might expect that practising straight leg raises, lying supine on a plinth, would carry over into stair climbing. But let's look at this example more closely. Undoubtedly, in order to ascend the stairs, one would require sufficient strength of the knee extensors. Hence, knee extension is necessary for stair climbing – but is it also sufficient? In stair climbing, one needs to use visual information to decide where to place the feet, while transferring weight from one foot to the next. The amount and timing of force produced by the knee flexors and extensors is controlled in concert with contracting hip flexors and extensors, which contract concentrically on the way up, and eccentrically on the way down. Meanwhile, hip abductors play an important role in stabilising the body in the transverse plane. Now let's compare this dynamic activity with the straight leg raising exercise, where the only degree of freedom to be controlled is hip flexion, where the knee extensors work isometrically and little visual guidance is required. Even from this incomplete analysis, we can already see that climbing the stairs requires more than the ability to contract one muscle group! This is not to say that practising straight leg raises is not useful; a study by Saunders et al. (2008) showed that leg extensor power is correlated with the ability to climb stairs in people with stroke. Hence, muscle power is necessary for functional activity. But, as our example showed, training muscle power per se does not address the coordination required for carrying out the functional task, and is therefore not sufficient.

There are numerous studies that have come to similar general conclusions: transfer from one movement (or skill) to the next is often very limited; a general finding that has become known as the **specificity of learning principle**. More formally, the specificity of learning hypothesis (e.g. Barnett et al. 1973, Proteau et al. 1992) predicts that skill acquisition is enhanced when conditions of practice match those during retrieval in terms of movement components – as well as the environment.

This hypothesis may be explained at different levels of analysis. Firstly, at the level of Schmidt's model of motor control, one would observe a number of crucial differences in the GMPs of the two actions (refer back to the example of straight leg raises and stair climbing used above), i.e. the order, relative timing and relative force are entirely different.

The specificity of learning hypothesis may also be explained at the neuronal level of analysis. As set out in Chapter 5, the contemporary model of the central nervous system is that of a functionally organised, distributed hierarchical circuit, where information is processed in a parallel-distributed manner (Kolb and Whishaw 2009). Many behavioural functions or skills are thus represented by specific maps in the brain and may be served by dedicated neural pathways (Kandel et al. 2000). This implies that a particular function is mediated through a specific neural network and that if this function is to be improved, training is required that targets that specific neural network.

The specificity of learning hypothesis – and the evidence supporting it – is the basis for **task-specific training** that is currently at the centre of attention, right across the various professions in neurological rehabilitation research, with examples such as constraint-induced movement therapy (Wolf et al. 2006), and ADL practice (Steultjens et al. 2003).

Summary

A key aim in rehabilitation is for therapists to facilitate the acquisition of skills that are relevant to the patient to support their activities and participation in their chosen environment. Given the specificity of learning hypothesis, therapists need to use the goals that have been agreed with the patient as a target and ensure that the content of their intervention transfers into the intended activities.

Furthermore, rather than focusing on immediate performance gains, long-term retention should be aimed for. This implies that learning strategies may need to be employed that may seem to be counterintuitive (e.g. random practice and reduced feedback).

It is important to remember that most of the research on skill acquisition has been undertaken with young, healthy populations, often using abstract tasks in laboratory settings. We have also tacitly assumed that the process of 'learning' is similar to that of 're-learning', but much research is still required to examine whether this assumption is valid in people

with conditions affecting the brain. For these reasons, generalisation to clinical populations should be undertaken with due caution and therapists should utilise the available evidence base, but integrate this with their clinical judgement of individual patients.

SELF-ASSESSMENT QUESTIONS

Following this chapter, can you:

1. Compare and contrast motor performance and learning?
2. Give an outline of the information processing approach to motor learning and define its key concepts, strengths and limitations?
3. Describe each of the three stages of learning and explain the role of cognition during each stage?
4. Explain why covert and overt action may be placed on a continuum?
5. Describe, compare and contrast various practice schedules and explain their effect on performance and learning?
6. Describe, compare and contrast various feedback strategies and explain their effects on performance and learning?
7. Discuss the importance of the concept of 'transfer' and explain how transfer may be enhanced between therapy sessions and patient's ADL?

Further reading

Cramer, S.C., Nudo, R.J. (Eds.), 2010. Brain Repair After Stroke. Cambridge University Press, Cambridge.

Edmans, J. (Ed.), 2010. Occupational Therapy and Stroke, second ed. Wiley-Blackwell, Oxford.

Kosslynn, S.M., Thompson, W.L., Ganis, G., 2006. The Case for Mental Imagery. Oxford University Press, Oxford.

Levin, H.S., Grafman, J. (Eds.), 2000. Cerebral Organisation of Function After Brain Damage. Oxford University Press, Oxford.

Raine, S., Meadows, L., Lynch-Ellerton, M. (Eds.), 2009. Bobath Concept: Theory and clinical practice in neurological rehabilitation. John Wiley, Chichester.

Stokes, M., Stack, E. (Eds.), 2010. Physical Management for Neurological Rehabilitation, third ed. Churchill Livingston Elsevier, Edinburgh.

References

Adams, S.G., Page, A.D., Jog, M., 2002. Summary feedback schedules and speech motor learning in Parkinson's disease. J. Med. Speech-Lang. Pa. 10, 215–220.

Baddely, A., Wilson, B.A., 1994. When implicit learning fails: amnesia and the problem of error elimination. Neuropsychologia 32, 53–68.

Bandura, A., 1986. Social Foundations of Thought and Action: a social cognitive theory. Prentice Hall, Englewood Cliffs NJ.

Barnett, M.L., Ross, D., Schmidt, R.A., et al., 1973. Motor skills learning and the specificity of training principle. Res. Q. Exerc. Sport 44, 440–447.

Battig, W.F., 1979. The flexibility of human memory. In: Cermak, L.S., Craik, F.I.M. (Eds.), Levels of

Processing in Human Memory. Erlbaum, Hillsdale, NJ, pp. 23–44.

Birkenmeier, R.L., Prager, E.M., Lang, C.R., 2010. Translating animal doses of task-specific training to people with chronic stroke in 1-hour therapy sessions: a proof-of-concept study. Neurorehabil. Neural. Repair. 24, 620–635.

Brazzelli, M., Saunders, D.H., Greig, C.A., et al., 2011. Physical fitness training for stroke patients. Cochrane Database Syst. Rev 11, CD003316. doi:10.1002/14651858.

Chiviacowsky, S., Wulf, G., 2005. Self-controlled feedback is effective if it is based on the learner's performance. Res. Q. Exerc. Sport 76, 42–48.

Croce, R., Horvat, M., Roswal, G., 1996. Augmented feedback for enhanced skill acquisition in individuals with traumatic brain injury. Percept. Mot. Skills 82, 507–514.

De Wit, L., Putman, K., Dejaeger, E., et al., 2005. Use of time by stroke patients: a comparison of four European rehabilitation centres. Stroke 36, 1977–1983.

Dick, M.B., Hsieh, S., Dick-Muehke, C., et al., 2000. The variability of practice hypothesis in motor learning: does it apply to Alzheimer's disease? Brain Cogn. 44, 470–489.

Di Pellegrino, G., Fadiga, L., Fogassi, L., et al., 1992. Understanding motor events: a neuropsychological study. Exp. Brain Res. 91, 176–182.

Donovan, J.J., Radosevich, D.J., 1999. A meta-analytic review of the practice distribution effect: now you see it, now you don't. J. Appl. Psychol. 84, 795–805.

Durham, K., van Vliet, P.M., Sackley, F.B. C., 2009. Use of information feedback and attentional focus of feedback in treating the person with a hemiplegic arm. Physiother. Res. Int. 14, 77–90.

Escolano, C., Ramos Murguialday, A., Matuz, T., et al., 2010. A telepresence robotic system operated with a P300-based brain-computer interface: initial tests with ALS patients. In: 32nd Annual International Conference of the IEEE EBMS, Buenos Aires, Argentina, pp. 4476–4480.

Fasoli, S.E., Trombly, C.A., Ticle-Degned, L., et al., 2002. Effect of instructions on functional reach in persons with and without cerebrovascular accident. Am. J. Occup. Ther. 56, 380–390.

Feltz, D.L., Landers, D.M., 1983. The effects of mental practice on motor skill learning and performance: a meta-analysis. J. Sport Psychol. 5, 25–57.

Fitts, P.M., Posner, M.I., 1967. Human Performance. Brooks/Cole, Belmot, CA.

Gentile, A.M., 2000. Skill acquisition: action, movement and neuromotor processes. In: Carr, J., Shepherd, R. (Eds.), Movement Science. Foundations for physical therapy and rehabilitation. Aspen Publishers Inc., Gaithersburg, MD, pp. 111–187.

Hanlon, R.E., 1996. Motor learning following unilateral stroke. Arch. Phys. Med. Rehabil. 77, 811–815.

Hashimoto, Y., Ushiba, J., Kimura, A., et al., 2010. Change in brain activity through virtual reality-based brain-machine communication in a chronic tetraplegic subject with muscular dystrophy. Br. Med. J. Neurosci. 11, 117.

Jeannerod, M., 2005. Levels of representation of goal-directed actions. In: Freund, H.J., Jeannerod, M., Hallet, M. et al., (Eds.), Higher-order Motor Disorders. From neuroanatomy and neurobiology to clinical neurology. Oxford University Press, Oxford, pp. 159–182.

Jeannerod, M., 2006. Motor Cognition. What actions tell the self. Oxford University Press, Oxford.

Kandel, R.R., Schwartz, J.H., Jesell, T.M., 2000. Principles of neural science, fourth ed. McGraw-Hill, New York.

Kessels, R.P.C., de Haan, E.H.F., 2003. Implicit learning in memory rehabilitation: a meta-analysis on errorless learning and vanishing cue methods. J. Clin. Exp. Neuropsychol. 25, 805–814.

Kessels, R.P.C., Olde Henskens, L.M.G., 2009. Effects of errorless skill learning in people with mild-to-moderate or severe dementia: a randomized controlled pilot study. NeuroRehabilitation 25, 307–312.

Kolb, B., Whishaw, I.Q., 2009. Fundamentals of Human Neuropsychology, sixth ed. Worth Publishers, New York.

Lang, C.E., MacDonald, J.R., Reisman, D.S., et al., 2009. Observation of the amounts of movement practice provided during stroke rehabilitation. Arch. Phys. Med. Rehabil. 90, 1692–1698.

Laufer, Y., Rotem-Lehrer, N., Ronen, Z., et al., 2007. Effect of attention focus on acquisition and retention of postural control following ankle sprain. Arch. Phys. Med. Rehabil. 88, 105–108.

Lee, T.D., Genovese, E.D., 1988. Distribution of practice in motor skill acquisition: learning and performance effects reconsidered. Res. Q. Exerc. Sport 59, 277–287.

Levack, W.M.M., Taylor, K., Siegert, R. J., et al., 2006. Is goal planning in rehabilitation effective? A systematic review. Clin. Rehabil. 20, 739–755.

Magill, R.A., 2007. Motor Learning and Control. Concepts and applications, eighth ed. McGraw Hill, Boston.

McNevin, N.H., Shea, C.H., Wulf, G., 2003. Increasing the distance of an external focus of attention enhances learning. Psychol. Res. 67, 22–29.

Mount, J., Pierce, S.R., Parker, J., et al., 2007. Trial and error versus errorless learning of functional skills in patients with acute stroke. NeuroRehabilitation 22, 123–132.

Nieuwboer, A., Kwakkel, G., Rochester, L., et al., 2007. Cueing training in the home improves gait-related mobility in Parkinson's disease: the RESCUE trial. J. Neurol. Neurosurg. Psychiatry 78, 134–140.

Page, S.J., Levine, P., Leonard, A., 2007. Mental practice in chronic stroke: results of a randomized, placebo-controlled trial. Stroke 38, 1293–1297.

Playford, E.D., Siegert, R., Levack, W.M.M., et al., 2009. Areas of consensus and controversy about goal setting in rehabilitation: A conference report. Clin. Rehabil. 23, 334–344.

Proteau, L., Marteniuk, R.G., Lévesque, L., 1992. A sensorimotor basis for motor learning: evidence indicating specificity of practice. Q. J. Exp. Psychol. A 44, 557–575.

ReSCUE project, 2002/3. Improving mobility for people with Parkinson's Disease: the ReSCUE project. Available online from: http://www.rescueproject.org/ (accessed 26.12.2011).

Rizzolatti, G., Fadiga, L., 2005. The mirror neurone system and action recognition. In: Freund, H.J., Jeannerod, M., Hallet, M. et al., (Eds.), Higher-order Motor Disorders. From neuroanatomy and neurobiology to clinical neurology. Oxford University Press, Oxford, pp. 141–158.

Royal College of Physicians, 2008. National Clinical Guideline for Stroke, third ed. Intercollegiate Stroke Working Party. Royal College of Physicians, London.

Saunders, D.H., Greig, C.A., Young, A., et al., 2008. Association of activity limitations and lower-limb explosive extensor power in ambulatory people with stroke. Arch. Phys. Med. Rehabil. 89, 677–683.

Schmidt, R.A., 1988. Motor Control and Learning. A behavioral emphasis. Human Kinetics, Champaign, IL.

Schmidt, R.A., Wrisberg, C.A., 2008. Motor Learning and Performance. A situation-based learning approach, third ed. Human Kinetics, Champaign, IL.

Schmidt, R.A., Lange, C.A., Young, D.E., 1990. Optimizing summary knowledge of results for skill learning. Hum. Mov. Sci. 9, 325–348.

Scottish Intercollegiate Guidelines Network, 2010. Guideline 118: Management of patients with stroke: rehabilitation, prevention and management of complications, and discharge planning: a national clinical guideline. Scottish Intercollegiate

Guidelines Network (SIGN), Edinburgh. Available online at: http://www.sign.ac.uk/guidelines/fulltext/118/index.html (accessed 27.12.2011).

Shea, J.B., Morgan, R.L., 1979. Contextual interference effects on the acquisition, retention, and transfer of a motor skill. J. Exp. Psychol. Hum. Learn. Mem. 5, 179–187.

Stelmach, G.E., 1969. Efficiency of motor learning as a function of intertrial rest. Res. Q. Exercise Sport 40, 198–202.

Steultjens, E.M., Dekker, J., Bouter, L.M., et al., 2003. Occupational therapy for stroke patients: a systematic review. Stroke 34, 676–687.

Summers, J., 2004. Historical perspective on skill acquisition. In: Williams, A.M., Hodges, N.J. (Eds.), Skill Acquisition in Sport. Research, theory and practice. Routledge, London, pp. 1–26.

Swinnen, S.P., Schmidt, R.A., Nicholson, D.E., et al., 1990. Information feedback for skill acquisition: Instantaneous knowledge of results degrades learning. J. Exp. Psychol. Learn. Mem. Cogn. 16, 706–716.

Talvitie, U., Reunanen, M., 2002. Interaction between physiotherapists and patients in stroke treatment. Physiotherapy 88, 77–88.

Thorndike, E.L., 1905. Cited in: Sternberg, R., 2003. Cognitive Psychology, third ed. Wadsworth/Thomson, Belmont, CA.

van Vliet, P.M., Wulf, G., 2006. Extrinsic feedback for motor learning after stroke: What is the evidence? Disabil. Rehabil. 28, 831–840.

Winstein, C.J., Gardner, E.R., McNeal, D.R., et al., 1989. Standing balance retraining: Effect on balance and locomotion in hemiparetic adults. Arch. Phys. Med. Rehabil. 70, 755–762.

Wolf, S.L., Winstein, C.J., Miller, J.P., et al., for the EXCITE Investigators, 2006. Effect of constraint-induced movement therapy on upper extremity function 3 to 9 months after stroke: the EXCITE randomized clinical trial. J. Am. Med. Assoc. 296, 2095–2104.

Wulf, G., Prinz, W., 2001. Directing attention to movement effects enhances learning: a review. Psychon. Bull. Rev. 8, 648–660.

Wulf, G., Lauterbach, B., Toole, T., 1999. The learning advantages of an external focus of attention in golf. Res. Q. Exerc. Sport 70, 120–126.

Wulf, G., McConnel, N., Gartner, M., et al., 2002. Enhancing the learning of sport skills through external-focus feedback. J. Mot. Behav. 34, 171–182.

Wulf, G., Landers, M., Lewthwaite, R., et al., 2009. http://www.ncbi.nlm.nih.gov/pubmed/19074619 External focus instructions reduce postural instability in individuals with Parkinson disease. Physical Therapy 89, 162–168.

Disorders of attention and memory

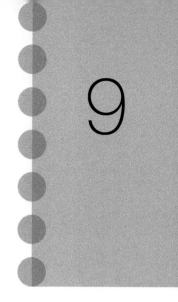

LEARNING OUTCOMES

At the end of this chapter, you should be able to:

- define attention and memory
- describe the potential effects of cortical, as well as subcortical lesions on attention and memory
- describe the main clinical manifestations of some common disorders of attention and memory
- demonstrate an understanding of the role of attention and memory in learning
- explore the implications that disorders of attention and memory may have for patients with a neurological condition
- define unilateral neglect, describe and explain the common clinical manifestations of this syndrome
- provide different explanations for unilateral neglect
- demonstrate an understanding of the possible implications of neglect for neurological rehabilitation
- demonstrate an understanding of the role of the multi-disciplinary team in the management of patients with neglect
- explore how you would adapt the general theory of motor learning for patients with impaired attention/memory as a result of a neurological condition.

Introduction

In the Introduction to this book, we explained how rehabilitation can be interpreted as a learning process; patients may need to learn (or relearn) how to carry out functional tasks, find new strategies for communication and self-care or develop more ergonomic ways for moving and handling. In order to store this information into long-term memory, the learner needs to be able to focus and maintain their attention on relevant information for long enough. However, attentional deficits are common in a number of patient groups, e.g. those with dementia or severe pain, and are widespread in people with neurological conditions such as traumatic brain injury or stroke.

Given the prerequisite of attention for learning, and the finding that attentional deficits are common in a number of clinical populations, it is important that health-care professionals have a sufficient understanding of the normal function of attention, the impact of specific health conditions on this function, and the impact that attentional deficits may have on the rehabilitation process. Consider Case study 9.1.

The case study above illustrates the importance of understanding a patient's attentional difficulties as a result of their health condition. Clearly, the health-care professional will need to tailor their intervention strategies to their patient's needs.

The aim of this chapter is to provide you with an understanding of attention and memory, an overview of the areas of the nervous system that are involved in these cognitive functions, and the role they play in learning. We will discuss a number of attentional and memory deficits that are common in neurological rehabilitation. At present, there are no definitive strategies for managing these, however, where possible, we will put forward some suggestions for clinical practice.

Attention

Attention described

As you are reading this, your attention may be focused on the text for some time, then shift towards your laptop as a signal indicates an incoming email. At the same time, you may be aware of a conversation between your friends, studying next to you. Then you

Case study 9.1

Unilateral neglect following stroke

Around 18 months ago, Mrs C. had a severe, total anterior circulation stroke affecting her right cerebral hemisphere. Her recovery was minimal and she is now severely disabled, using a wheelchair both in- and outdoors. Due to severe hemiparesis and spasticity, she has very limited voluntary movement in her left arm and leg. She indicates that she is more or less resigned to being in a wheelchair, but is more concerned about her affected arm. She would like to regain more function in order to undertake some personal self-care tasks for which she now requires her husband's assistance. Mr and Mrs C. own their own company and Mrs C. used to be responsible for undertaking all managerial and administrative tasks. However, since her stroke, the company has been struggling. Mrs C.'s husband is very keen for his wife to receive the best possible treatment. Mrs C.'s GP has referred her for further community-based rehabilitation.

During your first clinical examination, you observe that Mrs C. is looking slightly towards the right, away from the affected side of her body. In fact, her whole posture is asymmetrical, being inclined towards the right. When you position yourself on Mrs C.'s left hand side, she takes some time to react to you. Observing Mrs C.'s affected arm, you notice some bruising. When you point this out Mrs C. explains that her arm must have 'got caught against the door post again' – apparently she often bumps into obstacles that she has not noticed (although her eyesight

has recently been tested and is normal for her age). She says that she has had this problem since her stroke, but that it has got better over time. However, her husband has to remind her frequently when her affected arm is in an awkward position – she herself is usually unaware of this.

Further clinical examination reveals reduced sensation and proprioception in the affected arm, especially the hand. Limited passive range of movement in all upper limb joints, and increased resistance to passive movement, particularly affecting the flexors of the wrist, fingers and thumb, is also apparent. However, there is clearly potential for increasing voluntary movement and work towards functional activity – even if dextrous tasks are unlikely to be achievable. You ask Mrs C. to what extent she involves her left hand in daily activities, to which she responds that she has become entirely right handed since the stroke.

Testing Mrs C.'s spatial perception further, you ask her to indicate the midpoint of a horizontal line, placed straight in front of her. Mrs C. indicates to the right of the actual midpoint, and repeats this on three occasions.

Taken together, it is becoming clear that Mrs C. has potential to develop some functional activity involving her affected arm, but also has a very limited awareness of her affected side. How can this latter phenomenon be explained and what are the implications for her predicted outcomes? How will Mrs C. remember to involve her affected arm in daily activity?

refocus again on the text, blocking out your friends' conversation, until a hunger pang interrupts your concentration... In the span of less than a minute, your attentional system has automatically gone through its range of functions, i.e. to:

- focus
- divide
- disengage, shift and re-engage
- sustain.

In normal circumstances, attention operates in such an automatic manner that we hardly notice it; we effortlessly shift from one source of information to the next, as illustrated in the example above. But when asked to define 'attention', we may be stuck for words. The famous founder of psychology William James (1890) made the following statement about attention:

> *'Everyone knows what attention is. It is the taking posession by the mind, in clear and vivid form, of one out of what seems to be simultaneously possible objects or trains of thought'.*

James' interpretation of attention resembles that of a torch that illuminates certain objects and discerns them from a background of competing stimuli. In a similar vein, van Zomeren and Spikman (2003) more recently compared attention to a 'spotlight', which provides both intensity and selectivity.

Additionally, for this 'spotlight' to work, one needs to have a sufficient level of arousal, defined by Stuss and Benson (1986) as:

> *'the ability to be awakened, to maintain wakefulness and to follow signals and commands'*

Taken together, attention could be interpreted as illustrated in Figure 9.1, which may help to understand the range of difficulties that patients with impaired attention may experience.

Clinical manifestations of attentional deficits

Disorders of attention are common in neurological populations (Geschwind 1982), especially in patients with head injuries and frontal lobe lesions (Hécaen and Albert 1978). Common signs and symptoms of attentional difficulties include those associated with impaired arousal, ranging from coma, drowsiness, a lack of concentration, through to hypervigilance and panic. Patients may lack a general awareness of what goes on around them, e.g. they may be oblivious to a

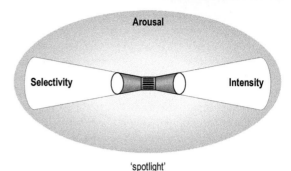

'spotlight'

(based on van Zomeren & Spikman, 2003)

Fig. 9.1 • Dimensions of attention. Using the analogy of a lighting system, "arousal" provides ambient illumination, while "selectivity" and "intensity" together function as a spotlight that focuses attention

dispute between fellow patients. Fatigue (see Chapter 14) is a common problem in patients with conditions affecting the CNS, which therapists need to take into account; sessions that may not place a notable cardiovascular or biomechanical load on patients may still induce fatigue due to attentional demands. Overall processing speed may be reduced, which may manifest itself as a learning difficulty. Patients may complain that the usual conversations with their family are too fast, and that they are unable to follow the news on TV. Attentional capacity may be more limited, restricting the amount of information they can take in. In terms of selectivity, patients may have difficulty focusing and sustaining their attention, and as a result they may be easily distracted. This can pose a particular challenge in a busy therapy department (see Clinical box 9.1), where there is a constant source of diversion in the form of other people,

---

Clinical application box 9.1

You are a senior therapist working in a busy therapy department. What measures could you take to accommodate patients with attentional deficits?
  Consider the following questions:
- How could you help a patient to concentrate on their tasks?
- How could you help a patient to focus their attention on relevant information?
- How would you handle fatigue?
- How would you adapt your instructions for a patient with attentional deficits?

moving objects and – in some situations – music. Multi-tasking, which requires attention to either be divided or switched between one task and the next, may be impossible. Some patients will stop talking when concentrating on a task, or stop practising while talking to their therapist. In terms of intensity, some patients may find it difficult to generate sufficient attention and this apparent apathy may be misinterpreted as a lack of motivation. Other patients may show perseveration, which means that they continue a task even if it has been completed, signalling difficulty with disengaging attention.

In summary, attentional difficulties are common in patients with conditions affecting their central nervous system. The next section will focus on underlying neural structures that normally support the various functions of attention.

Attention and the brain

Given the different dimensions of attention, it is perhaps not surprising that there is a range of areas within the nervous system that play a role in attention (see Kolb and Whishaw, 2009). Neuro-imaging and clinical studies have shown that the following areas play a major role:

- The reticular formation
- The right cerebral hemisphere – more so than the left
- The posterior parietal lobe
- The posterior temporal lobe
- The frontal lobe.

We will now look at each of these areas in turn.

Reticular formation

The reticular formation (from the Latin *reticulum*: network, see Chapter 2) is an extensive neural network that connects the thalamus with the cerebrum. Its main functions include regulating the level of arousal, the sleep–wake cycle, and motor activities that involve motivation and reward. It follows that damage to this network (e.g. through a traumatic brain injury, which may cause diffuse axonal tearing) may result in abnormal levels of arousal (e.g. coma, drowsiness), disturbances in sleep–wake rhythm (e.g. the patient may be sleepy during the day, but active at night), or lack of response to incentives.

Right cerebral hemisphere

For a reason not readily understood, the right cerebral hemisphere plays a dominant role in attention.

Neuroimaging studies have shown that if a person directs their attention to the left visual field, only the right cerebral hemisphere is activated. In contrast, if a person focuses on stimuli in their right visual field, both left and right hemispheres are activated. It follows that if a person sustains a lesion to the left hemisphere, their right hemisphere can continue to focus their attention on the left visual field, and compensate for the damaged left hemisphere when focusing attention on the right visual field. Thus, despite the left hemisphere lesion, there may not be a noticeable attentional deficit. But what happens when the right hemisphere is affected? The patient will still be able to direct their attention to their right visual field, but they will now have difficulty focusing on their left visual field (Fig. 9.2). This scenario is known as **hemi-inattention**, other terms being hemispatial neglect or unilateral neglect (see later).

Refer back to the case study at the start of the chapter: Mrs C. clearly demonstrated hemi-inattention; she lacked awareness of the affected side of her body, was positioned to the right of her midline, while the line bisection test confirmed that her midline had been displaced away from the affected side. It was as if her affected side no longer featured in her body image. Unaware of that side of space, she would then bump into obstacles. Unaware of that side of her body, she would not notice the bruises of such collisions, or the awkward position her arm may have been in.

Posterior parietal lobe

The posterior parietal lobe is especially involved in focusing attention on a particular location. Refer back to Chapter 5 on the relationship between the brain and behaviour: we saw there that the posterior parietal lobe was responsible for integrating information for planning action in user-centred space. More specifically, this part of the brain is involved in disengaging, moving and re-engaging attention to a particular location. Lesions of this part of the brain (e.g. due to a tumour or stroke) may result in **unilateral neglect** (i.e. having difficulty shifting attention towards the affected side). More about this syndrome will be discussed later in this chapter.

Posterior temporal lobe

Chapter 5 explained the role of the temporal lobe in object recognition. More specifically, this part of the brain is involved in focusing attention on particular

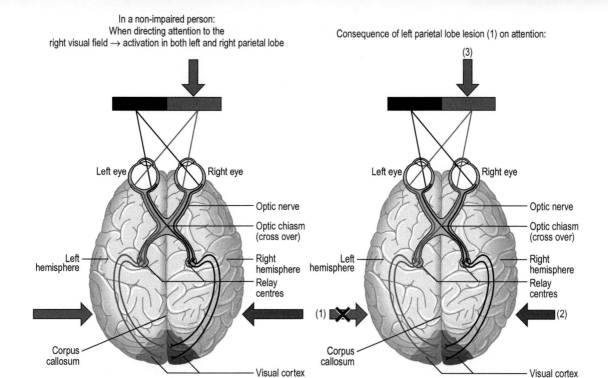

In a non-impaired person:
When directing attention to the
right visual field → activation in both left and right parietal lobe

Left eye   Right eye

Optic nerve
Optic chiasm
(cross over)
Left
hemisphere
Right
hemisphere
Relay
centres
Corpus
callosum
Visual cortex

Consequence of left parietal lobe lesion (1) on attention:

(3)

Left eye   Right eye

Optic nerve
Optic chiasm
(cross over)
Left
hemisphere
Right
hemisphere
Relay
centres
(1)   (2)
Corpus
callosum
Visual cortex

Right hemisphere compensates (2) → patient can still shift attention to
right visual field (3) → both visual fields remain represented

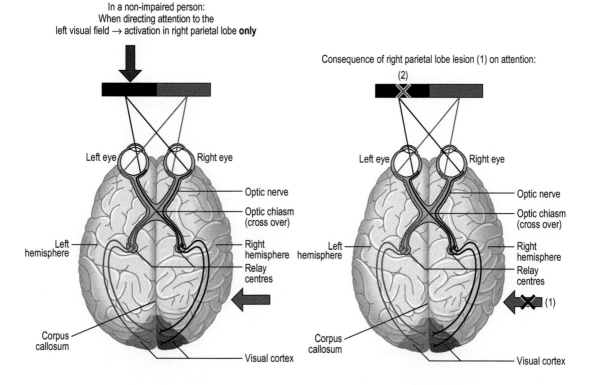

In a non-impaired person:
When directing attention to the
left visual field → activation in right parietal lobe **only**

Left eye   Right eye

Optic nerve
Optic chiasm
(cross over)
Left
hemisphere
Right
hemisphere
Relay
centres
Corpus
callosum
Visual cortex

Consequence of right parietal lobe lesion (1) on attention:

(2)

Left eye   Right eye

Optic nerve
Optic chiasm
(cross over)
Left
hemisphere
Right
hemisphere
Relay
centres
(1)
Corpus
callosum
Visual cortex

→ no compensation → representation of left visual field is lost (2).
Right hemisphere parietal lesion causes more neglect than
left hemisphere parietal lesion

Fig. 9.2 • Impact of lesion side on attention. See text for details.

features of an object. Damage to this part of the brain, therefore, often leads to difficulties recognising objects, a condition known as **visual agnosia**.

Frontal lobe

The frontal lobe is involved in short-term memory, in the sense that it keeps track of what has just been done. It is also involved in prospective memory (i.e. keeping track of what needs to be done next) and in selecting appropriate actions. Lesions to the frontal lobe (e.g. due to head injuries) impair this process, causing a person to 'lose track' of what they are doing and rendering their behaviour disorganised. This type of disorder, which is part of '**executive dysfunction**' or 'dysexecutive function', will be discussed in more detail in Chapter 12.

Taken together, building on Figure 9.1, a simple way to remember the various main brain areas involved in attention is illustrated in Figure 9.3.

Clinical implications of attentional deficits

In Chapter 8, we have seen how attention is a prerequisite for learning; attention is a major control process in the passing of information through to memory – a function that will be discussed in the next section. It is not surprising, therefore, that attentional deficits can present a real bottleneck for rehabilitation. Given the complexity of attention, which comprises a number of different functions, it is not possible to provide a standard protocol for managing attentional deficits. van Zomeren and Spikman (in Halligan et al. 2003) suggest the following pointers:

- Indicate priority
- Avoid or reduce time pressure
- Offer structure
- Avoid distraction.

Think about whether any of these pointers may help you to answer the questions in the clinical application in Box 9.1–and why they might be effective.

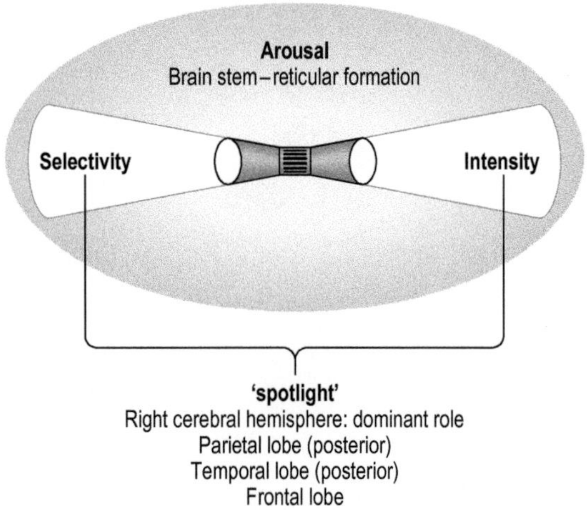

Memory

Memory: a definition

Memory can be described as a function involved in processing information resulting in a relatively permanent change in knowledge and behaviour. In this process, the following stages can be discerned (Fig. 9.4).

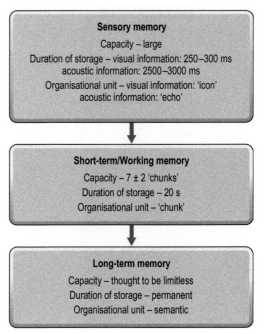

Fig. 9.3 • Dimensions of attention and main areas of the brain involved in attention.

Fig. 9.4 • Outline of the stages of memory

Sensory memory

Let's use an example to illustrate the process of storing information in memory; a patient working with a speech and language therapist in a busy treatment room, with a number of other patients and staff also present. A range of stimuli will be captured by the sensory systems, including visual, acoustic and proprioceptive information, which will be encoded and transmitted to the relevant parts of the central nervous system. Visual information will be the most fleeting; within one-third of 1 second an icon will have disappeared. Acoustic information, however, will linger a bit longer, i.e. up to 3 seconds. Sensory memory enables us to capture a wealth of information from around us. For example, the patient will use their sensory memory to read successive letters and remember them for long enough to capture a whole word. However, should this process be slowed down (e.g. due to a condition such as dementia, or pharmacological agents such as the antiepileptic drug, carbamazepine), the information may be lost before a whole sentence has been read.

Working memory

Working memory is like the RAM of a computer; involved in the recollection of 'last sentence', addition of numbers, composition of a sentence, and following directions. However, working memory has limited capacity, both in terms of the amount of information it can hold, and the duration of storage (see Fig. 9.4). Hence, within a very short period of time, the sensory information from sensory memory must be *organised* (i.e. grouped into coherent chunks of information) or else it is likely to be lost. Being an experienced reader, the patient will probably not be required to read every letter to remember a word; the information is 'chunked' into a more meaningful unit. However, this process is vulnerable to interference; additional information may compete with this process, leading to a loss of information. For example, the patient who is trying to read an instruction may be disrupted by acoustic information from other conversations around her. Furthermore, the amount of information that can be processed at this stage is limited, i.e. 7 plus/ minus two chunks. Therefore, the better one's capacity to chunk information, the more information one can store.

Long-term memory

Information that has been compressed and organised in chunks can then progress to long-term memory, where allegedly it is stored permanently. However, the success of being able to *retrieve* this information depends on how well it has been *stored* (i.e. organised and linked to other information) and *maintained* (i.e. how frequently the information has been used). Compared to short-term memory, the mode of memory in long-term memory is based on the meaning of the information rather than its literal detail. Retrieving information can involve recall (i.e. spontaneously retrieved information without prompting) or recognition (i.e. information retrieved following a prompt).

In general, three different categories of memory may be distinguished:

- Semantic memory: this refers to memory of facts and figures about the world (e.g. facts related to human anatomy). This category of memory is also known as 'declarative' memory in that it is possible to declare (i.e. verbally state) the information.
- Episodic memory: this comprises memories of personal episodes, or events, in one's life (e.g. remembering your first anatomical dissection class). Together, semantic memory and episodic memory comprise the entire database of the facts, figures and names, as well as experiences and conscious memories you learn in your lifetime. A key structure in 'filing' new memories is the hippocampus, as the case study on H.M. will demonstrate.
- Procedural memory: this refers to memory of how to undertake skills and procedures, including all actions and habits learned by repetition (e.g. cycling, eating with chop sticks or palpating a muscle group on the living body). In this case, it is more effective to demonstrate one's knowledge rather than declaring it. Procedural memory is the most durable category of memory; even if you haven't played a piece of music for years, your 'fingers' usually remember the piece. The cerebellum plays an important role in this category of memory, whereas the hippocampus is not much involved.

As we will see later, different areas of the brain and different neural networks support each of these three categories of memory.

Although our long-term memory is quite impressive (e.g. your 83-year-old patient may vividly remember the price of different food stuffs during the war), it is important to note that remembering information is not a process of 'replaying' the information. According to Barlett (1932), memory is *not a process of revival, but one of reconstruction*. This may explain why, years later, your recollection of a family event may be entirely different from the memory shortly after the event took place; your reflections upon the event and further personal experiences since may be drawn into the reconstruction, giving it a different meaning. In fact, Elizabeth Loftus (1997) has specialised in what is known as 'false memories', demonstrating that memories that are entirely synthetic can be 'implanted', causing participants to vividly remember events that never took place. The fallacy of our memory is an important issue in court cases, where the judiciary process relies on accuracy of witnesses' memories.

What are the processes that may cause us to forget information? Normal processes of forgetting include:

- A lack of attention: especially with respect to sensory memory, not paying attention to information may result in the data not making it through to short-term memory
- Decay: information 'fades' away if it is not rehearsed – this can occur in short-term memory, if information is not sufficiently maintained
- Interference:
  ○ in short-term memory, information overload may lead to data being displaced (e.g. someone asking you a question while you try to remember a number plate)
  ○ in long-term memory, interference may be pro-active or retro-active. In pro-active interference, old information impairs the storage of new information (e.g. having previously learned the highway code, you find it difficult to remember new regulations). In retro-active interference, new information impairs the retrieval of old information (e.g. having recently taken part in an Italian class, you have trouble remembering your French).

What strategies may be helpful to reduce forgetting?

This section provides some suggestions for helping patients remember important information.

Focus

Enable patients to focus their attention, e.g. by giving clear pointers, and reduce distractions where required. This allows patients to select the relevant information to be processed in sensory memory.

Chunk

Chunking information enables the patient to combine more information together into larger clusters, thereby extending the amount of information that can be stored in short-term memory. Compressing information is also useful, e.g. providing a demonstration of a procedure rather than extended verbal instructions.

Rehearse

Allow the patient time to repeat relevant information. This facilitates information to be processed in short-term memory. Some patients may need to verbally repeat instructions, using self-talk. This is often seen when the patient is in the cognitive stage of learning (Chapter 8).

Engage

To enhance storage of information in long-term memory, patients could be encouraged to think about what the information means to them. Relating it to their previous knowledge is also helpful to link new information to information already stored. Elaboration refers to expanding on the information, e.g. by questioning and applying. The function of relating new with existing information, as well as elaboration, are to extend the 'semantic network'; a network of related concepts.

Retrieve

Check whether the patient is able to actually retrieve the information! Considering the distributed neural networks involved in different categories of memory (see section Memory and the brain), it is important to consider how we ask the patient to demonstrate what they have learned. If we really want to check whether they can reproduce a procedure, asking if they 'know what they are doing' is not sufficient!

A considerable body of research has shown that people are better able to retrieve information in a situation that is similar to the one in which they originally learned the information. For example, if you have learned your clinical skills in a class room, you will probably find it easier to retrieve the information in a classroom than in a hospital ward. Processing information in a way where the encoding (i.e. learning) process matches the retrieval process is known as **transfer-appropriate processing**. This is an important phenomenon if we consider the issue of transfer (or carry-over) from a patient's clinical setting to their home situation. In Chapter 8, we pointed out that transfer from one skill to another or to a different environment is often limited. For example, a patient with a recent hip replacement who has been taught how to move safely out of bed in a hospital ward may not necessarily be able to transfer this skill to their own home situation. The entire spatial configuration, e.g. the position of the bed in relation to walls and other furniture, may require a different solution than that learned on the ward. Additionally, the home environment offers no prompts that help retrieve the information acquired in the hospital environment. This phenomenon, where memory depends on the context in which it was acquired, is known as **context-dependency**.

What does this mean for health-care professionals? Ideally, if a patient is taught new skills or information that is intended to be utilised in a different environment, the therapist should check that the patient is actually able to retrieve the required information in the required setting.

Additionally, a phenomenon known as **state-dependency** may manifest itself. This is a situation where it is easier to remember information if the acquisition and retrieval take place when the person is in a similar psychological condition. For example when patients learn new information when they feel depressed, they will remember this information better when they feel depressed again, compared to when they feel more optimistic.

In summary, memory is a process involving the encoding, organisation, storage and retrieval of information from sensory, to short-term and finally to long-term memory. The organisation and maintenance of the information are key to the successful retrieval of information. Memory may involve semantic, episodic or procedural categories of information, each of which is supported by different neural networks. Memory is a reconstructive process, which means that recall of events may change with experience.

Clinical presentations of memory disorders

Having given an overview of the functions of normal memory, it is time to look at signs and symptoms of disorders of memory.

A common scenario for memory loss, or **amnesia**, is in the case of a traumatic brain injury as a result of a road traffic accident (RTA). Usually, the person remembers little from before the impact – this is

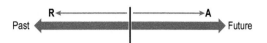

Amnesia: memory loss

- **Retrograde amnesia (R)**
  Memory loss for *previously learned* information
- **Anterograde amnesia (A)**
  Inability to form *new memories* following brain trauma

Fig. 9.5 • Anterograde and retrograde amnesia

known as **retrograde amnesia** (i.e. the memory loss pertains to information prior to the accident) (see Fig. 9.5). The person may also experience **anterograde amnesia**, i.e. a loss of memory related to events after the accident.

The period of retrograde amnesia may range from several weeks to just a few seconds before the accident. Normally, this period reduces over time; however, the person may never remember the actual accident. This is thought to be attributable to neural networks involved in storing this information being physically disrupted at the time. Anterograde amnesia is related to difficulty storing new information following the accident this could be due to lesions in the neural networks involved in storing new information. See Case study 9.2.

Memory functions and the brain

H.M.'s case study has been crucial in developing our understanding of memory – and appreciating that 'memory' is a collection of different functions, each of which may be affected independently.

In recent years, the picture has emerged that areas that are involved in certain forms of perception or action are also involved in the memory of these specific forms of perception or action. This notion is based on pioneering work by Donald O. Hebb (1949), as described in his work *The Organization of Behavior*. Pursuing the quest of the memory trace (or engram), Hebb set out to investigate *where* memories were stored in the brain. According to Hebb, when presented with a stimulus (say, that of a face), a network of neurons would respond together. Hebb named this collective a '**cell assembly**'. This neural activity would continue as long as the stimulus was present, and 'resonate' for some time after its removal. Following repeated exposure to the same stimulus, the network of neurons would be activated more readily each time, through a physiological process known as '**Hebbian modification**'. This network strengthening process would eventually

Case study 9.2

In 1957, Scoville and Milner published a paper entitled 'Loss of recent memory after bilateral hippocampal lesions'. It was to become a groundbreaking study in memory research. The authors described a surgical technique (bilateral medial temporal lobe resection – see Fig. 9.6) to alleviate symptoms of psychosis and epilepsy in patients severely affected by their condition and not responding to conventional medical treatment. Of the 10 patients described in the paper, the case study of H.M. has become a classic in the literature of neuropsychology.

H.M., a 29-year-old male motor winder at the time of his operation, suffered intractable epilepsy from the age of 10, initially starting with minor seizures. At the age of 16, he also developed major seizures that increased in frequency and intensity, eventually affecting him to such an extent that he was unable to work. H.M.'s seizures did not respond to maximum dosage of a range of anti-epileptic medications, and eventually it was agreed that the patient would undergo a surgical procedure so far only performed on patients with severe psychosis. This would involve the bilateral removal of the uncus, the anterior hippocampus and hippocampal gyrus in the medial temporal lobe. The rationale for the removal of these structures was that these were known to be prone to generating electrical abnormalities – even though in H.M.'s case, EEG failed to indicate any specific epileptinogenic locations. Together with these structures, the amygdala were removed on both sides as well.

Following the operation, H.M.'s seizures were reduced considerably and, although they returned to some extent after about a year, their severity was much reduced. There appeared to be no side effects in terms of deterioration in the patient's intelligence, or changes in personality. One side effect, however, was noted in all 10 cases described in the paper, including H.M.:

'There has been one striking and totally unexpected behavioural result: a grave loss of recent memory in those cases in which the medial temporal-lobe resection was so extensive as to involve the major portion of the hippocampal complex bilaterally.'

(Scoville and Milner 1957, p. 12).

In H.M.'s case, his memory loss was apparent when, following the operation, he was unable to recognise staff in the hospital where he was being treated, or find his way around. At follow up, his inability to remember seemingly simple things, e.g. the location of the house they had moved to recently, a conversation he had just had with someone, or even the fact he had just had lunch, was striking. Crucially, following his operation, H.M. failed to learn any new information. Formal psychological testing confirmed the discrepancy between his intelligence, which had been preserved and even improved, and recent memory. H.M. also had retrograde amnesia, comprising a period of about 3 years, while childhood memories seemed to have been preserved. Motor skills were intact, and so were his reasoning and perceptual skills.

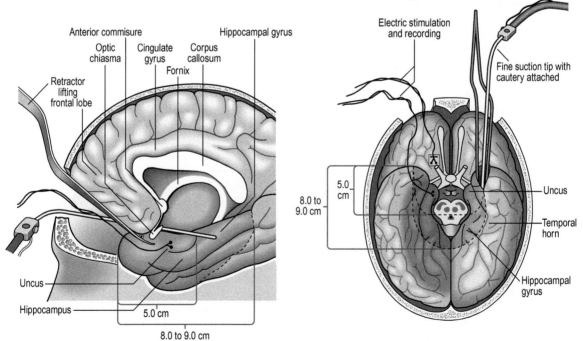

Fig. 9.6 • Bilateral medial temporal lobe resection, as detailed by Scoville and Milner in their classic 1957 paper, with permission from the British Medical Journal Group.

H.M.'s case, and that of the others described in the paper, led the authors to conclude that *'the anterior hippocampus and hippocampal gyrus, either separately or together, are critically concerned in the retention of current experience. It is not known whether the amygdala plays any part in this mechanism,* *since the hippocampal complex has not been removed alone, but always together with uncus and amygdala.'* (p. 21). A more precise report of H.M.'s brain structures can be found in Corkin et al. (1997), the first MRI study to examine H.M.'s brain at the age of 66 years.

ensure that, even if only part of the stimulus were provided (e.g. by covering part of it, or showing it under poor illumination), the whole cell assembly would respond, and result in recall of the entire stimulus. In other words, Hebb proposed that the memory (or engram) of a stimulus is represented internally by a specific neural network, i.e. by the neurons involved in the *sensation* and *perception* of the stimulus. Thus, memories could be stored in different locations in the brain, depending on the type of sensory information involved. Further, a particular memory would likely be stored in a distributed way, with multiple sources of sensory information contributing to the same memory (e.g. think of Scottish haggis, with its distinctive taste, texture, smell and colour).

Hebb's ground breaking theory explains a number of important phenomena; it explains our ability to recognise information, even if this has been degraded (e.g. a text with spelling mistakes or a foreign accent) – a finding explained as top-down processing in the next chapter. Also, the previous chapter on skill acquisition discussed the specificity of learning principle and how learning one skill does not necessarily carry over to another skill – unless the same motor programme is activated. A motor programme is another term for an engram and represents a specific memory, a formula, for producing movement. For example when we compared the activity of straight leg raising while lying supine with that of stair climbing, we reasoned that the two activities had to involve different motor programmes. Following Hebb's thinking, we can also reason that each activity will be represented by a different neural network and constitute a different 'motor memory'.

Additionally, Hebb's interpretation of memory supports the principle of redundancy, explained in Chapter 5. This means that if a patient loses some brain tissue due to injury or disease, a memory may still be preserved if the cell assembly representing that memory is distributed. 'Tapping into intact' memories really means finding which aspects of a memory, or which modality, has been preserved.

Thus, multiple neural networks and brain areas support memory functions.

Areas that are involved in **declarative memory** include:

- cortical areas:
  - parietal cortex
  - temporal cortex
  - frontal cortex
- subcortical areas:
  - hippocampus
  - thalamus
  - amygdala.

Compare and contrast these areas with those involved in procedural memory, detailed below. The case study of H.M. highlighted the special role of the hippocampus in memory, which is worth exploring in more detail.

The hippocampal formation

The hippocampal formation (see Fig. 9.7) consists of the hippocampus, the dentate gyrus and the subicular cortex and it is widely known that these areas play a key part in learning and memory functions. Over the years, a large amount of literature has been gathered concerning human and animal studies, all of which indicate a role for the hippocampal formation in learning processes.

The phenomenon of spatial learning (spatial memory) has been associated with the hippocampal formation, with evidence being gathered from a number of studies (both animal and human). These studies have involved the use of the rat 'Y-Maze' or 'radial maze' tests, in which the rat can learn to enter the correct arm of the maze in order to gain a food reward. However, following a hippocampal lesion in the same rat, there is a consistent failure to approach the correct arm.

Some of the human studies have involved studying patients who are suffering from Korsakoff's syndrome. Korsakoff's syndrome, which is typically associated with the toxic effects of alcohol (or from vitamin B deficiency), results in damage to the neurones in the hippocampal circuits. The patients with this syndrome display both anterograde and retrograde amnesia. As a result, the affected

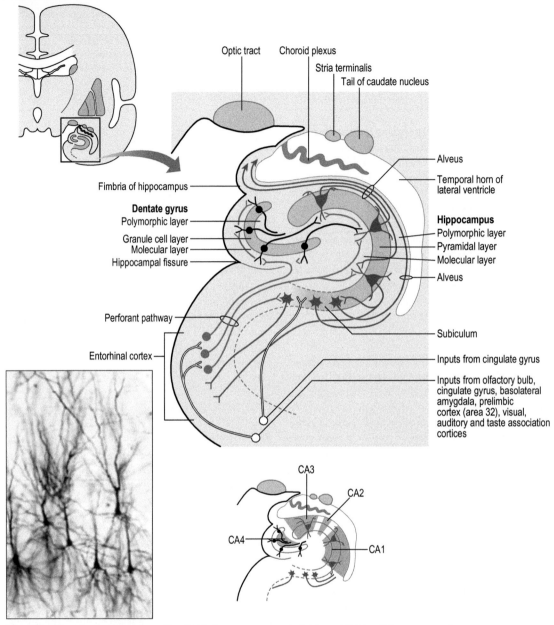

Fig. 9.7 • The hippocampal formation (CA1-4: cornu ammonis fields; subfields of hippocampus). From Haines 2005, with permission

individual experiences a marked difficulty with three distinct aspects of memory:

1. Recalling events in the recent past
2. Handling and retaining new information
3. Remembering those events that took place in the distant past

Further human studies have revolved around investigations of patients who have received a hippocampal lobectomy. Such a procedure will cause short-term memory disorders and anterograde amnesia (there is some retrograde amnesia, but it is less severe). Although the memory is impaired, the studies have shown that there is little loss of intellectual ability. One interesting aspect of the short-term memory disorder is the fact that the individual may also have a difficulty with reading, which arises from being unable to remember the line of text which they have previously read.

In a patient who has received a bilateral temporal lobectomy, where much of the hippocampal formation on both sides has been removed in order to eliminate the spread of severe seizure activity (see earlier section on H.M.), memory is also impaired. Such a patient may be able to remember where they lived many years earlier, but would not necessarily remember where they moved to since receiving the surgery. As for the unilateral lobectomy, although the memory is impaired, other forms of intellectual ability remain intact.

One major point that arises from all of the studies mentioned is that one of the functions of the hippocampal formation is to play a part in the transfer of memories from short-term to long-term storage, i.e. the **consolidation** of memory. Although we know that the location of these consolidatory processes is the hippocampus, exactly how this process takes place is yet to be fully understood.

Although some detail may be lacking, it is reasonable to suggest that the hippocampal formation must receive, process and categorise sensory information during learning. As an example, think of the various strategies you may use when trying to revise for an exam. You may read and re-read notes, re-write lecture material, draw your own diagrams, etc. – all of which result in sensory input as a way of learning. It can then be seen that any lesion with the circuitry of the hippocampal formation would upset such processes and further interfere with the attentional mechanisms required for processing and storage of sensory events.

The mechanism process as a model for the memory consolidation process is that of **long-term potentiation**, or LTP. LTP represents a change in synaptic strength as a manifestation of synaptic plasticity, a specific form of neuroplasticity. Synaptic plasticity is the mechanism whereby the brain is able to adapt in response to a change in use, i.e. the more you stimulate a particular pathway the better the synapse will respond and function. LTP can be produced by stimulating the neurones that make excitatory connections with the hippocampal pyramidal cells. Experiments have shown that short bursts of high-frequency stimulation of neuronal inputs to the hippocampal cells over a period of time results in an increased efficiency of the CA1 pyramidal cell response. Such an increase in excitatory response potency in these pyramidal cells (lasting anything from minutes to weeks) may provide us with a possible cellular mechanism through which learning occurs. The neurotransmitter that

has been proposed to facilitate this synaptic mechanism is glutamate, which is the major excitatory neurotransmitter in the brain. Glutamate is thought to act on the N-methyl-D-aspartate (NMDA) receptor, as experiments have shown that the use of an NMDA receptor antagonist can block the long-term potentiation.

Interestingly, this overview indicates that memory is linked with brain areas that also serve **emotion** (e.g. the amygdala). From personal experience, you will know that events which had an emotional impact on your life are better remembered than those that have left you indifferent, e.g. you may vividly remember your first day at school, which may have been coloured by excitement (and apprehension perhaps), while you are less likely to remember what you did three days ago, on a routine day at university. From an evolutionary perspective, it is important that we remember events that instilled intense emotions such as fear, joy and pleasure, as these may be linked with behaviours that mediate our survival.

Areas involved mainly in **procedural memory** (i.e. skills and operations) include:

- cortical areas:
  - pre-motor cortex.
- subcortical areas:
  - basal ganglia
  - ventral thalamus
  - cerebellum.

It is worth pointing out that this overview demonstrates that brain areas supporting declarative memory are distinct from those serving procedural memory. This explains why patients may have deficits in one domain (e.g. in semantic dementia, the person may be unable to differentiate between different animals), but be perfectly preserved in other domains such as playing football, or dressing oneself. Furthermore, this information would suggest that if a therapist wishes to verify whether a patient is competent in a specific procedure, that taking someone's word for it may not be valid!

Kolb and Whishaw (1996, p. 366) describe memory as '...*a process of neural activity rather than as a site to be found*'. In other words, memory is not like a filing cabinet where different 'items' are stored; instead, specific information is constantly encoded, stored, integrated with existing information, and retrieved from dedicated and often distributed areas. An important question for health-care professionals is how they can optimise this process.

Implications for rehabilitation

As stated before, an important aim of rehabilitation is to enable patients to learn new information and behaviours that will serve them – not just in the short term, but especially in the longer term, following discharge. As health-care professionals, we are, therefore, concerned with optimising processes involved in attention, learning and memory. Each patient will have different needs in this respect, which must be clearly identified and tailored where possible. Based on an information processing approach, the following general principles may be useful:

- Make learning *meaningful* to the patient in order to enhance motivation, attention and memory.
- Ensure that the learning experience is *enjoyable* where possible.
- *Target* the learning experience to specific functions in order to train the specific networks subserving these functions.
- Create plenty of opportunities for learning; ideally *over-learning is* required to forge long-term neuroplastic changes.
- Tap into intact memory systems; encourage *association* between information that is new and what is familiar.
- Reduce information if required; less may well be more. When providing instructions or feedback: *prioritise* information, present it succinctly and in a language that is readily understood.
- *Verify a patient's understanding* of information; if the information is procedural, ask for a demonstration.
- Use *prompts* and prosthetic memory (e.g. notices, reminders).
- Ensure similarity between the environment where information is to be retrieved and where it is practised (i.e. ensure *transfer-appropriate processing*)

Hemi-inattention/unilateral neglect

Having introduced the topics of attention and memory, it is time to refer back to our case study at the start of this chapter. Remember that Mrs C. had difficulty orienting her attention towards the affected side of her body, difficulty responding to stimuli from, and initiating action towards that side. These are some of the classic signs of what is known as **unilateral neglect**. Other terms, denoting the same syndrome, include contralateral neglect, hemi-spatial neglect, visual neglect and hemi-inattention.

Unilateral neglect is described as referring to:

'. . . *a difficulty in detecting, acting on, or even thinking about information from one side of space.*'

(Manly and Robertson 2003, p. 92).

Clinical manifestations of unilateral neglect include:

- having little or no notion of the affected side of the body
- being unaware of anything being "wrong" with the affected side (anosognosia)

In addition, on the side of the body, contralateral to the brain lesion:

- failing to report visual, auditory and/or somatosensory stimulation
- forgetting food on plate
- forgetting to shave one side of one's face
- unable to recall buildings
- difficulty reading or using the computer.

A person with unilateral neglect might see the above description of neglect as follows, complaining it does not make sense at all!:

ng, acting on, or even thinking
ne side of space.'

(Manly and Robertson 2003, p. 92).

Unilateral neglect is common, particularly in patients with right-hemisphere lesions. A study by Stone et al. (1993) with 171 acute stroke patients demonstrated that 82% of patient with right-hemisphere lesions and 65% of patients with left-hemisphere lesions had signs of visual neglect. In many cases, the severity of neglect reduced spontaneously in 10 days, and came to a plateau in about 3 months. In the chronic stage after stroke, those still experiencing unilateral neglect were primarily those with right hemisphere lesions.

The impact of unilateral neglect on rehabilitation outcomes can be considerable, especially in patients who are lacking in awareness of their condition. Referring to the case study above, Mrs C. indicated that she had become entirely right-handed since her stroke. In other words, she has become habituated to not using her affected left hand. This is a process known as **learned non-use**, whereby the perceived slowness and awkwardness, associated with using the affected side, conditions the patient to avoid that side and rely on the non-affected side instead. Patients with an intact awareness of this situation can be taught to self-prompt into using their affected side more. However, you can see that in patients lacking such awareness, a situation known as **anosognosia**, this is much more of a challenge.

The term anosognosia requires a little elaboration; stemming from the Greek 'nosos' (illness) and gnosein (to know), a-noso-gnosia refers to a situation where the patient is not aware of their condition. This can lead to some challenging situations, where a patient is clearly severely disabled, but maintains they are 'fine', or where they will not accept that a disabled body part is actually their own (enthusiasts might like to read the case study –The man who fell out of bed (Sacks 1985)). Those recovering from unilateral neglect may report stimulation of their affected side as if their non-affected side were stimulated (this is known as **allesthesia**). In some cases, such denial might signal a defence reaction, but in patients with a brain lesion, there may (additionally) be an organic foundation for such a reaction. This brings us to possible explanations for neglect.

Taking an information processing approach, unilateral neglect may be explained as follows:

- Attentional/orientational neglect: if attentional networks have been affected, the patient may not be able to focus or maintain their attention on their affected side. Especially in cases where the right hemisphere has been affected (see above), patients are more vulnerable to neglect. In fact, most patients with unilateral neglect have difficulty sustaining their attention with any task (Halligan et al. 2003).
- Sensory/perceptual neglect: this would explain unilateral neglect as a result of a deficit in processing sensory information from the affected side. For example, if the primary sensory cortex has been affected, somatosensory information from the affected side of the body may not be registered; as a result a patient may not be aware that their affected leg has slipped off the footplate of their wheelchair and is at risk of injury.
- Representational neglect: this is a form of neglect that indicates deficits in spatial cognition. Bisiach and his colleagues (1978, 1981) designed an elegant experiment, whereby they asked their patients to imagine that they were positioned at a place known to be familiar to them, i.e. the cathedral square in Milan. Patients were instructed to imagine they were facing the cathedral from the other end of the square and then asked to describe the buildings they could 'see'. Patients with left-sided neglect typically identified buildings on their right side, but omitted buildings on their left side. Patients were then asked to take up the position on the opposite side of the square and imagine looking in the direction where they had previously been positioned. Interestingly, patients now reported the buildings on their right that they had previously omitted, but failed to report buildings, now situated on their imaginary left side – which they previously had identified. Thus, patients systematically failed to mention imaginary objects positioned on their affected side. Their memory of these objects per se was clearly intact; however, the problem concerned the *representation* of these objects in relation to their body.
- Motor neglect refers to the difficulty patients may have in initiating action towards or in the affected hemi-space (Riddoch et al. 1995).

In conclusion, unilateral neglect is a complex condition that may involve attention, sensation/perception, spatial cognition and action.

A number of therapeutic strategies have been explored for unilateral neglect, including scanning towards the affected side, in some cases with cueing (e.g. flashing lights or auditory prompts) (Bowen and Lincoln, 2007). Prism spectacles have been used, in an attempt to move the patient's midline (which in unilateral neglect is often shifted away from the affected side) back to normal, although the effects of such an intervention are usually short term. A considerably body of evidence suggests that prompting the affected limb to move in the contralesional hemispace (e.g. left arm moving in left hemispace) may reduce neglect, and that interventions encouraging such activity may transfer to functional activities.

Summary

In summary, attention is necessary for learning – and learning is a prerequisite for memory. One of the key aims of rehabilitation is to enable patients to remember useful information and skills for the longer term. However, disorders of attention and memory are common, especially in populations with conditions affecting the central nervous system. It is important that health-care professionals do not misinterpret patients who have difficulty paying attention, or who are forgetful, as 'lacking in motivation', or 'uninterested'. Together with a multidisciplinary team, it is crucial that any deficits in attention or memory are identified correctly, as such difficulties may form a major obstacle in regaining independence, and that educational strategies are tailored accordingly.

SELF-ASSESSMENT QUESTIONS

Following this chapter, can you:

1. Define attention and memory
2. Describe the potential effects of cortical, as well as subcortical lesions on attention and memory
3. Describe the main clinical manifestations of some common disorders of attention and memory
4. Demonstrate an understanding of the role of attention and memory in learning
5. Explore how you would adapt the general theory of motor learning for patients with impaired attention/memory as a result of a neurological condition
6. Define unilateral neglect, describe and explain the common clinical manifestations of this syndrome
7. Provide different explanations for unilateral neglect
8. Demonstrate an understanding of the possible implications of neglect for neurological rehabilitation
9. Demonstrate an understanding of the role of the multidisciplinary team in the management of patients with neglect

Further reading

Bliss, T.V.P., Collinridge, G.L., 1993. A synaptic model of memory: long-term potentiation in the hippocampus. Nature 361 (6407), 31–39.

Cooke, S.F., Bliss, T.V.P., 2006. Plasticity in the human nervous system. Brain 129, 1659–1673.

Kandel, E.R., 2006. In Search of Memory. The emergence of a new science of mind. W.H. Norton and Co, New York.

Luria, A.R., 1968. The Mind of a Mnemonist: A little book about a vast memory. Basic Books, New York.

Luria, A.R., 1972. The Man with a Shattered World. The history of a brain wound. Harvard University Press, Cambridge, Massachusetts.

References

Bartlett, F.C., 1932. Remembering: a study in experimental and social psychology. Cambridge University Press, Cambridge.

Bisiach, E., Luzatti, C., 1978. Unilateral neglect of representational space. Cortex 14, 129–133.

Bisiach, E., Capitani, E., Luzzatti, C., et al., 1981. Neuropsychologia 19, 543–551.

Bowen, A., Lincoln, N., 2007. Cognitive rehabilitation for spatial neglect following stroke. Cochrane Database Syst. Rev 2, CD003586. doi:10.1002/14651858.

Corkin, S., Amaral, D.G.R., Gonzalez, G., et al., 1997. H. M'.s medial temporal lobe lesion: findings from magnetic resonance imaging. J. Neurosc. 17, 3964–3979.

Geschwind, N., 1982. Disorders of attention: a frontier in neuropsychology. Philos. Trans. R. Soc. Lond. B Biol. Sci. 298, 173–185.

Haines, D.E., 2005. Fundamental Neuroscience for Basic and Clinical Applications. Churchill Livingstone Elsevier, London.

Halligan, P.W., Kischka, U., Marshall, J.C. (Eds.), 2003. Handbook of Clinical Neuropsychology. Oxford University Press, Oxford.

Hebb, D.O., 1949. The Organization of Behavior. John Wiley, New York.

Hécaen, H., Albert, M.L., 1978. Human Neuropsychology. John Wiley & Sons, New York.

James, W., 1890. The Principles of Psychology, vol. 1. Henry Holt, New York.

Kolb, B., Whishaw, I.Q., 1996. Fundamentals of Human Neuropsychology, fourth ed. W.H. Freeman and Co, New York.

Kolb, B., Whishaw, I.Q., 2009. Fundamentals of human neuropsychology (6th ed.). Worth Publishers, New York.

Loftus, E.F., 1997. Creating false memories. Sci. Am. 277, 70–77.

Manly, T., Robertson, I.H., 2003. The rehabilitation of attentional deficits. In: Halligan, P.W., Kischka, U., Marshall, J.C. (Eds.), Handbook of Clinical Neuropsychology. Oxford

University Press, Oxford, pp. 89–107.

Riddoch, M.J., Humphreys, G.W., Luckhurst, L., et al., 1995. 'Paradoxical neglect': spatial representations, hemisphere-specific activation and spatial cueing. Cognitive Neuropsych. 12, 569–604.

Sacks, O., 1985. The Man Who Mistook his Wife for a Hat. Pan Books, London.

Scoville, W.B., Milner, B., 1957. Loss of recent memory after bilateral hippocampal lesions. J. Neurol. Neurosurg. Psychiatry 20, 11–21.

Stone, S.P., Halligan, P.W., Greenwood, R.J., 1993. The incidence of neglect phenomena and related disorders in patients with an acute right or left hemisphere stroke. Age Ageing 22, 46–52.

Stuss, D.T., Benson, D.F., 1986. The Frontal Lobes. Raven Press, New York.

van Zomeren, E., Spikman, J., 2003. Assessment of attention. In: Halligan, P.W., Kischka, U., Marshall, J.C. (Eds.), Handbook of Clinical Neuropsychology. Oxford University Press, Oxford, pp. 73–88.

Disorders of sensation and perception

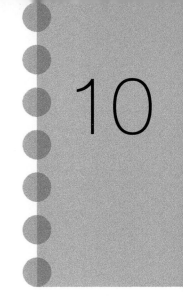

10

CHAPTER CONTENTS

LEARNING OUTCOMES

At the end of this chapter, you should be able to:

- detail the processes involved in sensation, and compare and contrast these with perception
- explain the terms bottom-up, top-down and network processing, and apply these to human perception
- explain how a neurological condition could impact on sensation and perception, and give rise to perceptual disorders
- define the concept of pain, describe the processes involved in pain perception, and explain how a neurological condition, such as stroke, may impact on this
- detail some of the difficulties associated with the assessment of pain in people with neurological conditions.

Introduction

The senses that we possess (sight, hearing, touch, taste, smell and proprioception) are used by us all continuously throughout each day of our life. Their apparently flawless function makes that their essential contribution to our existence is rarely appreciated. Consider the example where, in your university cafeteria, you have made your selection of food and drink and placed this on your tray. Joining the queue at the cash till, you meet one of your lecturers. You engage in a lively debate about the lecture you just had, while balancing your tray on which there is a bowl, filled to the brim, with hot soup. Although the balancing is a seemingly effortless task, the fact that you perform it without conscious awareness does not render this a simple problem. While conducting your conversation your proprioceptors – the sensors in your muscles, tendons and joint capsules that provide information about your posture and movement – as well as various sensors in your skin, continuously detect changes in joint position and orientation, speed, pressure and shear forces in your skin. This afferent information is relayed to the spinal cord, where it feeds into various reflex loops under higher cortical and cerebellar influence (Chapter 6). The resulting motor output is geared towards maintaining a level position of your tray to ensure your soup does not spill over and create a mess, as well as preserve your posture.

People with the – albeit rare – condition of sensory neuropathy would probably not be able to do this; they would be unable to feel the position of themselves – or the tray – in space. With afferent information being corrupted or lacking altogether, the postural reflex mechanisms are unable to produce the required output, and the person would be likely to drop the tray. A fascinating study can be found in Sacks (1985), where he describes the case of a so-called 'disembodied lady'. Bereft of proprioception due to a rare infection, she does not 'feel' her body, and lacks the unconscious control to stabilise her posture. Through the process of rehabilitation, she learns to compensate for the lack of automatic posture control by using vision, and by consciously focusing her attention, e.g. by looking at her tray. But the moment her attention is distracted and she looks elsewhere, her posture collapses. Such profound isolated impairments of proprioception are rare; however, case studies such as this highlight the important role of sensory information in our daily activities and illustrate how senses can compensate for each other to a certain degree.

The aim of this chapter is to compare and contrast 'sensation' with 'perception', detail the various stages involved in information processing, and explain the impact that a neurological condition, e.g. stroke, may have on this. We will focus on pain perception in particular, as an analysis of this phenomenon demonstrates how sensation, perception, as well as cognition interact in creating this unpleasant experience. Studying the process of 'central post-stroke pain' also helps to deepen our understanding of the impact that a lesion of the central nervous system may have on signal processing (Case study 10.1). Finally, interesting work has been carried out in the domain of pain assessment, which highlights some further complications in people with a neurological condition such as stroke.

Sensation

As explained in Chapter 9, attention is a major factor in the processing of information, as it helps us to direct our sensory systems towards relevant information, select appropriate information, allocate energy to process the information and regulate our attention to allow us to complete a task. Sensory information that is not attended to is poorly remembered, and, therefore, attention is a major component in the process of learning.

Case study 10.1

A case of central post-stroke pain

A 68-year-old man suffered a 'lacunar' stroke due to a blocked cerebral artery (i.e. infarction) 6 weeks previously. This has caused a left-sided face, arm and leg weakness. He is not yet walking, but has increasing muscle tone in his arm and leg. Since the stroke he has described his left arm as feeling 'dead', but for the last week has been complaining that it aches before his therapy sessions. After therapy, however, the pain seems to be better. The medical team have prescribed ibuprofen. The therapist considers whether the pain is due to spasticity, especially as there is some glenohumeral mal alignment (i.e. shoulder subluxation). However, careful passive external rotation of the humerus does not make the pain any worse and the elbow easily straightens with a slow stretch. Palpation of the shoulder does not reveal any tenderness. The patient remarks that the pain is worse when they wear a long sleeved shirt and sometimes there is an uncomfortable tingling feeling between the mid upper arm and forearm. In this area the therapist finds reduced sensitivity to temperature; using a cold teaspoon while lightly

touching the skin recreates the paraesthesia. Also, after some careful questioning, it emerges that the increase in pain before therapy may be related to anxiety; when practising transfers (e.g. moving from sit to stand), the patient experiences pain, which is probably caused by the weight placed on the affected arm. The fear associated with anticipating pain causes anxiety, which increases autonomic activation, which in turn aggravates the neuropathic pain prior to treatment sessions – even though other aspects of the intervention reduce the pain.

Based on this information, the medical team decides that this is possibly a case of central post-stroke pain. After discussion with the medical team, amitriptyline is prescribed and a pain record is kept by the nursing staff using a 0–10 rating scale. After 7 days the pain sensations are becoming less intense and less frequent. As the patient's apprehension about transferring during therapy sessions improves, the association between pain and therapy also disappears.

When we talk about sensation, what we are really referring to is the process of information coming in from the environment (internal or external) through the sense organs and being relayed to the central nervous system. The various sense organs (eyes, ears, nose, tongue, skin and proprioceptors) possess dedicated mechanisms that allow them to receive a specific form of energy from the environment (e.g. electromagnetic wavelengths of a specific range) and transduce this into nerve impulses. Transduction is the key component of sensation, as it is only after this has taken place that the nervous system can begin to process information in the form of action potentials. It is important to remember that sensory information, when it is first encountered, is in its rawest form and inherently meaningless. Assigning meaning to information requires the process of perception, which will be outlined in the next section. To be able to appreciate the complexity of sensation, we will take one example by going through the processes involved in vision. Although readers are referred to other texts (e.g. Kindlen 2003) for a description of the anatomy of the various other sense organs, and the sensory processes involved in each of these, what you should aim to remember from the section on vision are the generic principles involved in information processing.

Vision

Sight is the sense through which we are able to perceive electromagnetic radiation in the form of light waves. The light waves pass into the eye through the cornea (see Fig. 10.1), which starts to curve the light waves before they pass through the lens of the eye, where further curvature results in the light being focused onto the surface of the retina.

Retina

The retina can be considered to be the major structure within the eye since it is the location of the key process of transduction. Transduction is the process by which light energy gets converted into electrical energy (in the form of action potentials), thereby allowing the signal to be processed up through the various levels of the brain.

The retina (see Fig. 10.2) is a thin film of tissue lining most of the inside of the eyeball and contains blood vessels, nerve cells, photoreceptors and

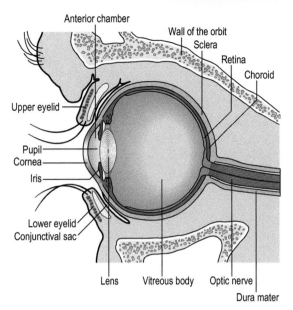

Fig. 10.1 • Structure of the eyeball. From Kindlen 2003, with permission

pigment cells. It is orangey-red in colour when viewed through an ophthalmoscope because of its blood supply and pigments. In one part of the retina a whitish patch (optic disc) can be seen, which consists of the axons of the optic nerve, i.e. the site where these axons leave the eyeball. The disc appears white because the axons here are myelinated.

Photoreceptors

Two types of photoreceptors can be found in the retina – the rods and the cones – both of which are responsible for the conversion of wave energy into electrical energy. There are approximately one hundred million rods per retina and they are responsible for 'shades of grey' vision. The rods exhibit high sensitivity and low acuity, are more numerous in the periphery and are utilised primarily for night vision.

The cones on the other hand, of which there are only three million per retina, are responsible for colour vision and exhibit a low sensitivity and high acuity. The cones are utilised for day vision and can be found concentrated in the fovea.

The photopigments found in the pigment cells of the retina consist of retinal, a vitamin-A derivative, coupled to one of several lipoproteins (opsins). In the human eye there are four different lipoproteins creating four different photopigments: rhodopsin in the rods, and erythrolabe, chlorolabe, and cyanolabe

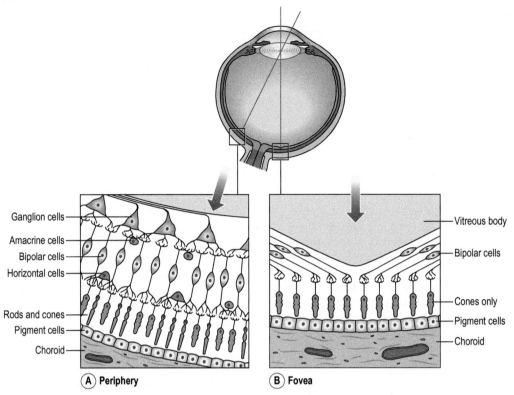

Fig. 10.2 • Structure of the retina. From Kindlen 2003, with permission

in the cones. Only one type of photopigment is present in each cone and each pigment is best at absorbing light rays of a particular range of wavelengths. These ranges overlap and, as a result, the rays of one wavelength are absorbed by more than one photopigment, but to differing extents, e.g. 580 nm rays are absorbed by both erythrolabe and chlorolabe, but not by cyanolabe. The sensation of colour is created by the blend of signals generated by the three different types of cone. If one or more types of cone are absent from the retina, or lack photopigment, then our perception of colour changes (colour blindness), e.g. some colours may not be seen at all, while others are confused. Stacked, flattened membrane discs contain large amounts of the photopigment molecules. Each rod cell contains about 2 000 stacked discs, studded with 100 million molecules of the photopigment **rhodopsin**. Rhodopsin consists of an opsin protein and retinal, a light-absorbing vitamin A derivative existing as isomers.

If we take rhodopsin as an example, we can look in some detail at the biochemical cascade of events that takes place when light strikes the retina and stimulates a photoreceptor (see Fig. 10.3).

The whole process occurs within 0.2 s of the photon reaching the rod cell and similar processes occur within the cones. In the cones, the variation in pigment is produced by different forms of opsin each with their own specific interaction with 11-cis-retinal. As a result of this there are different absorption sensitivities in the cone system:

- B cones at 420 nm (blue)
- G cones at 531 nm (green)
- R cones at 558 nm (red).

Visual pathways

The optic nerves from each eye meet up at the optic chiasma (see Fig. 10.4) where the nerve fibres carrying signals from the nasal half of the retina cross over to the other side so that information about objects on the right-hand side of the scene we are looking at (right visual field) is carried over to the left side of the brain and vice versa. If injury occurs to the visual pathway on one side of the brain after the chiasma, there will be loss of vision in one half of the visual

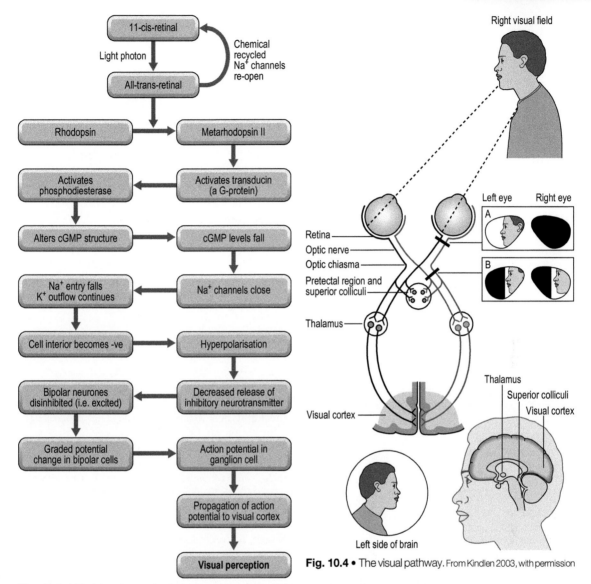

Fig. 10.3 • The visual transduction process. From Kindlen 2003, with permission

Fig. 10.4 • The visual pathway. From Kindlen 2003, with permission

field of both eyes, which is known as a homonymous hemianopia (see Chapter 5).

From the chiasma, impulses are transmitted to the midbrain (to evoke several visual reflexes) and to the thalamus and the visual cortex in the cerebral hemispheres, to give rise to the sensations of light, colour and movement. After the optic chiasma, some fibres branch off the optic tract to go to parts of the pretectal region and to the superior colliculi. These areas are concerned with several visual reflexes including the pupillary light reflex and reflex eye and head movements.

The pupillary light reflex

When light is shone into either, or both, of the two eyes, the pupils normally constrict. As this reflex is coordinated in the midbrain and not further along the visual pathway, it can be evoked in someone who has cortical brain damage. If the visual cortex itself is damaged, someone is unable to see even though the pupillary light reflex is present. The reflex is controlled from the Edinger-Westphal nucleus and a descending signal is sent to the muscles surrounding the pupils of both eyes. In this way both pupils will constrict in response to bright light, even if one of the eyes is closed. This acts in a protective way should we look at a bright light while closing one eye.

Cerebral hemispheres

Axons of the retinal ganglion cells pass to the thalamus in each cerebral hemisphere and from there another set of nerve fibres carry the signals to the visual cortex in the occipital lobe of each hemisphere (Chapter 5). The visual cortex comprises a number of different areas, each of which plays a different role in the processing of impulses from the eyes. Each area receives information from both eyes (binocular vision) creating a three-dimensional (3D) mental picture of what we see.

One area of the visual cortex, referred to as V4, creates the sensation of colour, while another creates an awareness of movement. The primary visual cortex, or striate cortex, is primarily concerned with the shape of objects. Normally these areas are interlinked, and so the features they represent are fused in our minds. If they become disconnected, or if one area is damaged, there can be curious disturbances of perception, such as seeing objects but not properly following their movement. Such deficits in visual perception are known as **visual agnosias**, which were mentioned in Chapter 5. Examples are prosopagnosia (difficulty recognising faces), visual form agnosia (difficulty recognising line drawings of objects), and apperceptive agnosia (an inability to recognise, copy or match shapes). Further details and case studies on visual agnosia can be found in Kolb and Whishaw (2009).

In each of the different areas, adjacent cells receive signals from adjacent areas of the retina, so that each area of the visual cortex is like a map of the retina (retinotopic representation). This map is not to scale, because it relates to the number of receptors in the retina and the way they are innervated. As the fovea is richly innervated with nerve fibres, a disproportionately large area of the visual cortex is devoted to it.

Binocular vision

When we look at an object close to us, the image of it seen by each eye is not exactly the same. The differences are minimised by the way in which our two eyes are caused to swivel inwards, as part of the near response so that the image falls on the fovea in each eye. These differences are not eliminated because each eye views the object from a slightly different perspective, so we actually see both pictures, although we think we are only looking at one. As a result we gain the impression of depth and perceive three dimensions rather than two.

The process of vision, described above, demonstrates key stages in the process of sensation in general, which can be summarised in the following way:

1. A stimulus (i.e. energy) impacts on a sense organ.
2. The sense organ transduces the energy into neural activity.
3. The sensory nerve conducts the signal to the central nervous system (spinal cord, brain).
4. The thalamus processes and relays the signal.
5. The cortex receives the signal.
6. Sensation occurs.
7. Perception (i.e. interpretation of the sensation) occurs.

Perception

As explained above, all of the information coming in through the various sense organs would be meaningless if we were not able to interpret it in a coordinated way. We use our prior and existing knowledge and understanding of the world around us to process the input in a meaningful way. This processing of information can be carried out in one of three ways: bottom-up, top-down and network processing.

The **bottom-up** approach starts with raw data to make sense of the world around us. In this approach the stimulus leads to feature detection, followed by feature combination and, finally, pattern recognition. For example, feature detection could involve seeing a corner, feature combination would be the detection of three corners in close proximity that are facing each other, and pattern recognition would be the recognition of a triangle. Or consider the following analogy: this is your first assessment of a patient with Parkinson's disease on clinical placement. Being an inexperienced clinician, you are likely to begin by systematically noting the individual's features. You observe a shuffling gait with a short stride length, limited range of motion in ankle, knee and hip joints, limited trunk rotation and arm swing, a tremor of the hands, flexion of the hips and spine, and – when you finally look up – a lack of facial expression. Using the bottom-up process of combining all these individual components, you arrive at the overall picture of 'Parkinson's disease'.

In the **top-down** approach, we start from previous knowledge and experience, and make inferences about sensory information to make sense of the world. For example, if we are doing geometry, and observe a figure with two corners and one faded feature (there is a blotch of coffee on the page, right there), we are likely to deduce that the other feature is also a corner and that what we are looking at is a triangle. In this case, we have used previous knowledge to fill in the gaps. The more experience and knowledge we have, the easier it is to recognise a particular pattern. Aspects of our cognition that can influence our perception include knowledge and experience, expectancy, context, as well as motivation. Continuing with our example of assessing a person with Parkinson's disease, once you have seen a few patients with this condition, there is a chance that you will be able to spot this from a distance, without having to actually see each sign and symptom. Having been through the experience time and again, you have developed a **schema**, or template, of this phenomenon. And once this is stored in memory, all you need is a single feature (e.g. the sound of the shuffling gait, or the tremor), to elicit the entire 'Gestalt' of Parkinson's disease. This form of memory is made possible by a process known as a **Hebb's cell ensemble** (Chapter 9). Being a more experienced clinician, you now rely on top-down processing. However, could this have pitfalls? Relying exclusively on top-down processing may cause you to miss important features that could point to a different conclusion. Relying too much on what you have seen in a textbook, without careful observation of actual signs and symptoms, may lead you to make premature conclusions, e.g. the patient may have a form of parkinsonism instead, and require a different form of intervention. So there is a case to be made for combining bottom-up with top-down processing.

Network processing involves the integration of top-down and bottom-up processing at the same time; feature detection is combined with existing memories, knowledge and expectations, in order to interpret and make sense of information. For those whose first language is not Greek, learning the Greek alphabet is likely to start with bottom-up processing, where you learn to detect relevant features for each letter. With more experience, you will recognise these faster, until you are able to understand a whole sentence, even if some of the visual information is degraded, or if there are spelling mistakes. In clinical practice, the analogy is that we assess patients, using bottom-up processes, and combine our observations with our knowledge. This integrated information is used to form an hypothesis about the patient's

condition, on the basis of which a treatment plan is instituted. We then require bottom-up processing again to observe whether the expected changes have actually taken place (note that our expectations can cause us to miss important information!). Should the predicted improvements not have materialised, we need to observe again, and perhaps use further knowledge to adjust our hypothesis, and so on. You will remember from Chapter 5 how extensive neural networks are both within and between hemispheres, and from caudal to cranial, supporting this type of parallel distributed information processing.

An example we will now turn to is the perception of pain. Pain is a complex and fascinating phenomenon, on which there is an extensive and growing body of literature, a comprehensive discussion of which is beyond the scope of this chapter. What we would like to highlight in the following sections is the integration of both bottom-up and top-down processing in the perception of pain. This will form the basis for exploring how a neurological condition such as stroke may give rise to disordered pain perception.

Pain and analgesia

According to the International Association for the Study of Pain, pain is defined as 'an unpleasant sensory and emotional experience associated with actual or potential tissue damage, or described in terms of such damage' (IASP 2008). Pain is primarily a protective mechanism that brings about our conscious awareness that tissue damage may be occurring, or is about to occur. It never occurs on its own, but is normally accompanied by motivated behavioural responses (e.g. withdrawal or defence) and emotional reactions (e.g. crying, fear, cursing!!).

Pain receptors

As with all sensations, the stimulus as it occurs cannot be detected by the central nervous system without being converted into electrical impulses (action potentials). We, therefore, need to have a detection system that can 'sense' the painful stimulus and convert it to neuronal impulses – once again, transduction has to take place. The detection systems for sensing pain are known as the nociceptors and they exist as three separate types:

- **Mechanical nociceptors** which respond to mechanical damage such as cutting, crushing or pinching

- **Thermal nociceptors** which respond to temperature extremes
- **Polymodal nociceptors** which respond equally to all kinds of damaging stimuli.

Although these nociceptors are known as pain receptors, none of the types has a specialised receptor structure (as you would find for the receptor for a particular neurotransmitter, for example). Rather the nociceptors are all naked nerve endings. Unlike transmitter receptors, the nociceptors do not adapt to sustained or repetitive stimulation. This is of great value in terms of our survival, since we would not want the nociceptors to become desensitised to repeated stimulation and respond less well to the same level of stimulation. All nociceptors can be sensitised by the presence of prostaglandins (part of the inflammatory response) and this explains why aspirin, which inhibits prostaglandin synthesis, acts as both an anti-inflammatory and analgesic.

When you think of pain you may feel that there is only one type – it is either sore or not sore. Yes, there may be more severe pain, but it is all the same type. However, there are in fact two types of pain signals – fast pain and slow pain. **Fast pain** occurs upon stimulation of mechanical and thermal nociceptors and the signals are carried by large myelinated A-δ fibres. Fast pain produces a sharp, prickling sensation, is easily localised and occurs first. **Slow pain**, on the other hand, occurs upon stimulation of the polymodal nociceptors and in this case the stimulus is carried by small unmyelinated C fibres. Slow pain produces the dull, aching, burning sensation and is poorly localised. Although it is perceived second, slow pain persists for longer and is more unpleasant. Slow pain is activated by chemicals, including bradykinin, a chemical which is normally inactive, but becomes activated by enzymes released into the extracellular fluid from damaged tissue. These chemicals provoke pain by stimulation of polymodal nociceptors and also contribute to the inflammatory response to tissue injury.

Pain pathways

Ascending pain pathways: bottom-up processing

When we perceive pain, it is not just about the awareness of the pain itself, but also about locating the source and responding emotionally and behaviourally

to it. All of the different responses occur due to the widespread journey that the pain signal impulses take upwards through the nervous system (Fig. 10.5).

The primary afferent fibres synapse with second-order interneurones in the dorsal horn of the spinal cord, where a unique neurotransmitter, substance P, is released. The spinal cord interneurones connect with reflex mechanisms (e.g. the withdrawal reflex), which are aimed at moving away from the noxious stimulus.

The actual destinations of the pain pathways are not fully understood, but they are known to include the thalamus, reticular formation and somatosensory cortex. The specific role of the **cortex** in pain perception is not entirely clear, but it probably plays an important part in localisation, identification of the type and possible causes of the pain. It should be noted that pain can still be perceived in the absence of the cortex, probably by the **thalamus**. The **reticular formation** (introduced in Chapter 9 as a regulator for arousal levels) increases the level of alertness associated with the noxious encounter. Interconnections from the thalamus and reticular formation travel to the **hypothalamus** and the **limbic system**, areas that elicit the appropriate behavioural and emotional responses to accompany the painful experience. This explains why 'pain' is a whole-body experience, involving sensation, perception, emotion, behaviour and autonomic responses. This multimodal experience is encapsulated in a commonly used clinical measure for pain, the McGill Pain Questionnaire (Melzack 1983). This tool represents the sensory, affective and evaluative properties of pain, as well as pain intensity and other pain properties. It is via the complex mechanism described above that the pain accompanying peripheral injury serves – in most cases – as a normal, protective mechanism.

Descending pain pathways: top-down processing

Our central nervous system contains a neuronal system that can suppresses or amplifies (i.e. modifies) pain (Fig. 10.6), but our knowledge of this system is still fragmentary. The system comprises neural mechanisms that are able to modify the transmission in the pain pathways as they enter the spinal cord, and at each relay station within the central nervous system. Melzack and Wall proposed the – then groundbreaking – **Gate Control Theory** of pain perception in 1965, which postulated a mechanism in the spinal cord that acted as a gate, blocking or

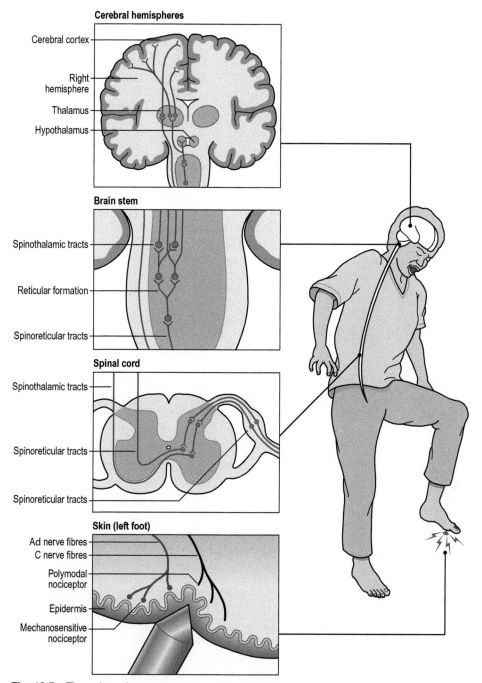

Fig. 10.5 • The pain pathway. From Kindlen 2003, with permission

permitting pain signals to travel through to the brain. The explanation in the original version has now been updated, but the phenomenon of 'gating' is based on a substantial body of research, including studies showing that stimulation of the periaqueductal grey matter (PAG) or reticular formation results in profound analgesia. Part of a descending pathway (shown in Fig. 10.6) blocks, by presynaptic inhibition, the release of substance P from the afferent pain fibre terminals.

135

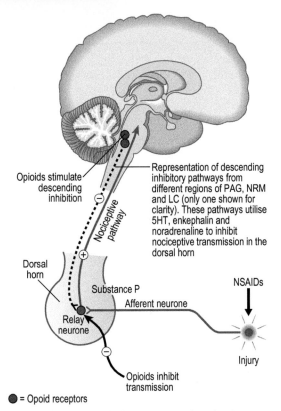

Opioids stimulate descending inhibition

Representation of descending inhibitory pathways from different regions of PAG, NRM and LC (only one shown for clarity). These pathways utilise 5HT, enkephalin and noradrenaline to inhibit nociceptive transmission in the dorsal horn

Nociceptive pathway

Dorsal horn

Substance P

Afferent neurone

NSAIDs

Relay neurone

Injury

Opioids inhibit transmission

● = Opoid receptors

Fig. 10.6 • The intrinsic (or endogenous) analgesic system. From Waller 2005, with permission

This built-in analgesic system is dependent upon the presence of opiate receptors on which our **endogenous opiates** (endorphins, enkephalins, dynorphin) can act. These endogenous opiates serve as analgesic neurotransmitters. They are released from descending pathways and bind with opiate receptors on the afferent pain fibre terminal. When they suppress the substance P release, they block transmission of signals.

Pain and network processing

From the previous sections on the processing of pain signals, it is clear that 'pain' is the result of complex network processing. Cases where people continue to fight in battle, despite serious injuries, highlight how effective the top-down drive to survive can be in suppressing pain signals – at least until the person is out of immediate danger, when the gating ceases to be effective. Another example of pain modulation is body piercing during religious ceremonies, where people apparently tolerate what would normally appear to inflict excruciating pain (e.g. from a trident piercing one's cheeks).

Pain expectations also influence the pain experience, e.g. people who were given threatening information about an experimental pain stimulus are more likely to expect tissue damage, to tolerate less pain, to have difficulty coping with the pain, and catastrophise more than people who were not given this information (Jackson et al 2005). 'Catastrophising' is a term used to indicate emotional and cognitive processes that involve fearing and thinking the worst (e.g. I'm going to get frostbite and lose my hand), and is known to amplify pain reports (Campbell et al 2010).

Interestingly, a systematic review has shown that virtual reality, which can be interpreted as a distractor, can be effective in reducing both experimental and clinical pain associated with burns (Malloy & Milling 2010).

How can this knowledge inform health-care professionals? Clinicians can make effective use of opportunities to exert analgesic effects on their patients, e.g. by reducing anxiety and offering patients reassuring information on the causes of their pain and on what can be done about it, while suggesting distraction from pain where this is judged to be appropriate. Taken together, the previous sections on pain processing demonstrate the complexity of this multimodal experience. Students who are interested in reading more about this topic are referred to Wall & Melzack's *Textbook of Pain*.

Disorders of perception: pain syndromes

The IASP definition of pain, provided earlier, indicates that, although pain may be associated with tissue damage, this phenomenon may also be experienced in the absence of actual damage. There is evidence to indicate that in some cases 'pain' is – or over time has become – dissociated from 'damage'. Chronic pain is the type of pain that continues when the causative stimulus is no longer present, and the features of chronic pain may include *hyperalgesia* (more pain felt for a given amount of noxious stimulation), *allodynia* (pain caused by an innocuous stimulus) and spontaneous *pain spasms* (pain felt in the absence of any stimulation). It is speculated that the experience of pain in the absence of detectable tissue lesion arises from abnormal *signalling* within pain pathways in the absence of typical painful stimuli, e.g. strokes that damage ascending pain pathways may lead to a persistent painful sensation.

Central post-stroke pain (CPSP) occurs in an estimated 2–8% of stroke patients (Andersen et al 1995) and has been defined by the International Association for the Study of Pain (IASP) as: '…pain initiated or caused by a primary lesion or dysfunction in the central nervous system…' (Klit et al 2007, p. 12). CPSP is often described as a burning sensation, paradoxically with an ice-cold quality, while other descriptors include aching, stabbing, shooting or tearing pain. Factors that may exacerbate CPSP include movement or touch. CPSP may occur immediately after stroke, or sometimes even months later. What causes this pain experience is not fully understood. Previously, the term 'thalamic syndrome' was used to indicate CPSP. However, there have been suggestions that lesions to the dorsal horn in the spinal cord, ascending pathways, brainstem, thalamus, subcortical white matter and cerebral cortex can all give rise to CPSP (Nurmikko 2000). A more recent study correlating neuroimaging findings with clinical pain scores also found that there was no difference in clinical pain scores between patients with thalamic and extra-thalamic lesions (Kalita et al 2011), casting further doubt on the appropriateness of the term 'thalamic syndrome'. Clinical box 10.1 elaborates on the challenges associated with the assessment and treatment of pain after stroke.

Pharmacological treatment options for pain

The complexity of the pain pathway can be used to our advantage by giving us a number of different sites to target when trying to achieve analgesia. The major analgesics include:

- the opioid analgesics (morphine, heroin, codeine), which act on the endogenous system of pain control (see Box 10.1)
- the non-steroidal anti-inflammatory drugs (NSAIDs: aspirin, ibuprofen), which reduce the production of inflammatory mediators that sensitise nociceptors to bradykinin + 5-HT
- local anaesthetics (lidocaine), which block AP conduction.

More detail on the mechanism of action of these various agents can be found in any standard pharmacology or neuropharmacology text.

Summary

The aim of this chapter was to explain the information processing stages involved in sensation and perception. We used examples from vision to illustrate the detailed processes involved in sensation.

Clinical box 10.1

Assessing pain after stroke

In clinical practice there are two main challenges in the assessment of pain after stroke:
1. Determining whether treatments are effective in cases where patients have cognitive, communication and/or visuospatial deficits (e.g. after a stroke or head injury)
2. Distinguishing pain which has a mechanical element from non-mechanical or central post-stroke pain.

A common method to assess pain intensity in clinical practice uses the visual analogue scale (VAS). Patients make a mark on a 100 mm line anchored at either end by 'no pain' and 'worst pain imaginable' and the distance along the line represents the pain intensity. However, it has been shown that visuospatial deficits significantly hamper the reliability of the scale as patients are unaware of the whole line, even when turned vertically. An alternative is the 0–10 numerical rating scale, which asks patients to select a number to represent pain intensity. Although this lacks the sensitivity of the VAS and is still difficult for patients with language and numeracy impairments,

it does appear to be more reliable (Price et al 1999). Vascular lesions causing stroke can interrupt the spinothalamic pathway and thereby trigger neuropathic pain (also known as central post-stroke pain). Typically patients will complain of intermittent 'shooting', 'burning' or 'electrical' sensations which are worse with anxiety or sometimes just light stimulation. To recognise central post-stroke pain it is important to listen to the patient's description of their pain and note that movement is often not a particular exacerbating factor compared to other mechanisms such as spasticity. The area affected by pain has often lost sensitivity to pain and temperature. The pain can start at any time after stroke, but often develops some weeks after the acute event, which can lead to delayed recognition. Analgesic agents treating local inflammation will not be effective, whereas those which act on central pain processing (such as amitriptyline) and counter-stimulation measures (such as electrical stimulation) may be helpful.

Box 10.1

Opiate pharmacology

Although our knowledge is still somewhat fragmented, it is known that our body possesses a central, neuronal system that suppresses pain – this is known as the **intrinsic analgesic system.** As the pain signal is passing up through the brain, a descending pathway releases neurotransmitters (noradrenaline (norepinephrine), serotonin and the endogenous opioids) at the spinal cord to block the release of substance P at the afferent pain fibre terminals. This built-in analgesic system is dependent on both the endogenous opioids (endorphins, enkephalins and dynorphin) and the fact that the human body contains opiate receptors. When these endogenous opiates are released from the descending pathway and bind with opiate receptors on afferent pain fibre terminals they suppress substance P release and, subsequently, block/reduce the transmission of the spinothalamic pain up to the brain. It can, therefore, be seen that these endogenous opioids have no effect at the source of the pain, but only on the transmission of the signal from the level of the spinal cord onwards. It is this intrinsic analgesic system that is utilised by the drugs that are known as the opioid analgesics when they bind to the same receptors as the endogenous molecules.

The opioid analgesics include such drugs as morphine, diamorphine (heroin), codeine and pethidine and can be considered as exogenous analgesics. Full details on the use and dosage of these agents can be found in the British National Formulary Section 4.7.2 (BNF 2012). The aforementioned exogenous analgesics produce their effects by acting as agonists at the opiate receptor. There are three classes of opiate receptors: μ (mu), κ (kappa) and δ (delta) and each receptor has subtypes that have distinctive regional distributions.

The precise mechanism of action of the exogenous opioid drugs is not clearly understood, although it is thought that the effect is mediated, at least in part, via an interaction with the same opiate receptors that the endogenous opioids work on. The main receptor sub-type mediating the analgesic effect is thought to be through an agonist action on the μ-receptor; however, the κ receptor has also been implicated in the spinal phase of pain transmission.

The opiate receptors are members of the G-protein coupled receptor (GPCR) family (see Chapter 4) and they produce their effect by decreasing cAMP production. What happens next is dependent upon the location of the receptor. If it is found in the spinal cord there will be a decreased firing of presynaptic neurones brought about by reduced Ca^{2+} influx, whereas if the receptor is located in the CNS, there will a decreased firing of postsynaptic neurones as a consequence of increased Na^+ efflux. Either way, noxious stimuli emanating from the source of the pain are no longer perceived.

The mechanism of action of the various opioid analgesics can be seen in Table 10.1.

Table 10.1 Opioid analgesic drugs (from Kester et al 2007-with permission)

Drug	Mechanism of action	Indication	Side effects/comment
Morphine	Strong opiate; μ-agonist	Analgesic	Poorly bioavailable. Side effects shared by most opioid drugs: respiratory depression, nausea, vomiting, dizziness, confusion, constipation, abuse potential
Meperidine	Strong opiate; μ-agonist	Analgesic	Treatment for postoperative shivering
Methadone	Strong opiate; μ-agonist	Analgesic, heroin recovery	Used in maintenance therapy for recovering opiate addicts because it has a long half life ($t_{1/2}$)
Fentanyl	Strong opiate; μ-agonist	Analgesic	100 times more potent than morphine
Oxycodone	Moderate μ-agonist	Analgesic	Excellent bioavailability; significant abuse liability
Codeine	Moderate μ-agonist	Cough suppressant, analgesic	Frequently combined with aspirin or acetaminophen
Pentazocine	κ-agonist and partial μ-agonist	Analgesic	Lower abuse potential than others
Buprenorphine	Partial μ-agonist and weak κ-agonist	Analgesia and treatment for opiate addiction	Partial agonist with weak analgesic activity; alleviates symptoms of opiate withdrawal

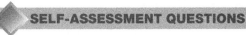

Next, we explored the perception of pain and focused on the effects of a stroke on pain perception, which highlighted the complexity of signal processing. An understanding of signal processing in pain may inform decisions on treatment options, which were outlined briefly.

So what we can see from this chapter is that our senses allow us to perceive what is going on around us. Without perception we would be unable to appreciate the complexity of human life. However, the down side is that with the good (the sight of your partner, the taste of your favourite food, the smell of your favourite flower, etc.) comes the bad (pain, negative emotional responses to particular sights, noise, etc.). That said, it is the presence of such ups and downs that give us depth in our lives. To do without pain, we would have to do without the rest.

SELF-ASSESSMENT QUESTIONS

1. Describe the general process of sensation, and compare and contrast this with perception.
2. Use an example to explain the differences between bottom-up, top-down and network processing, and the errors that might occur during each type of processing.
3. Identify the biochemical processes that occur during visual transduction at the level of the retina.
4. Describe the phenomenon of homonymous hemianopia and explain how this might interfere with the assessment of pain after stroke if a horizontal VAS (visual analogue scale) is used.
5. Explain the different processes involved in the processing of fast and slow pain.
6. Describe the mechanism of action of an opiate analgesic, such as morphine.

Further reading

Bruce, V., Green, P.R., Georgeson, M.A., 2003. Visual Perception: Physiology, psychology and ecology, fourth ed. Psychology Press, New York.

Girard-Powell, V., 2009. Pain, Analgesia and Anesthesia, an issue of perioperative nursing clinics (The Clinics: nursing). Saunders, Philadelphia.

McMahon, S.B., Koltzenburg, M. (Eds.), 2005. Wall & Melzack's Textbook of Pain, fifth ed. Churchill Livingstone, Edinburgh.

Sacks, O., 1984. A Leg to Stand On. Picador, London.

Sacks, O., 2007. Musicophilia. Tales of music and the brain. Picador, London.

Snowdon, R., Thompson, P., Troscianko, T., 2006. Basic Vision: An introduction to visual perception. Oxford University Press, Oxford.

Yassin, G., Dawson, J., 2007. Crash Course: Pharmacology. Mosby, St Louis.

Zeki, S., 1999. Inner Vision. An exploration of art and the brain. Oxford University press, Oxford.

References

Andersen, G., Vestergaard, K., Ingeman-Nielsen, T.S., 1995. Incidence of central post-stroke pain. Pain 61, 187–193.

BNF: British National Formulary. 2012. http://bnf.org/bnf/index.htm.

Campbell, C.M., Witmer, K., Simango, M., et al., 2010. Catastrophizing delays the analgesic effect of distraction. Pain 149 (2), 202–207.

IASP: International Association for the Study of Pain, Proposed taxonomy changes. 2008. http://www.iasp-pain.org/AM/Template.cfm?Section=Home&Template=/CM/ContentDisplay.cfm&ContentID=6633..

Jackson, T., Pope, L., Nagasaka, T., et al., 2005. The impact of threatening information about pain on coping and pain tolerance. Br. J. Health Psychol. 10, 441–451.

Kalita, J., Kumar, B., Misra, U., et al., 2011. Central post stroke pain: clinical, MRI, and SPECT correlation. Pain Med. 12, 282–288.

Kester, M., Vrana, K.E., Quraishi, S.A., Karpa, K.D., 2007. Elsevier's Integrated Pharmacology. Mosby, UK.

Kindlen, S. (Ed.), 2003. Physiology for Health Care and Nursing. Churchill Livingstone, Edinburgh.

Klit, H., Finnerup, N.A., Jensen, T.S., 2007. Clinical characteristics of central post stroke pain. In: Henry, J.L., Panju, A., Yashpal, K. (Eds.), Central Neuropathic Pain: focus on poststroke pain. ASP Press, Seattle, pp. 27–41.

Kolb, B., Whishaw, I.Q., 2009. Fundamentals of Human Neuropsychology, sixth ed. Worth Publishers, New York.

Malloy, K.M., Milling, L.S., 2010. The effectiveness of virtual reality

distraction for pain reduction: a systematic review. Clin. Psychol. Rev. 30 (8), 1011–1018.

Melzack, R., 1983. The McGill Pain Questionnaire. In: Melzack, R. (Ed.), Pain Measurement and Assessment. Raven Press, New York, pp. 41–47.

Melzack, R., Wall, P.D., 1965. Pain mechanisms: a new theory. Science 150, 971–979.

Nurmikko, T.J., 2000. Mechanisms of central pain. Clin. J. Pain 16, S21–S25.

Price, C.I.M., Curless, R.H., Rodgers, H., 1999. Can stroke patients use visual analogue scales? Stroke 30, 1357–1361.

Sacks, O., 1985. The Man Who Mistook his Wife for a Hat. Picador, London.

Waller, D.G., Renwick, A.G., Hillier, K., 2005. Medical Pharmacology and Therapeutics, second ed. WB Saunders, UK.

Communication disorders

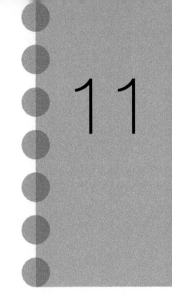

CHAPTER CONTENTS

LEARNING OUTCOMES

At the end of this chapter, you should be able to:

- demonstrate an appreciation of the importance of good communication in clinical practice
- demonstrate an understanding of the importance of having a sound working knowledge of common speech and language problems in neurological rehabilitation
- compare and contrast 'aphasia' with 'dysarthria'
- describe, compare and contrast Broca's, Wernicke's and conduction aphasia
- identify the key brain areas involved in each of these three types of aphasias
- demonstrate an understanding of the integration between various cortical areas in speech and language. Explain why categorising aphasia as 'expressive' or 'receptive' is too simplistic. Explain the strengths and limitations of categorising aphasia as 'Broca's' or 'Wernicke's'
- demonstrate a basic awareness of how communication may be facilitated in people with speech and language impairment.

Introduction

The spoken language used between one human and another is, without a doubt, one of the most important and complex interactive tools that we use. That said, we must remember that non-verbal communication is also widely used by us through gesture, body posture and facial expression. Patients with speech problems gave early researchers the first clues about the involvement of the brain in language. It was the Ancient Greeks who noticed that brain damage could cause language function to be impaired (aphasia). They noticed that if the brain was damaged by a physical trauma (e.g. a head injury in battle) then the speech function of the individual concerned could be affected.

Communication difficulties are common in people with neurological conditions and are often encountered in those with a head injury, stroke and progressive neurological conditions such as Parkinson's disease and dementia, to name but a few. In patient-centred health care, good communication between patient and health professional is essential, e.g. to establish initial rapport with a patient and their family, obtain information about a patient's health status, accurately assess a patient's abilities and difficulties, negotiate treatment goals, clarify information about interventions or monitor pain. For these reasons, it is essential that health professionals have a sound understanding of the speech and language disorders they are most likely to come across.

The aim of this chapter is to explain the concept of language disorders (known as **aphasia**) and speech disorders (such as **dysarthria** and **apraxia of speech**), explore their underlying neural mechanisms and discuss the impact that speech and language disorders may have on a person's ability to communicate. There are many different types and subtleties in speech and language disorders, which is unsurprising given the complexity and scope of human communication. This chapter is designed to give you an introduction to this topic to enable you to develop your understanding of some of the most common issues in communication disorders, and assist you in problem solving when working with people with speech and language impairments.

An overview of speech and language processes

What is language? It is a complex form of communication involving written or spoken words used to symbolise objects and convey ideas. Reading, writing, drawing, gesturing, making eye contact and facial expression, speaking and listening, adjusting one's tone of voice, are all part of our 'toolkit' for communication. It involves 'expression' and 'comprehension', with each aspect being related to a specific neural network – as we shall see later on in this chapter.

Before we examine impairments in speech and language, it may be useful to consider what is involved in normal communication. Think for a moment about a situation where you wish to express yourself, e.g. you have a question about what you have just read. Firstly, you need to formulate an idea

in your mind, using knowledge and understanding you have stored already. People with cognitive impairments may have difficulty at this stage. Next, you need to formulate your question, and find the right words with the right meanings and place these in the appropriate logical order using the correct grammatical coding (e.g. correct tense). Aphasia is the collection of impairments at this level of communication. You must then select the correct motor program in order to articulate your actual question and use your articulatory muscles (for example your tongue and lips) to speak. Problems at these final levels are known as apraxia of speech and dysarthria respectively. Figure 11.1 gives an overview of the various functions required for communicating an idea, and examples of common disorders where these functions may be found to be impaired.

In this chapter we are going to go into more detail about aphasia, apraxia of speech and dysarthria. You may hear aphasia being referred to as dysphasia. While **aphasia** literally means total loss of language, **dysphasia** means partial loss of language. However, nowadays the two terms are used interchangeably to indicate a damaged language system. It is important to understand that aphasia is a *language* problem; a higher order communication impairment. Our society tends to consider the ability to communicate through speech and writing to be signs of intelligence. However, while language difficulties that arise as a result of aphasia may hinder a

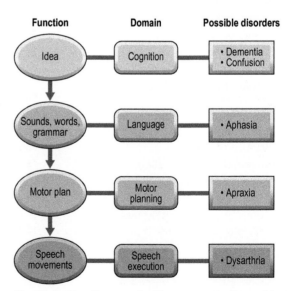

Fig. 11.1 • Functions required for communicating an idea, and examples of common disorders where these functions may be found to be impaired (Yorkston et al. 1999, with permission from Pro-ed, Austin, Texas, USA).

person's understanding or expressing themselves in the spoken and/or written medium, it does not affect their ability to think, feel, remember and plan, and, therefore, intelligence is not considered to be affected by aphasia.

Dysarthria or apraxia of speech are *motor speech* problems. Speech in people with dysarthria often sounds slow and laboured, with consonants often having a 'slurred' quality and vowels may sound distorted. Intonation and voice quality may also sound 'abnormal'. In contrast to those with higher order communication impairments, however, people with dysarthria have no problems with comprehension and no problems thinking of what they want to say, selecting the correct words, sequencing them in the correct order or selecting the right motor programme (which is a problem for people with apraxia of speech). The problem here is the tone and coordination of the muscles involved in speaking, for example, tongue, lips, soft palate, vocal folds and respiration system. Because of the slurred aspect of this motor speech disorder, many people with dysarthria find that some members of the public treat them as if they have a learning disability or assume that they have been drinking alcohol. Although aphasia often coexists with motor speech problems, it is important for health-care professionals to be aware of this distinction to avoid misinterpretation and poor communication.

Aphasia: brain–behaviour relationship

Perhaps one of the single most important discoveries in speech and language research was made by the French neurologist, Marc Dax. In 1836, at a conference in Montpellier, Dax described a group of patients who had difficulties speaking and he further reported that all of the patients had left-sided brain damage. Although Dax's paper on left hemispheric dominance for spoken communication was written and published in 1936, a year before his death, the left-sided localisation of speech and language is often attributed to Paul Broca, who we shall discuss shortly.

Although the language centres are located in the left hemisphere in approximately 95% of the population, it was thought that if damage to the brain occurs within the first 3 years of life, language acquisition follows normal development after an initial delay, with some of the function being transferred to the

right hemisphere. This transfer, however, may be at the expense of other non-verbal skills. Up to the age of 10 years, language ability is often re-established following brain damage, with permanent impairment often observed if damage occurs beyond the early teens. There is an unconfirmed hypothesis that cerebral plasticity ceases by the age of 10 as a result of the establishment of cerebral dominance of language function. However, research indicates that even for some children under 10 years of age who have had brain damage and in whom language appears to have fully recovered, subtle but persistent deficits (e.g. literacy problems), still persist. Findings such as these suggest that the brain regions involved in language comprehension and expression are permanently assigned before adolescence. So the majority of patients who experience brain damage to the left hemisphere may experience language disorders, in fact it is thought that one-third of patients who have a stroke experience aphasia. We will discuss the intricacies of aphasia a little later, but first let's go back to Broca's work.

Broca's area

As mentioned earlier, the French neuroanatomist/ anthropologist Paul Broca is often credited with the localisation of language function, specifically the motor aspects of speech production, in the left hemisphere of the brain. This is despite the fact that Marc Dax had published a paper on left hemispheric dominance for language some 25 years before Broca. There is actually little doubt that Broca was aware of the work of Dax, but he steadfastly refused to acknowledge the original theoretical contribution – 'I do not like dealing with the questions of priority concerning myself. That is the reason why I did not mention the name of Dax in my paper'. Not only did he fail to acknowledge Dax, he actually claimed to be the first to discuss the theory of left hemispheric dominance! An interesting article was written by the authors Cubelli and Montagna (1994) who state that 'the weight of evidence reported . . . . suggests that the theory of the left hemisphere dominance for speech must be attributed equally to Dax and Broca, and henceforth should be called the theory of Dax-Broca'. Let us leave this debate behind and examine the work of Broca a little more closely.

Broca (1861) examined a man, who was able to understand what was said to him but was unable to pronounce any words other than 'tan' over and over

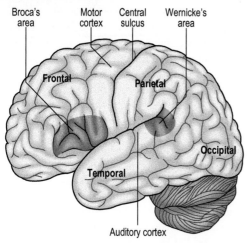

Broca's area | Motor cortex | Central sulcus | Wernicke's area

Frontal | Parietal | Occipital | Temporal | Auditory cortex

Fig. 11.2 • Localisation of Broca's and Wernicke's areas

again. Although he was referred to as 'Tan', the unfortunate individual was a M. Leborgne who died a mere 6 days after examination. His death gave Broca the chance to examine the brain which revealed that the area damaged was a small region towards the front left hand side of brain – a region that became known as Broca's area (Fig. 11.2).

Broca's area is often referred to as the motor-speech area and it is located adjacent to the precentral gyrus of the motor cortex in the frontal lobes (see Fig. 11.2). This area controls the movements required for articulation, facial expression and phonation. Broca's patients generally had good overall comprehension but their speech was often limited in their vocabulary and grammar which contained inaccurate pronunciation of words or parts of words which often made their speech unintelligible. More about the clinical presentation of people with Broca's aphasia can be found below.

Wernicke's area

Karl Wernicke, a Prussian physician, discovered a different kind of speech and language problem a few years later, which uncovered damage to a completely different region of the brain – unsurprisingly thereafter called Wernicke's area. Wernicke's patients generally possessed good articulation, but their speech often didn't make sense, with words jumbled together in an incoherent sequence. They frequently used 'made-up' words with no meaning (**neologisms**).

Wernicke's area, which includes the auditory comprehension centre, lies in the posterior superior temporal lobe near the primary auditory cortex at the junction of the parietal, temporal and occipital lobes (see Fig 11.2). Wernicke's area plays a critical role in understanding both spoken and written messages (See Clinical application box 11.1), as well as being responsible for formulating coherent speech patterns. These 'commands' formulated in Wernicke's area are transferred via a fibre tract, the **arcuate fasciculus**, to Broca's area. Wernicke's receives input from both the visual cortex in occipital lobe (an important pathway in reading, comprehension and describing objects seen) and the auditory cortex (essential for understanding spoken words).

Wernicke suggested that this joining of Broca's and Wernicke's areas by the arcuate fasciculus results in the formation of a complex network, rather than language simply being produced by two independent language centres. He further proposed that damage to this connection would lead to **conduction aphasia**, which will be discussed later on. Damage to specific brain regions can lead to selective language disturbances and these clinical presentations will be discussed in more detail in the following sections.

Clinical application box 11.1

To give us some idea of the complexity of these pathways let us consider a couple of everyday processes:

1. Speaking the written word

    The information must first get to the primary visual cortex where it is then passed to the posterior speech area, including Wernicke's area. From there it will travel to Broca's area via the arcuate fasciculus and on to the primary motor cortex (for initiation of the appropriate motor speech commands).

2. Speaking the heard word

    The information must first get to the primary auditory cortex where it is then passed to the posterior speech area, including Wernicke's area. From there it will travel to Broca's area via the arcuate fasciculus and on to the primary motor cortex (for initiation of the appropriate motor speech commands).

    It is important at this stage to differentiate between repetition (where you would not have to understand the words) and speaking aloud (where you would understand the words). There will be patients who can repeat what is said to them and mislead the therapist into thinking that they understand them.

Aphasia: clinical presentation

As mentioned earlier, communication is a very complex human skill. Damage to the language component of communication, i.e. aphasia, can therefore affect some or all modalities of language processing: expression and comprehension of speech, reading and writing, gesture and the use of language (i.e. pragmatics). The severity can also vary between individuals, so someone may have occasional problems thinking of a word (which means that there will be some pauses or some errors when they are speaking to you), whereas other people may be more severely affected and unable to put their ideas and intentions into spoken and/or written language, having no intelligible communication. As aphasia also affects the understanding of language it can affect the ability of a person to understand even simple sentences or single words. Aphasia can also affect the ability to understand and use various methods of communication other than speech, for example, gesture. And the severity of aphasia can also fluctuate from one day to the next where an individual may have many word-finding problems one day and on another they may speak much more fluently.

So with such an array of complexities how is it possible to describe your patient's type of aphasia? This is not a new problem. As more information was discovered over the years about the various complexities of language, researchers devised a large number of ways of describing and classifying the different types of aphasia. However, as we mentioned above it is important to remember that the aphasic population is heterogeneous in nature and any number and variations of the characteristics of aphasia can affect individuals. Therefore, it is important for health professionals to understand that aphasia is variable and different for each individual. In saying that, it is very useful to be able to discuss a patient with colleagues, e.g. during a multidisciplinary team (MDT) meeting, in terms of the general type of aphasia a patient presents with, using terminology that is understood. Some of the ways that people with aphasia are classified include: expressive versus receptive aphasia; fluent versus non-fluent aphasia and the Boston Classification approach (who have a localisationalist viewpoint) including Broca's, Wernicke's and conduction aphasia. It is likely that this is the terminology that you will come across in a patient's medical notes and, therefore, they will be described below.

You must remember though that these are only some of the ways to describe aphasia and there are often various issues in determining the exact boundaries between one type of aphasia and another.

Expressive versus receptive aphasia

The division of patients into 'expressive' or 'receptive' aphasia is a very broad classification which was proposed by Weisenberg and McBride (1935).

Patients with **expressive aphasia** (also called motor aphasia) have difficulty translating their ideas into meaningful sounds resulting in non-fluent speech with pauses between words and or phrases. Expressive aphasia is associated with damage involving the anterior language centre of the dominant hemisphere, i.e. Broca's area (see Fig. 11.2). It must be noted that people with expressive aphasia may also present with mild comprehension difficulties.

Receptive aphasia (also called sensory aphasia) is associated with damage to the posterior language area of the dominant hemisphere, i.e. Wernicke's area (see Fig. 11.2). Patients with receptive aphasia present with difficulty in the comprehension of language. While their speech is normally fluent it is full of errors. For example, it may contain **jargon** (made-up words) or substitutions of words (**paraphasias**) amongst others.

Fluent versus non-fluent aphasia

The division of aphasia into fluent and non-fluent aphasia was based on a number of characteristics of their spontaneous speech, i.e. verbal expression.

Patients with **fluent aphasia** are generally considered able to select the correct sounds and put them in the correct order. However, depending upon the exact site of brain damage, some people present with word or sound substitutions and typically have difficulty finding the words that they want to say. The rate of their speech sounds and intonation patterns (i.e. melody and rhythm) are normal or near normal and they tend to use a variety of different grammatical structures, including function words (e.g. pronouns such as 'he-him', 'she-her'; articles such as 'the' and 'a' etc.) and grammatical inflections (e.g. plurals such as dog-dogs; verb tense such as sing-sang-sung, mouse-mice, etc.). However, fluent speech is not the same as meaningful speech. Patients with fluent aphasia vary in the number and type of paraphasias in their speech, their ability to repeat what they hear and the presence of auditory receptive impairments, depending upon the exact site of the damage.

In contrast, the speech of people with **non-fluent aphasia** is generally slow and often laboured and they find it difficult to select the correct sounds and put them in the correct order. Their speech sounds 'choppy' and 'awkward' and there is often less than three or four words in a breath. Their range of intonation may be reduced or even absent. Unlike people with fluent aphasia the variety of grammatical structures in non-fluent speech is often restricted and they may often leave out function words or grammatical inflections mainly relying on nouns to communicate their message. These patients appear to be better at comprehension rather than expressions of speech and language. See case study box 11.1.

Describing a patient's aphasia using the terms expressive/receptive aphasia or fluent/non-fluent has some usefulness; however, none of these terms adequately explains the various aspects of specific difficulties a person has, for example, how much can they actually understand? Can they understand single words or simple grammatical sentences only? How do they manage conversing with someone they know or is there more difficulty speaking to a stranger, or on the telephone? While some people present with 'pure' aphasia (e.g. pure motor or pure sensory

aphasia) this is not common and most of the patients you will see will have symptoms of both of these types. In addition, not all people with aphasia can be classified as fluent or non-fluent and, with the exception of children who acquire aphasia (who tend to be non-fluent and do not present as fluent), some patients' aphasia starts out as non-fluent for a period of time and then becomes fluent. It is evident that aphasia needs to be described in more detail than these broad descriptors.

Boston Aphasia Classification

One major classification system that has gained some degree of clinical acceptance in recent years is the Boston Aphasia Classification system, which was developed in the Veterans Administration Hospital in Boston. This group focused on classifying and describing aphasia in terms of the location of their brain damage and their language problems. So they looked at the speech and language abilities of people who had roughly the same types of speech and language difficulties and classified them into one of eight clinically recognisable aphasia 'syndromes' (see Table 11.1). So each patient is allocated to one of these syndromes according to the speech and language difficulties they experience.

Case study box 11.1

Can you identify which patient has fluent aphasia from their narration of the Cinderella story?

Patient A

Cinderella em....Princess em.....Princess em......fall down... right... sleep... right... em....by..em..... birds.....trees......sun...em...fine..em...sleep.... man........... girl....... Princess......laugh....... haaaaaaaa.....fall down......apple.....pear.... apple..... fall down..... sleep.. ha ha ha ha....finished em....man....Prince eh....kiss kiss....sleep....ooh oh Prince.

Patient B

Cinderella was a step mother had two daughters and Cinderella was the orphan and buttons helped her. She was in the kitchen and...... eh.... the wood eh the garden up the sticks and he she eh come came across a don't know was a prince but he was inconik...incognito.

Table 11.1 Classification of aphasia

Aphasia syndrome	Expressive/ receptive	Fluent/ non-fluent
Broca's aphasia	Expressive	Non-Fluent
Wernicke's aphasia	Receptive	Fluent
Conduction aphasia	Receptive	Fluent
Global aphasia	Expressive and receptive	Non-fluent
Transcortical motor aphasia	Expressive	Non-fluent
Transcortical sensory aphasia	Receptive	Fluent
Mixed transcortical aphasia	Expressive and receptive	Non-fluent
Anomic aphasia	Expressive	Fluent

Before we discuss a selection of these aphasia syndromes a few things must be noted:

- Only 30% of patients fit neatly into these syndromes.
- There are a wide variety of opinions regarding the precise anatomical locations of these syndromes and some studies have shown exceptions to the rule where patients present with the same type of aphasia but have a different lesion site.
- The symptoms in each cluster don't always occur together.
- Patients don't have to present with all of the symptoms in a syndrome to be allocated to that syndrome.

On the other hand, this classification system is still widely used and you are likely to find reference to these syndromes in your patients' medical notes, discussed in MDT meetings and in referral letters from doctors.

The remainder of this chapter is going to explore four of the eight aphasia syndromes – Broca's, Wernicke's, conduction and global aphasia. If you wish to go into more detail about the remaining syndromes, see the reference list at the end of this chapter for suggested reading.

Broca's aphasia

As mentioned in the previous section on Broca's area, in Broca's aphasia the patient's comprehension is usually relatively preserved. In contrast, language production is often seriously impaired as a result of damage to the motor association cortex of the frontal lobe. In severe cases, the premotor and prefrontal areas may also be damaged resulting in a range of deficits of language production, i.e. from complete muteness to a slowed, deliberate speech using very simple word forms. Speech of a patient with Broca's aphasia is slow and effortful with pauses occurring between words and phrases. They may have '**perseveration**' where they use the same words repeatedly in the same conversation (even if the word is not the correct word). Such patients may express nouns in the singular, verbs in the infinitive or participle, and eliminate articles, adjectives and adverbs, e.g. 'I saw some large black cats' – > 'see black cat'. This can result in what is known as **telegraphic speech**. Patients may try and compensate for their word-finding problems by **circumlocution,** i.e. talking around the word they are trying to express. For example, if they were trying to say the word 'knife', they

might say something like 'bread and butter, cut, sharp'. Such patients are generally aware of errors.

Further deficits can result in difficulty reading aloud while reading comprehension is usually similar to auditory comprehension. Writing problems are usually similar to speech impairments and typically contains spelling errors, omission of letters and individual letters tend to be oversized and poorly formed. This is exacerbated by the fact that people with Broca's aphasia often present with concomitant right hemiparesis following their stroke and have to use their non-dominant left hand to write. As Broca's area is located near the motor cortex and the internal capsule, the aphasia is often accompanied by right-sided paresis and a loss of vision, though visual field deficits occur less frequently in Broca's aphasia than other aphasia syndromes.

Although the key problem in Broca's aphasia is verbal expression, it is important to appreciate that comprehension of language (spoken and written) may also be impaired to some extent. Listen carefully to your patients for indications that they have difficulty for example, following the news (e.g. this may be too fast), or a conversation in a group of friends in a noisy pub (e.g. background noise coupled with parallel conversations). Complex messages may also not be entirely understood and subtleties in communication, or jokes, may be missed. Health-care professionals should, therefore, ensure that their communication is clear and unambiguous – and check it is understood!

It is also important for health professionals to try and understand the impact of aphasia on the patient and their family. Imagine being in a situation where you have experienced a devastating brain injury, and on top of that you are struggling to express yourself. You try, but you are only too aware of your limitations and mistakes, while people around you fail to understand you. It is perhaps not surprising that anxiety and depression, as well as sudden emotional outbursts (so-called 'catastrophic reactions') are common in people with Broca's aphasia (See chapter 13).

Wernicke's aphasia

Wernicke's aphasia often represents a major deficit in comprehension, and damage may comprise superior parts of the temporal lobe if the lesion is extensive. This can lead to a severe impairment of the comprehension of both auditory and written language input. The patient may present with fluent speech (although this can have a tendency to be verbose – **logorrhoea**), with sentences of normal length, normal rate and melody, but can often experience difficulty finding the right word. As a result they tend to use the wrong words/combination of words (**verbal paraphasia**) or parts of words (**literal paraphasia**) and have a tendency to add syllables to words and additional words to phrases. They may also make up new words (**neologisms**) which result in the patient failing to convey the ideas that they have in their mind, i.e. 'empty speech' (e.g. if asked 'Where do you live?' patient states 'I came there before here and returned there'). Importantly, such patients are unable to monitor their own speech as the impairment of comprehension also affects understanding of their own speech. They are unaware of the fact that, although they speak in full sentences, the sentences don't make any sense to the listener. As a result patients may get very frustrated if the person they are communicating with fails to understand them; as in their own mind they are making perfect sense and think that the problem lies with the person who is listening. This makes it very difficult to carry out speech and language therapy with such patients as they often don't feel that they need therapy as they do not consider themselves as having a communication problem.

Visual field deficits (Chapter 5) are also present in some patients with Wernicke's aphasia (quadrantanopsia, i.e. ¼ of the visual field) which needs to be taken into account and while this may impact to some degree on the patient's ability to read, it is important to note that reading aloud and reading comprehension are both severely impaired in patients with Wernicke's aphasia (though reading comprehension may be better than reading aloud). While handwriting is usually legible in terms of motor ability with well-formed letters (Wernicke's patients rarely have concomitant hemiplegia), as with their spoken language the content is also devoid of meaning, in some cases mirroring their paraphasic spoken language.

Conduction aphasia

As was mentioned earlier in this chapter, the idea of conduction aphasia was put forward by Wernicke when he proposed the pathway between Broca's and Wernicke's areas. Clinical studies have verified that lesions sparing both areas could nevertheless disconnect the two by lesions located at the **arcuate fasciculus**, thus leading to conduction aphasia.

The spontaneous speech in patients with conduction aphasia is relatively fluent and generally grammatically correct, although less fluent in language production than patients with Wernicke's aphasia. Patients with conduction aphasia usually have relatively good comprehension of what they hear and read but have a disproportionate impairment in *repeating* what they hear relative to their spontaneous speech and comprehension. Patients with conduction aphasia have problems choosing and sequencing their speech sounds, therefore, their speech is filled with many paraphasic errors (mainly literal paraphasias with the incorrect word sounds within words) while the intonation and rhythm of speech is often also affected. This affects both their spontaneous speech and reading aloud. In addition, there may be frequent pauses between words as they try to find the correct word. Unlike Wernicke's aphasia, patients with conduction aphasia will be aware of their errors and will repeatedly try to correct them (*conduite d'approche*), sometimes successfully, sometimes not. Written spontaneous language is similarly impaired to spoken spontaneous language. While the motor aspects of handwriting are normally preserved, spelling is impaired with letters reversed, omitted or substituted. Words in sentences are frequently interchanged or omitted.

Global aphasia

Global aphasia occurs following widespread brain damage, including extensive left hemisphere lesions involving both Broca's and Wernicke's areas. This results in both expressive and receptive language functions being seriously impaired. A range of concomitant neurological signs usually accompany global aphasia such as hemianopia, hemiplegia, sensory loss, attention, memory and other cognitive impairment. Where global aphasia is severe, the patient is unable to communicate at all and their verbal output is limited to repetitive utterances which lack meaning. At times these repetitive utterances will sound quite fluent with intonation and associated emotional expression which conveys some meaning. People with global aphasia have severely impaired comprehension and expression of speech and writing; however, it is generally considered that comprehension is better preserved that expression. As a health-care professional you need to be sure that such patients really do understand your interaction with them, for example, they may have become more skilled at interpreting non-verbal communication such as gesture, facial expression or your intonation, but not actually understand the words you are saying.

Other types of aphasia

In the section above, we have selected and described four different types of language disorders. There are many more aphasic syndromes (see Table 11.1 for examples), and further details can be found in other texts (see reference list at the end of this chapter for suggestions). As previously mentioned, aphasia is not to be confused with motor speech impairments (dysarthria or apraxia of speech) which are caused by a defect in the mechanical aspect of speech, e.g. weakness or incoordination of the muscles controlling the speech apparatus. Aphasias are disorders of *language* which interfere with other cognitive functions and occur frequently as a consequence of a stroke.

It is important at this point to caution against a simplistic approach to this complex topic. As already mentioned, these are only a selection of approaches that are used to describe the various complex presentations of aphasia that your patient may present with. Also remember that these approaches are not an exact science and, therefore, it is important to liaise with the speech and language therapist on your team who will provide an in-depth assessment to help identify the exact nature of your patients' difficulties.

Given the complexity of communication, it is essential to remind ourselves of the principles of **parallel distributed processing** (Chapter 5). Communication requires multiple skills, i.e. attention and memory, semantic (word meaning) and phonological (word sounds) knowledge, and pragmatic skills (the use of language), together with using appropriate body language (such as gesture and facial expression) and listening skills, often used simultaneously. It is, therefore, not surprising that there is no simple one–one relationship between the brain and communication. Even anatomical areas which were thought to be precisely located and associated with specific aphasias (e.g. Broca's) no longer stand up to the scrutiny of more advanced anatomical investigation. It is, therefore, important that, independent of the diagnosis of a patient, health-care professionals carefully look out and listen for any signs and symptoms indicative of difficulties with speech and language, in order to tailor their communication appropriately.

The role of the right hemisphere in communication

So far, we have highlighted the dominance of the left hemisphere in communication, which indicates **cerebral** asymmetry. Does the right hemisphere have any role to play in speech and language? A British neurologist, John Hughlings Jackson, was the first to propose that the right hemisphere does indeed have a role in language processing. While it has been a topic of controversy ever since, evidence of the important role of the right hemisphere in normal linguistic functioning has been accumulating in recent years. In particular it is thought that the right hemisphere helps in the processing of *non-literal language*, for example, in our understanding of jokes, stories and figurative language (such as irony or indirect requests) (Meyers, 1999). It also is essential in how we integrate complex linguistic information with the context in which it is spoken. Patients with right hemisphere damage may initially seem to be able to communicate competently with surface conversation; however, their problems become more evident when the communication interaction is more in-depth or complex.

So while such patients may have good comprehension of the individual words within a conversation and the grammar used, they may have problems in the pragmatics or use of language. For instance, they have problems extracting critical pieces of information in the conversation, often honing in on an insignificant piece of information while totally missing the main message from the conversation. In addition, they have a very literal interpretation of what they hear and do not seem able to fully appreciate abstract meanings such as jokes, idioms, proverbs and metaphors which they interpret literally. For example, if you asked them 'can you open the window?' they would reply 'yes' rather than performing the action. Also they can misread your tone of voice (intonation) and while they understand the actual words you are saying they may misunderstand the message you are trying to convey, e.g. the phrase 'you don't know?' can be spoken in a number of ways (e.g. teasing, accusatory). The meaning of an ambiguous phrase like this depends not on what you say but how you say it! In summary, if the right hemisphere has been affected, subtleties in the understanding of intonation, i.e. the musical aspect of language, may be missed and the patient may entirely misunderstand the meaning of the communication (despite comprehending the words).

When speaking to a person with right hemisphere damage they may initially sound like a competent communicator; however, you will notice that they will have a reduced range of intonation and tend to talk excessively and often go off the point.

However, it is important to note that not all patients with right hemisphere damage present with communication impairment. In those that do, communication impairment depends on the severity of the brain lesion, level of fatigue and type of communication taking place.

Motor speech disorders

Aphasia is one of the most complex communication disorders that people can experience following brain injury, which impacts on approximately one-third of patients who experience a stroke. However, there are other communication problems such as motor speech disorders that can co-occur with aphasia or occur in isolation, i.e. dysarthria and apraxia (of speech). We will describe them briefly but if you wish to look into them in more detail, further reading suggestions are given at the end of this chapter.

Dysarthria

In order for our speech to be executed precisely it requires the intricate coordination of five subsystems:

- Respiration (breath control)
- Phonation (vocal fold vibrations)
- Articulation (precise movement of tongue, lips, etc.)
- Resonance (vibrations in oral and nasal cavity that affect voice quality)
- Prosody (rhythm, rate and melody).

A weakness in any of the systems or any incoordination between these systems can cause dysarthria. Some of the causes of dysarthria include the following: stroke, traumatic brain injury, tumours and some progressive diseases such as Parkinson's and Huntington's disease, motor neurone disease and multiple sclerosis. There are a number of different types of dysarthria which can be classified according to defined neuropathological conditions (see Table 11.2).

The symptoms combine in varying degrees of prominence in the different types of dysarthria. However, some of the most common symptoms include: limited tongue, lip and jaw movement

Table 11.2 Aetiology of dysarthria

Dysarthria	Lesion site	Some aetiologies*
Flaccid	Lower motor neurones	Brain tumour Brainstem stroke
Spastic	Upper motor neurones	Stroke (most common) Traumatic brain injury Amyotrophic lateral sclerosis (ALS) Multiple sclerosis (MS)
Hypokinetic	Basal ganglia and associated brainstem nuclei	Parkinsonism Basal ganglia stroke Toxic metal poisoning
Hyperkinetic	Basal ganglia and associated brainstem nuclei	Huntington's disease Dystonia
Ataxic	Cerebellum and/or its connections	Toxic conditions Cerebellar stroke Traumatic brain injury
Mixed	Depending on the site of damage, e.g. flaccid-spastic – lower and upper motor neurone damage	ALS

* It is important to note that the aetiology examples above are not exhaustive and some of the dysarthrias can be caused by the same aetiology depending on the site of damage or the stage of a progressive disease for example, both spastic and ataxic dysarthria can be caused by traumatic brain injury.

resulting in 'slurred' speech and imprecise articulation, slow rate of speech; or depending on the type of dysarthria, rapid rate of speech with a mumbling quality; abnormal intonation; changes in vocal quality such as hoarseness/strained voice quality or breathiness/whispering voice. It is worth noting that many patients with dysarthria also have difficulties managing their saliva (often drooling) and some also have chewing and swallowing difficulties.

Apraxia of speech

While aphasia is caused by impairment at the level of language and dysarthria at the level of the execution of speech, a process occurs between the two levels which is the *programming* of the articulators to communicate the language (see Table 11.1 as a reminder). An impairment in the programming of movement is called **apraxia**, i.e. the inability to make purposeful movements despite having normal muscle tone and strength, reflexes, coordination and sensation in the absence of cognitive impairment (see also Chapter 7). So people with apraxia are unable to carry out a task when they are asked to but can often do it automatically, e.g. if someone is asked to open their mouth wide, they are unable to do it on demand, but they can do this movement when they are yawning. There are a number of different types of apraxia that you will come across in patients with neurological conditions:

- Swallow apraxia (inability to swallow volitionally)
- Gait apraxia (problems coordinating actions involved in walking)
- Limb apraxia (difficulty performing hand movements in the absence of impaired strength, i.e. weakness)
- Ideomotor apraxia (inability to correctly imitate hand gestures and voluntarily pantomime tool use, e.g. pretend to brush your teeth)
- Oral apraxia (difficulty performing oral movements on command or imitation, e.g. 'round your lips', 'protrude your tongue')
- Apraxia of speech (inability to program speech movements).

Thus, apraxia of speech is impairment in the ability to program speech movements, i.e. coordinate the timing, force production and sequencing of movements for the production of speech sounds. The speech of people with apraxia of speech contains distorted sounds, disordered stress patterns (the stress on the wrong syllable in a word so instead of saying DIScharge they say disCHARGE which has a very different meaning), abnormal rhythm of speech, and pauses between sounds and words as they try to get their muscles to carry out what they want to say. People with apraxia of speech are very aware of their errors and you can often see the person moving their mouths silently groping for the correct articulatory postures. The longer the word and the more complex the sound structure, the more difficult it is for the person to say the word accurately. People with apraxia of speech tend to perform better given repeated trials of a word. As some of the features of apraxia of speech can be found in some types of aphasia, an in-depth speech and language assessment will help with differential diagnostics.

Non-verbal communication

Much communication occurs without a single word being spoken. The way we look at another person, and the way he or she looks at us, conveys a lot of information, as does the body language involving posture and gesture. We convey feelings and attitudes such as those of happiness, expectancy and welcome, or of hostility, anger and withdrawal. We study one another's faces and read facial expressions.

Facial expression

The facial expressions adopted in emotions such as fear, anger, disgust, sadness, surprise and happiness are similar in different cultures and countries, suggesting that they are pre-programmed reflex patterns of muscle contraction triggered by our emotional state (see Chapter 13 on Emotion).

When we are surprised, we raise our eyebrows; when we are angry we lower them. When we are happy we pull up the corners of our lips by contracting the zygomatic muscles in order to smile and we screw up our eyes by contracting the outer part of the orbicularis oculi (see Fig. 11.3). We can pretend various emotions by voluntarily contracting the same muscles, but it is interesting that most people do not seem to be able to contract the outer part of the orbicularis oculi voluntarily. Only genuine happiness seems to act as the trigger.

If there is impairment of motor function, some of these natural forms of expression may be affected too, and the cues that tell us how that person is feeling may be lacking. A face may be expressionless, but that does not necessarily mean that the person behind the face has no feelings. In Parkinson's disease, for example, a patient may have an expressionless ('dead-pan') face. This is because of the patient's difficulty in initiating motor programs. Patients with facial cranial nerve (CNVII) damage post-stroke have a reduced ability to manipulate the fine muscles required to make their target facial expression, for example, when a patient with unilateral facial nerve damage smiles, the mouth does not move on the affected side or they may have difficulty frowning. This can make it difficult to discern the emotion that the patient is trying to convey.

Implications for rehabilitation

Communication difficulties impact on a patient's relationships, quality of life, social roles, and employment

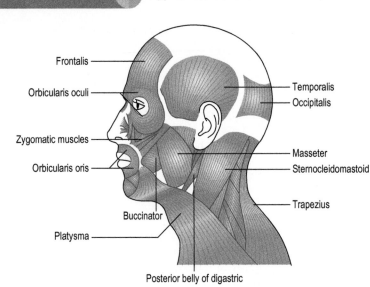

Fig. 11.3 • Muscles of the head and neck. From Kindlen, with permission

Frontalis

Orbicularis oculi

Zygomatic muscles

Orbicularis oris

Buccinator

Platysma

Posterior belly of digastric

Temporalis

Occipitalis

Masseter

Sternocleidomastoid

Trapezius

opportunities. Patients with speech and language impairments are often misunderstood and discriminated against in society, and some develop withdrawal symptoms and depression as a result. It is important for health-care professionals to be aware that speech and language problems are usually specific and not to assume that there is a global deficit (e.g. learning difficulties or dementia, however it is also important to note that these client groups will also have speech and language problems).

There are a number of ways that communication impairments could affect your intervention with a patient. You may find that their performance is variable and can change according to the time of day – some patients find that morning is better for them as they tire in the afternoon, while others find it difficult getting themselves focused until the afternoon. Their performance may also change according to what other activities they have been involved in that day, for example, if they have already seen a consultant, been for an X-ray and had some rehabilitation from another health-care professional, they may be less able to fully engage in your rehabilitation. Below are just some of the ways that aphasia may affect your intervention:

Comprehension impairments

- The patient may not understand some or all of the instructions you are giving them.

- The patient's non-verbal communication may suggest that they understand you but they may not. They may mirror your affect so, for example, if you speak to a patient smiling and nodding and ask questions they may smile and nod back so you think that they understand what you are saying to them, whereas in fact they are just mirroring your communication stance. This mirroring body language is something that we all do from time to time. Think about your body language in relation to someone who you are trying to create a rapport with. You (or they) will find that you tend to take on similar postures to the person you are speaking to.

- It is important to note that many assessments that evaluate the emotional status of patients are very difficult for someone with communication disorders to complete as they are language based. Therefore, if you are using such assessments with someone with communication impairment, you must be aware that the assessments may not be accurate.

Working with patients who have comprehension impairments will challenge you in your assessment of their abilities, for example, whether the patient is unable to carry out a physical movement because of muscle weakness or whether they were unable to fully understand your verbal instructions.

Expressive impairments

- Patients with aphasia often have difficulty finding the words they want to say which will affect their ability to answer your questions. While it may seem like a good idea to ask questions where a patient only has to answer either 'yes' or 'no', it is important to be aware that many people with aphasia have difficulty with 'yes' and 'no' and often say 'yes' when they mean 'no' and vice versa.
- While it may be uncomfortable for you it is essential that you do not 'pretend' or 'assume' that you know what a patient is saying, even if they look frustrated. It is better to tell them that you do not understand what they are saying but that you could come back to it another time.
- Some of the patients that you will work with will have problems speaking and may also have difficulties writing, drawing and/or gesturing, so you need to consider how best to help them communicate their health concerns, opinions and decisions to you in a way that you can understand.

When you are working with a patient with communication impairments it is important that you firstly establish if the person has been assessed by a speech and language therapist who will advise you on the best way to communicate with each person with aphasia. If not, make a referral for the person to be assessed and then find out the best method(s) of communicating with your patient. However, it is possible that you may see the patient before they have been assessed by the speech and language therapist, so here are a few ways to try to communicate with people with aphasia:

- Where possible, choose a *quiet place* with few distractions – background noise and more than one person speaking at once can make it very hard for the patient to follow a conversation.
- Get the person's *attention* before you speak and *keep eye contact* with them. This will ensure that facial expression and gestures will give a lot of clues about the message that you are trying to get across.
- Speak to the person *directly* and not over their head to a relative or other health professional.
- Allow plenty of *time* for the patient to absorb what you have said and to respond to you.

- Talk to your patient in a normal voice but *slightly slower speed* than usual
- Give only *one piece* of information at a time.
- Use *short* sentences with *simple* grammatical structures, for example, say 'is your arm sore?' rather than 'I was wondering if you are in pain as I can see that your arm is in spasm'.
- Use *familiar* words and phrases and avoid terminology that the person may not understand.
- *Let the patient know* when you are going to change the topic or this can confuse them.
- Make sure that your patient has *understood* what you've said to them.
- When you ask your patient questions, don't expect long detailed answers. It is easier for them to answer 'closed questions' rather than 'open questions' so for example, don't ask 'what would you like to drink?' but rather 'would you like tea or coffee?' You need to be aware that this will help some people with aphasia but others may respond with the wrong word so may say coffee (the last word they heard) when they meant tea. So always *double check*.
- Some people find 'yes'/'no' questions easy to answer but remember that this is often a problem for people with aphasia.
- *Avoid raising your voice* (this will not help as they are not deaf!)
- *Avoid interrupting* the person with aphasia as they may lose their train of thought.
- *Don't pretend* that you understand someone when you don't – your non-verbal communication will give it away!
- Have a *pen and paper* handy, as some people can read or write better than they can speak (while others cannot). Other people may be able to draw, point or gesture to express themselves.
- Do not assume that what works for one individual also works for another; *remember to ask*!
- *Keep trying*, unless both of you agree it is better to call it a day.

Summary

In this chapter, we have explored disorders of speech and language due to damage to the left and right hemispheres, and the associated problems of dysarthria and apraxia of speech. We have seen that aphasia is common in neurological rehabilitation with one-third of people who have a stroke experiencing aphasia. Aphasia can have a considerable impact on communication, quality of life, social roles as well as the outcome of rehabilitation. In this chapter, we have described a number of ways that are used to describe patients' communication problems and highlighted four different types of aphasia, i.e. Broca's, Wernicke's, conduction and global aphasia. However, we cautioned against a simplistic approach and indicated that the specialist area of speech and language disorders comprises many more categories and subtleties. Likewise, the relationship between the brain and behaviour in terms of communication is complex. Careful examination by a speech and language therapist, communication between members of the multidisciplinary team, as well as with the patient and their carer, is essential to identify each individual's communication abilities and support needs, and tailor interventions specifically to ensure optimum interaction and outcome in rehabilitation.

 SELF-ASSESSMENT QUESTIONS

1. Discuss the similarities and differences between aphasia and dysarthria.
2. Explain why categorising aphasia as 'expressive' or 'receptive' is too simplistic.
3. Describe the speech of a patient with fluent and non-fluent aphasia.
4. What are the main functional deficits found in Broca's, Wernicke's and conduction aphasia?
5. What communication difficulties could a person with right hemisphere damage have?
6. Consider the various ways in which a patient's communication impairment could impact on your assessment of them and their rehabilitation:
   ♦ Comprehension problems
   ♦ Expressive problems.
7. How can communication be facilitated in people with speech and language impairment?

Further reading

Bear, M.F., Connors, B.W., Paradiso, M.A., 2007. Neuroscience: Exploring the brain, third ed. Lippincott Williams & Wilkins, Baltimore.

Communication: Stroke Core Competencies for Health and Social Care Staff (the STARS project, Core competency 12). Available online from: http://www.strokecorecompetencies. org/node.asp?id=core.

Connect: the communication disability network. http://www.ukconnect.org/.

Kolb, B., Whishaw, I.Q., 2009. Fundamentals of Human Neuropsychology, sixth ed. Worth Publishers, New York.

Murdoch, B.E., 2010. Acquired Speech and Language Disorders: a neuroanatomical and functional neurological

approach, second ed. Wiley-Blackwell, Chichester.

Parr, S., Byng, S., Gilpin, S., 1997. Talking About Aphasia: living with loss of language after stroke. Open University Press, London.

Speakability.http://www.speakability. org.uk/.

West, P., 2008. The Shadow Factory. Lumen Books, Santa Fe, NM.

References

Broca, P.P., 1861. Perte de la parole, ramollissement chronique et destruction partielle du lobe antérieur gauche du cerveau. Bulletin de la Société Anthropologique 2, 235–238.

Cubelli, R., Montagna, C.G., 1994. A reappraisal of the controversy of Dax

and Broca. J. Hist. Neurosci. 3, 215–226.

Meyers, P., 1999. Right Hemisphere Damage: Disorders of communication and cognition. Singular Publishing Group Inc, London.

Weisenberg, T., McBride, K.E., 1935. Aphasia. A clinical and psychological

study. The Commonwealth Fund, New York.

Yorkston, K.M., Beukelman, D.R., Strand, E.A., Bell, K.R. 1999. Management of motor speech disorders in children and adults. Pro.ed, Austin, Texas, U.S.A.

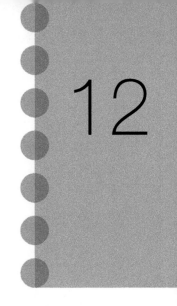

Executive dysfunction

> ### LEARNING OUTCOMES
>
> At the end of this chapter, you should be able to:
>
> 1. define *executive dysfunction* and describe common manifestations of this syndrome
> 2. identify the key brain areas and pathways that may be implicated in this syndrome and list common pathologies that may be associated with executive dysfunction
> 3. demonstrate an understanding of the possible implications of this syndrome for rehabilitation
> 4. demonstrate an understanding of the role of the multidisciplinary team in the management of people with executive dysfunction.

Introduction

An important aim of rehabilitation is to enable patients to contribute – wherever possible to the management of their condition. Eventually, most patients will need to be discharged from a health-care setting and, if left with a long-term condition such as multiple sclerosis (MS) or stroke, learn to live their lives as fully as possible. Self-management of one's long-term condition requires patients to be motivated and able to articulate appropriate goals, follow a plan, adjust their behaviour where necessary, and reflect on progress. Patients with clear and realistic goals, who are keen and driven, are often 'easy' to work with. In contrast, those with difficulty formulating appropriate goals, sticking to a plan, apparently lacking in motivation or displaying disruptive behaviour are much more of a challenge.

Case study 12.1 describes a person with executive dysfunction and indicates the challenges this may pose for the person themselves, their family and health-care professionals involved in their rehabilitation.

It is clear from this case study why one of the most important goals of Mr F.'s treatment plan is to address his challenging behaviour, as this affects his relationship with his wife, and could affect his recovery as well as prospects of community re-integration and return to work.

The behaviour of patients with executive dysfunction like Mr F. is often misinterpreted as 'unmotivated', 'un-cooperative' or 'disruptive'. This, in turn, may jeopardise their relationships with family, health-care professionals and colleagues.

Thus, executive dysfunction is one of the most persistent and disabling effects of brain injury (McDonald et al. 2002) and can be one of the most difficult problems to manage (Worthington 2003). It may present a real bottleneck for rehabilitation and participation in the wider community, as patients may have considerable and ongoing difficulties in forming and maintaining personal relationships and meeting job requirements (Burgess 2003).

This chapter on executive dysfunction aims to explain how a number of neurological conditions may

Case study 12.1

Mr F., a 26-year-old self-employed painter and decorator, has recently been discharged from neurosurgery, where he was treated for a traumatic brain injury (TBI) affecting mainly both frontal lobes (left more than right). Mr F. is the victim of an assault; he was attacked in the street by strangers after leaving his church. He sustained multiple head injuries, including a basal skull fracture, due to blows to his head.

Mr F. has just been admitted to an in-patient unit for further rehabilitation.

Mr F. has been married for 2 years and his wife is expecting their first child in 3 months' time. Before the accident, Mr F's hobbies were playing the flute in a local orchestra and organising charity events in his church. Mr F. was known to be kind and considerate and was respected for his excellent organisational skills.

Initial assessment by the multidisciplinary team yields the following information. The main effects of the TBI are: right-sided weakness, reduced motor control of his right arm, including loss of fine dexterity, reduced weight bearing on the affected leg and poor balance. During transfers and more complex activities of daily living, Mr F. demonstrates disorganised behaviour, e.g. he often forgets that he has already placed in a teabag in a cup when making tea, repeats this action even when a therapist

points out to him that he has already done so, and is easily distracted. Mr F.'s speech and swallowing have also been affected; Mr F. has difficulty expressing himself because of dysarthria and dysphasia. Marked changes have been observed in Mr F's overall behaviour since the accident; he is irritable, makes inappropriate jokes and has emotional outbursts. He seems to be unaware of how this affects others and does not seem to care. He appears to be unconcerned about his wife who is pregnant, and who has reported that her husband has been verbally aggressive towards her – a behaviour that is 'totally out of character'.

Mr F. is unable to undertake any activities of daily living independently, despite his physical recovery, and requires constant supervision from the occupational therapist to complete activities such as dressing and food preparation. Especially during his speech and language therapy sessions, Mr F. often gets frustrated and upset, and sometimes refuses to cooperate.

Mr F. has been referred for further in-patient specialist rehabilitation in order to reduce his impairments, improve his activities of daily living, address his communication needs and behavioural difficulties, and prepare him for discharge home in 3 months' time. Mr F.'s own goal is to go home next month and resume his business.

affect a person's ability to plan and govern their behaviour as well as their emotions, and deepen your understanding of these difficulties and the impact they may have. This chapter will introduce the concept of normal executive function, describe the signs and symptoms of executive dysfunction, outline the role of specific areas of the brain in executive function, and finally discuss the implications of executive dysfunction for rehabilitation.

Executive function

Daily life is governed by executive functioning. Consider the following scenario: you enter the hospital ward in the morning, where new patients have been admitted overnight – some of which require urgent care. One of your colleagues is off sick, hence you need to prioritise your workload, plan which patients you will see first, inform the consultant, keep track of time, consider how you could involve another colleague, talk to patients' anxious relatives while trying not to be distracted by other conversations around you, and ensure that your notes are up to date for the next colleague. All the time, you are

governing your behaviour, which involves a number of executive processes. There is debate on how many executive processes there are, with some models including just one and others including multiple. Smith and Kosslyn (2007) identify the following five executive processes:

- Selective attention focusing on achieving one's goal (i.e. executive attention)
- Switching executive attention from one activity to another
- Inhibiting/ignoring information that has already been registered
- Planning a sequence of activities
- Monitoring behaviour.

The notion of a **central executive** was proposed by Baddeley (1986), although Stuss and Alexander (2000) emphasised that there is no *unitary* executive (i.e. a 'homunculus', or 'ghost in the machine') that is solely responsible for this function, nor is there a single anatomical site in the brain where executive function resides. Instead, executive function is understood to comprise a number of different yet interrelated processes that enable us to engage in **metacognition**; a supervisory function that governs underlying cognitive functions of attention, thinking, problem solving and memory, and which enables us to reflect on processes themselves. Which processes and brain regions are involved in executive functioning depends on the task and its complexity, the intention and context in which it takes place (Stuss and Alexander 2007).

Executive function is particularly important in situations where one is learning a complex or new behaviour (Stuss 1992), as is often the case in adjusting to life after brain injury.

Taken together, executive function has been described as:

> '... the abilities that enable a person to establish new behaviour patterns and ways of thinking and to introspect upon them'
>
> (Burgess 2003, p. 302.)

The ability to introspect, or self-reflect, is necessary for self-awareness, as well as for being aware of other people's thoughts and emotions (Stuss and Levine 2002). Furthermore, self-awareness is necessary for **self-regulation**, which is the ability to orchestrate one's behaviour in the direction of one's goals, taking account of constraints (Stuss and Levine 2002). Stuss (1991, 1992) proposed a model that comprised executive function as part of the self: in his hierarchical model of interacting levels of information processing, the lowest level covers sensory and perceptual functions, the second level comprises executive functions, while the highest level represents self-reflection and meta-cognition.

Although executive function, self-awareness and self-regulation are different, all three are often found impaired in people with frontal lobe lesions (Stuss and Benson 1986), such as frontal lobe tumours, traumatic brain injury or the later stages of Alzheimer's disease.

Executive dysfunction

Terminology used in the literature for impaired executive function include: dysexecutive function, dysexecutive syndrome, and frontal (lobe) syndrome. Although there is robust clinical evidence that executive dysfunction is often associated with frontal lobe lesions, the term 'frontal (lobe) syndrome' has been criticised, because executive functions are likely to extend beyond the frontal lobe (e.g. executive dysfunction has been observed in cerebellar patients, see Case Study 12.3). Additionally, it is probably more useful to focus on a patient's behavioural

problems, rather than a presumed anatomical lesion site (Baddeley 1996). Furthermore, given the complexity and diversity of executive function described above, it is only logical that there is no such thing as a unitary 'executive dysfunction' (Stuss and Alexander 2007).

Many patients undergoing rehabilitation, especially those who have experienced a crisis in their life, or whose condition will make it unlikely that they will be able to return to their 'old way of life', are challenged to find new behaviours, solve new problems and reflect on these. In the case of Mr. F (case study 12.1) limited use of one side of his body means that transferring from bed to wheelchair presents an entirely new problem. This may be compounded if his problem-solving capacity has been reduced. Mr F. may 'get stuck' and become frustrated – especially if he is unable to communicate effectively. Unable to govern his behaviour and being unaware of what is appropriate in a certain situation, he may vocalise his frustration and cause disruption. To compound the situation even further, Mr F. may lack the ability to reflect on his behaviour, remaining unaware that he has caused upset to others. This apparent lack of sensitivity towards others may cause even more upset – particularly if family members are unaware of executive dysfunction. Education has, therefore, an important role to play in the rehabilitation of people with executive dysfunction.

Following discharge, new problems are likely to emerge: not only will Mr F. need to adapt to the new role of being a father (a challenge in itself!), but also he is likely to need a new job to match his changed abilities, and to adjust to living with these impairments, activity limitations and participation restrictions.

In some cases, where the person will not be able to go back to their former lifestyle, but needs to create a new identity with new roles and a new purpose in life, it might actually be more appropriate to use the term 'habilitation' (from the Latin *habilitat*, meaning 'made able', (Oxford English on-line Dictionary)) rather than 're-habilitation'. In these circumstances, executive behaviour is often challenged, and patients and their families need to be resourceful to be able to solve the many problems they are suddenly confronted with.

Signs and symptoms

In summary, executive dysfunction can be seen as a constellation of impairments in normal executive functioning. Taking a cognitive approach, these may be summarised as difficulties involving the concept of '**schema**' (Worthington 2003) – an abstract term to indicate generic categories of events or objects:

- Schema formation
- Schema activation
- Schema regulation.

Furthermore, in addition to affecting cognition, executive function is known to impact on behaviour as well as mood (Damasio 1994). Depending on the site and extent of the brain lesion, signs and symptoms of executive dysfunction may include difficulties with the following:

- Goal setting:

  Patients may come up with treatment goals that are entirely unrealistic (e.g. Mr F.'s goal to resume business as a painter and decorator in 1 month's time). Some patients will simply claim that they will be 'alright', when it is clear that they will not. Others may have vague goals (e.g. to have more therapy, or to be normal again), without any specific targets.

- Planning and organisation:

  Some patients have difficulty with time management and may not realise that their plans may be impossible to carry out. Others, such as Mr F., have difficulties getting the steps of a serial task in the right order (e.g. transferring from bed to wheelchair, removing bedclothes first. Some patients have a plan, but then deviate from it, e.g. by getting distracted, and never reach their intended goal. It may be difficult – if not impossible – to expect a patient to carry out an activity programme by themselves.

- Self-initiation:

  Some patients launch themselves into an activity, without having thought it through. This may be hazardous, especially in situations where they are undertaking activities in a space with equipment and other people around. Others, such as Mr F., may have difficulty getting started in the first place, and some patients miss therapy sessions. Evidently, problems with self-initiation will impact on a patient's ability to make progress with their rehabilitation – and ultimately it may affect their prospects of returning to work.

- Self-direction:

  Patients such as Mr F. may have difficulty persisting with their activities; without frequent prompting, they may not be able to complete a task. Others may make some progress, but may lose track after having been distracted. Again, such problems have a considerable impact on a patient's capacity to live independently.

- Self-inhibition:

  Patients with executive dysfunction are often more distractible than healthy people; they may find it difficult to ignore extraneous stimuli and stick to their plan. In contrast, other patients may find it difficult to disengage from an activity, even if they know they have completed it – they may repeat the same activity over and over again, a problem known as **perseverance**. Self-inhibition also refers to avoiding behaviours that are driven by impulse, but may cause offense or harm to others (e.g. vocalising, quarrelling, using expletives or engaging in inappropriate sexual behaviour). Some patients may relieve themselves in inappropriate places – yet seem unbothered by this. Some patients come into conflict with the law, due to their unruly behaviour (Fuster 2003). It is easy to see how this type of behaviour may lead to the breakdown of relationships, loss of employment, homelessness and sometimes even prison sentences.

- Using cues to guide behaviour:

  Patients with executive dysfunction may have difficulty following instructions or using feedback to change their behaviour, hence their capacity to learn and adapt may be reduced, which impacts on their rehabilitation outcomes. Some patients may demonstrate risk taking and rule breaking – even if they are aware that they are breaking a rule, they may not necessarily be able to stop themselves.

- Problem-solving:

  Difficulties with problem-solving are typical of executive dysfunction, as this requires all the abilities identified above, including insight in identifying a problem, logical thinking to come up with a solution, self-initiation and direction to execute the solution, as well as monitoring to check that the plan is going ahead as intended. Poor strategy formation may be apparent, e.g. a head-injury patient turned up to your outpatient appointment, accompanied by her carer and two children, to tell you she was unable to make the appointment. It is the difficulty with problem solving that may well form the bottleneck to successful rehabilitation, as this is central to independent living.

- Supervision/monitoring:
  Patients with executive dysfunction may not be able to monitor themselves adequately. They may not be able to judge whether their goals are realistic; or they may not realise when they lose track, or get distracted from their plan. They may fail to detect when their behaviour is inappropriate – and understand how this may affect others around them. This apparent lack of insight is perhaps one of the most difficult aspects of executive dysfunction, both for the patient, their family and health professionals involved. For the family, living with a person with executive dysfunction may place a considerable burden on their relationships. Typically, a considerably greater number of carers report problems such as poor planning, lack of insight or concern, shallow affect, social disinhibition, and aggression on behalf of the patient, compared to patients themselves (Burgess and Robertson 2002). This lack of insight can make it very difficult for the patient to learn to adapt their behaviour.
  In these circumstances, it is essential that health-care professionals work with family members or carers to provide education about the nature of executive dysfunction and strategies for its management.

Interestingly, Damasio (1994) in his excellent work highlighted that people with executive dysfunction usually do not have any specific cognitive impairments as such, but are often profoundly impaired in their judgement, planning and decision making. Patients may have entirely normal (or even supranormal) IQ tests, yet fail in personal relationships and employment, as their self-awareness as well as their ability to understand other people's thoughts and emotions are impaired, leading to difficulty empathising with others and often resulting in appropriate social judgements (Stuss and Benson 1986).

Executive dysfunction and the brain

As mentioned before, a number of different conditions are known to be associated with executive dysfunction, including traumatic brain injury, herpes simplex encephalitis, neoplasms, fronto-temporal dementia, subcortical infarcts (affecting the thalamus or internal capsule), basal skull fractures and conditions affecting the cerebellum (Worthington 2003). For example, in traumatic brain injury (TBI), sudden impact between a head moving in space and a stationary object (or vice versa) may cause acceleration-deceleration impact. Depending on the severity of the impact, diffuse axonal tearing, contusions and sometimes intracerebral haemorrhage may result, affecting the frontal and temporal lobes, as well as subcortical structures.

Referring back to Chapter 5 on the relation between the brain and behaviour, we saw that Luria characterised the frontal lobe as the 'action unit'. As we have seen already, the frontal lobe comprises the following main areas:

- Primary motor cortex (area 4)
- Premotor and supplementary motor cortices (area 6) and Broca's area (area 44)
- Frontal eye field (area 8)
- Prefrontal cortex (the remainder of the frontal lobe).

To recapitulate, the primary motor cortex is involved in executing actions and the premotor cortex is involved in selecting the actions to be executed, especially when this involves reacting to external stimuli (e.g. kicking a ball that is thrown towards one). The supplementary motor cortex is more involved in selecting activities that are self-paced or driven by internal cues (e.g. one may decide to kick a ball, just because one wants to).

The prefrontal cortex is involved in judging the appropriateness of actions to be selected, e.g. regarding their timing and context. This part of the brain is also involved in short-term memory, in the sense that it keeps track of what has just happened. The process in judging the appropriateness of behaviour is often based on external cues (e.g. the type of environment one is in, or explicit instructions from someone else) or internal cues (e.g. an understanding of how to behave in certain circumstances). For example, your behaviour (including facial expressions, body language and vocabulary) with friends in the local pub is probably quite different from your behaviour in a clinical setting, working with patients. Obviously, fine-tuning your social skills is of considerable importance to your acceptance by, belonging to, and standing in, your social networks. In primates – especially humans – social skills are highly developed and this is one explanation for the expansion of the frontal lobe as one ascends the evolutionary ladder.

It follows that lesions to areas in front of the primary motor cortex may result in difficulty with selecting appropriate responses and governing behaviour, which results in errors in social interactions, poor divergent thinking (e.g. problem solving), a lack of spontaneous behaviour including speech and facial expression. If short-term memory is affected, a patient may lose track of what they have just done, resulting in them getting lost in or persevering with an activity. A combination of reduced spontaneous behaviour, 'flattened' facial expression, an apparent lack of interest, concern for others and reduced motivation is known as '**pseudo-depression**' (i.e. the depression is not the actual problem but it may have the appearance of depression). In contrast, the behaviour of patients who behave impulsively, use inappropriate language and demonstrate inappropriate social and sexual behaviour is known as '**pseudo-psychopathy**' (again, psychopathy is not the primary problem). The latter type of behaviour is often seen in patients with orbitofrontal brain lesions (i.e. affecting the area around the orbit), as described in Case study 12.2 for a classic case study on executive dysfunction.

The prefrontal cortex comprises the following main areas, which when affected may give rise to the signs and symptoms described below.

Orbito-frontal region

The role of this part of the brain is to monitor behaviour and inhibit inappropriate actions – especially in the social domain. It also enables one to defer immediate reward for long-term gain. A person with a lesion in the orbito-frontal region (as described in Case study 12.2) is likely to have difficulty resisting urges to satisfy their needs (e.g. food, sex) even if the context is inappropriate. They may be easily distracted, as they find it difficult to ignore stimuli. Mood may be labile, the person may get themselves into unprovoked arguments, and may in some cases break the law. Inappropriate jokes and a more general lack of judgement also characterise the behaviour of people with lesions in the orbito-frontal lesion.

Lateral pre-frontal cortex

Normally, this part of the brain enables one to hold information 'in mind'. This is the 'recency' function of working memory, which helps to keep track of what has just been done and what needs to be done next, thereby enabling planning. A lesion to this part of the brain causes people to lose track of what they were doing, resulting in chaotic behaviour.

Case study 12.2

The story of Phineas Gage

Probably the most well-known case study on executive dysfunction is that of Phineas Gage, a dynamite worker in the late 19th century, who was first described by John Harlow in 1868 (Harlow 1993). Gage was working on the construction of a railway line, when a dynamite explosion caused an iron bar (dimensions approx. 3 cm by 1 m) to enter and exit his skull. Miraculously, Gage survived the blast – but others around him described how his personality changed as a result of this accident. Before, Gage was known to be energetic and organised, whereas afterwards his behaviour was described as lacking in balance between intellect and impulse – with the latter dominating the former.

Harlow (1993, p. 277) described his behaviour as follows:

'His contractors, who regarded him as the most efficient and capable foreman in their employ previous to his injury, considered the change in his mind so marked that they could not give him his place again. The equilibrium or balance, so to speak, between his intellectual faculties and animal propensities, seems to have been destroyed. He is fitful, irreverent, indulging at times in the grossest profanity (which was not previously his custom), manifesting but little deference

for his fellows, impatient of restraint or advice when it conflicts with his desires, at times pertinaciously obstinate, yet capricious and vacillating, devising many plans of future operation, which are no sooner arranged than they are abandoned in turn for others appearing more feasible. A child in his intellectual capacity and manifestations, he has the animal passions of a strong man'

It is quite clear that Gage's behaviour was often unacceptable, that he did not seem to have much consideration for his colleagues, and that he had problems completing any of his plans. Gage took to travelling and eventually died following epileptic seizures, some 12.5 years after the accident. It was not possible to conduct an autopsy to examine the condition of his brain; however, his family donated his skull to Dr Harlow, for the benefit of science.

Through physical examination of his skull, together with imaging and techniques at a later date (e.g. Ratiu et al. 2004) it was possible to reconstruct how the tamping iron had travelled through the skull, probably injuring just the left frontal lobe – although the precise damage it inflicted has been debated (see http://www.deakin.edu.au/hmnbs/psychology/gagepage/Pgdamage.php).

Medial/cingulate region

Key signs of this area being affected are a lack of drive, interest and spontaneity, both in verbal and non-verbal expression. This area has strong connections with the limbic system, which is involved in governing emotion.

In summary, the frontal lobe – especially the premotor and prefrontal areas – are involved in the formation, activation, regulation and supervision of plans. However, there is more to executive dysfunction than impairment in the 'planning department'; there is also a distinctive impact on **motivation and emotion**. This is mediated by the extensive neural connections between the frontal lobe and other areas of the brain (see McDonald et al. 2002 for a review). The prefrontal cortex is intimately connected with a wide range of other cortical and subcortical areas, including the association cortices of the other lobes, the brainstem, hypothalamus, thalamus, limbic system and basal ganglia (Fuster 2003). The cerebellum has also been implicated in executive dysfunction, through its connections with the cerebral cortex via the pons (Schweizer et al. 2008). These connections are reciprocal, indicating intensive integration between the executive part of the brain and areas involved in perception and action, memory, the regulation of homeostasis, as well as motivation and emotion. Thus, the prefrontal cortex receives extensive information about the external, as well as internal environment.

Furthermore, several important neurotransmitter systems converge onto the prefrontal area of the brain, including the dopamine system (which is involved in behaviour associated with reward), the noradrenaline (norepinephrine) and serotonine systems (involved in general arousal and attention), the cholinergic system (involved in attention and short-term memory), while GABA (gamma-aminobutyric acid) plays an important role in inhibition, through modulating attention and working memory (Fuster 2003).

In the next chapter, we will take a closer look at the links between the prefrontal area and brain structures involved in motivation and emotion.

Implications for rehabilitation

From the description of the signs and symptoms of executive dysfunction above, it is clear that this presents a major challenge to the patient, their family members, their social network, as well as the multidisciplinary health care team. The extent of executive dysfunction may not be entirely clear while a patient is in hospital, as the numerous routines and limited scope for independence may mask the signs and symptoms. It may be further down the line, when admitted to specialist rehabilitation – or discharged home – that the true extent of the problem emerges as life becomes more complex. There is currently little information on the natural recovery of executive dysfunction, which is probably compounded by the fact that this is an umbrella term for a range of difficulties, involving a number of different neural structures.

Given the diversity, extent and complexity of executive dysfunction, it will not be a surprise that there is no single solution for this problem, and there is a lack of consensus on how best to assess and treat it. Executive dysfunction is poorly defined and the scientific and theoretical underpinnings of normal executive function are highly complex and only partially understood. Attempts have been made to bridge the gap between neuropsychological theory and clinical practice, for which the reader is referred to Burgess and Simons (2005). A review of assessments for executive dysfunction can be found in Crawford and Henry (2005), while different treatment approaches are summarised in McDonald et al. (2002).

The input from a clinical psychologist is usually required for a comprehensive assessment and treatment plan, which then requires consistent implementation by the MDT, as well as the patient's family and carers, as appropriate. The value of assessments based on real-life situations is becoming more widely recognised, as the complexity of real-world situations cannot be easily replicated through neuropsychological testing (Chan et al. 2008). Occupational therapists are skilled in providing assessments of occupational performance in real-life complex situations and can use assessments of cognitive process skills, e.g. Assessment of Motor and Process Skills (Fisher 1993) or more specific executive function assessments (Baum et al. 2008) to guide and support the patient and their families and the multidisciplinary team.

Pharmacological interventions may be required to modulate arousal, impulsive behaviour and mood. Providing the required behavioural therapeutic input may be problematic, especially for patients lacking in insight. Problems with agreeing on appropriate goals may set the rehabilitation process off to a difficult start, while it cannot be assumed that the patient is able to engage in self-management. Care must be taken not to misinterpret behaviour, and guidance needs to be extended to the patient's important others. Close supervision may be required, especially for those with challenging behaviour. Specialist occupational therapy and/or social work may be necessary to explore the patient's opportunities to return to work and independent living. With the patient's consent, partnerships may need to be developed with employers and colleagues who may need to be educated in terms of the person's situation, as well as relevant employment legislation.

Worthington (2003) described non-pharmacological interventions for people with executive dysfunction under the following headings:

- Environmental modification: this is aimed at reducing the burden on executive functioning, e.g. by removing distracting stimuli including temptations (e.g. television), simplifying the environment to avoid confusion, or laying out objects required for a task in a particular order (e.g. for dressing). Environmental modification may also include the social environment, e.g. by using reinforcement techniques such as 'time-out' in social interactions to improve behaviour.
- Compensatory strategies: these are aimed at changing behaviour, without trying to tackle the underlying impairments. Examples are external aids such as notebooks, checklists and pagers, used for example to remind people to check if they are on track with an activity.
- Task-specific training: these are aimed at improving functional skills (e.g. meal preparation or using public transport), ranging from specific activities of daily living to more generic skills. Conditioning methods can be used such as shaping and positive reinforcement to progressively approximate intended behaviour. Most skills, taught in a rehabilitation setting, will need to be adjusted to be fit for purpose in the patient's own environment.
- Training in metacognitive skills: this is aimed at improving overall supervisory functions and self-awareness through self-monitoring, self-prompting and problem solving (e.g. telling oneself to 'wait' when perceived to be provoked, or to 'just do it' in order to prompt oneself into action). Evidence, summarised by Worthington (2003) indicates that task-specific prompting may be internalised and thereby transferred to other activities.

It is clear from the above that there is some degree of overlap between these four categories, e.g. meta-cognition training (e.g. using self-prompting) may be integrated with task-specific skills training.

Gordon et al. (2006) describe the Executive Plus Model, an intervention approach based on a synthesis of the literature on executive dysfunction. It proposes that problem solving, emotional regulation and attention all need to be addressed. Impaired problem solving is one of the hallmarks of executive dysfunction, and this can be facilitated or further hampered by emotional self-regulation. For example, low mood may lead an individual to avoid solving a problem, while failure in solving a problem may cause frustration and emotional outbursts.

Case study 12.3 describes the application of goal management training to the treatment of executive dysfunction. For further detailed case studies the reader is referred to Wilson et al. (2009).

Case studies such as the one above are undoubtedly of value to inform clinical practice. However, following a review of the literature, Evans (2005) expressed caution in his conclusion that treatment of executive impairments can be effective. This is because it is not entirely clear which processes mediate improvement; there is a paucity of research in many areas; only few studies provide evidence that treatment generalises to activities of daily living; and it is difficult to measure the effects of interventions because of the complexity of the behaviours involved. Worthington (2003) also highlighted the paucity of detail in the descriptions of therapeutic interventions in the published literature, and the need for more robust research in this important topic area in order to improve clinical practice for individuals affected by this debilitating syndrome.

Summary

In this chapter, we have seen that a wide range of neurological conditions, from more general conditions (e.g. fronto-temporal dementia) to focal conditions (e.g. a tumour), may impair a person's executive function. In many cases, the frontal lobe is involved, which acts as a 'supervisor', enabling the person to set goals, plan the way to goal achievement, and govern and reflect on their behaviour.

To others, the patient with executive function may appear to be a different person from before they had their condition. Individuals who used to be

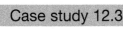

Case study 12.3

Effects of goal management training on executive dysfunction

Schweizer et al. (2008) evaluated the effects of goal management training (GMT), devised by Robertson (1996), in a male person with executive dysfunction, initiated at approximately 4 months following a right-sided cerebellar stroke. This 41-year-old patient experienced a rupture of an arteriovenous malformation in the right cerebellar hemisphere, resulting in focal cerebellar damage. Before this event, he had been employed as a high-level bank executive. Following neurosurgery, the patient was referred for 5 weeks of inpatient rehabilitation, concentrating on gait and speech. The patient was also referred for a neurobehavioural assessment, where executive dysfunction was noted. At follow-up, some 8 weeks after the acute event, the patient complained about dizziness upon sudden movement, slurred speech, and an inability to get back to work because of slowed thinking and impaired organisational skills. A detailed neuropsychological assessment was undertaken, following which GMT was instituted.

GMT uses task breakdown, self-prompting to halt automatic behaviours that impede progress, resuming control and monitoring progress with a task, to overcome disorganised behaviour. The intervention consisted of 2-hour sessions, once per week for 7 weeks. The effectiveness of GMT was assessed using a battery of standardised tests for attention and executive function, administered before, immediately after and 4 months after the completion of the GMT. Interestingly, before the treatment commenced, the patient's wife reported a greater number of difficulties than did the patient – an indication of the patient's lack of insight into his problems.

Following the intervention, improvements were noted in a number of outcomes, while there was an indication that the patient had become more aware of his difficulties. In functional terms, the patient was able to return to work, while his spouse noted that the symptoms of executive dysfunction had disappeared.

---

thoughtful, motivated and organised may appear to be aimless, lacking in motivation or drive, or have completely unrealistic expectations and vent their frustration without regard for others. It is clear that such challenging behaviour is a bottleneck in the rehabilitation process, in addition to putting a strain on relationships. It is, therefore, of great importance that health-care professionals working with such patients have a sound understanding of the physical substrate underlying executive dysfunction and appreciate that changes in the person's behaviour are primarily a consequence of the brain damage. However, this does not mean that behaviour cannot be modified. Input from the multidisciplinary team is, therefore, essential. Congruency in approach between different health-care professionals is essential to convey consistency to the patient and offer a progressive structure to enable the patient to regain their autonomy.

This chapter mentioned problems with motivation and emotion only briefly; the next chapter intends to concentrate on these important functions

and explore the intricate and important integration between emotion, motivation and executive function.

SELF-ASSESSMENT QUESTIONS

Following this chapter, can you:

1. Define *executive dysfunction* and explain why this is not a unitary concept?
2. Identify the most common signs and symptoms of executive dysfunction?
3. Identify the key brain areas that may be associated with this syndrome?
4. List common pathologies that may be associated with executive dysfunction?
5. Explain the possible impact of executive dysfunction on the affected person's rehabilitation outcomes, as well as their social relationships and prospects of reintegration into the community?
6. Outline the role of the multidisciplinary team in the management of people with executive dysfunction?

Further reading

Malia, K., Brannagan, A., 2005. How to do cognitive rehabilitation therapy. Brain Tree Training, Surrey, England.

References

Baddeley, A., 1986. Working Memory. Clarendon Press/Oxford University Press, New York.

Baddeley, A., 1996. Exploring the central executive. Q. J. Exp. Psychol. 49A, 5–28.

Baum, C.M., Connor, L.T., Morrison, T., et al., 2008. Reliability, validity, and clinical utility of the Executive Function Performance Test: a measure of executive function in a sample of people with stroke. Am. J. Occup. Ther. 62, 446–455.

Burgess, P.W., 2003. Assessment of executive function. In: Halligan, P. W., Kischka, U., Marshall, J.C. (Eds.), Handbook of Clinical Neuropsychology. Oxford University Press, Oxford, pp. 302–321.

Burgess, P.W., Robertson, I.H., 2002. Principles of the rehabilitation of executive dysfunction. In: Stuss, D. T., Knight, R. (Eds.), Principles of Frontal Lobe Function. Oxford University Press, Oxford, pp. 557–572.

Burgess, P.W., Simons, J.S., 2005. Theories of frontal lobe executive function: clinical applications. In: Halligan, P.W., Wade, D.T. (Eds.), Effectiveness of Rehabilitation for Cognitive Deficits. Oxford University Press, Oxford, pp. 211–232.

Chan, R.C.K., Shum, D., Toulopoulou, T., et al., 2008. Assessment of executive functions: Review of instruments and identification of critical issues. Arch. Clin. Neuropsychol. 23, 201–216.

Crawford, J.R., Henry, J.D., 2005. Assessment of executive dysfunction. In: Halligan, P.W., Wade, D.T. (Eds.), Effectiveness of Rehabilitation for Cognitive Deficits. Oxford University Press, Oxford, pp. 233–246.

Damasio, A., 1994. Descartes' Error. Emotion, reason and the human brain. Penguin Books, New York.

Evans, J.J., 2005. Can executive impairments be effectively treated? In: Halligan, P.W., Wade, D.T. (Eds.), Effectiveness of Rehabilitation for Cognitive Deficits. Oxford University Press, Oxford, pp. 247–256.

Fisher, A.G., 1993. The assessment of IADL motor skills: An application of many faceted Rasch analyses. Am. J. Occup. Ther. 47, 319–329.

Fuster, J.M., 2003. Functional neuroanatomy of executive process. In: Halligan, P.W., Kischka, U., Marshall, J.C. (Eds.), Handbook of Clinical Neuropsychology. Oxford University Press, Oxford, pp. 753–768.

Gordon, W.A., Cantor, J., Ashman, T., et al., 2006. Treatment of post-TBI executive dysfunction: application of theory to clinical practice. J. Head Trauma Rehabil. 21, 156–167.

Harlow, J.M., 1993. Recovery from the passage of an iron bar through the head. Hist. Psychiatry 4, 274. doi:10.1177/0957154X9300401407. Available online from:http://hpy.sagepub.com/content/4/14/274.citation (accessed 19.03.2011).

McDonald, B.C., Flashman, L.A., Saykin, A.J., 2002. Executive dysfunction following traumatic brain injury: neural substrates and treatment strategies. Neurorehabilitation 17, 333–344.

Oxford English on-line Dictionary. Available online from: http://oxforddictionaries.com/ (accessed 18.03.2011).

Ratiu, P., Talos, I.F., Haker, S., et al., 2004. The tale of Phineas Gage, digitally remastered. J Neurotrauma 21, 637–643. Available online from: http://www.nejm.org/doi/full/10.1056/NEJMicm031024 (accessed 18.03.2011).

Robertson, I.H., 1996. Goal Management Training: A clinical manual. PsyConsult, Cambridge.

Schweizer, T.A., Levine, B., Rewilak, D., et al., 2008. Rehabilitation of executive functioning after focal damage to the cerebellum. Neurorehabil. Neural. Repair. 22, 72–77.

Smith, E.E., Kosslyn, S.M., 2007. Cognitive Psychology, Mind and Brain. Pearson Prentice Hall, Upper Saddle River NJ.

Stuss, D.T., 1991. Self, awareness and the frontal lobes: a neuropsychological perspective. In: Strauss, J., Goethals, G.R. (Eds.), The Self: Interdisciplinary Approaches. Springer Verlag, New York, pp. 255–279.

Stuss, D.T., 1992. Biological and psychological development of executive functions. Brain Cogn. 20, 2–23.

Stuss, D.T., Alexander, M.P., 2000. Executive functions and the frontal lobes: a conceptual view. Psychol. Res. 63, 289–298.

Stuss, D.T., Alexander, M.P., 2007. Is there a dysexecutive syndrome? Philos. Trans. R. Soc. Lond. B Biol. Sci. 362, 901–915.

Stuss, D.T., Benson, D.F., 1986. The Frontal Lobes. Raven Press, New York.

Stuss, D.T., Levine, B., 2002. Adult clinical neuropsychology: lessons from studies of the frontal lobes. Annu. Rev. Psychol. 53, 401–433.

Wilson, B.A., Gracey, F., Evans, J.J., et al., 2009. Neuropsychological Rehabilitation. Theory, models and outcome. Cambridge University Press, Cambridge.

Worthington, A.D., 2003. Rehabilitation of executive deficits: effective treatment of related disabilities. In: Halligan, P.W., Wade, D.T. (Eds.), Effectiveness of Rehabilitation for Cognitive Deficits. Oxford University Press, Oxford, pp. 257–270.

Problems of emotion and motivation

CHAPTER CONTENTS

LEARNING OUTCOMES

At the end of this chapter, you should be able to:

1. explain the difficulty of defining the concept of 'emotion'
2. discuss the importance of having a working knowledge of emotional difficulties in people with a neurological condition
3. discuss the main theories related to depressive disorders and detail the mechanism of action of the major classes of anti-depressant medication
4. describe the most common emotional problems in people with stroke, traumatic brain injury (TBI), Parkinson's disease (PD) and Alzheimer's disease (AD)
5. outline the basic principles of our current understanding of the relationship between the brain and emotion
6. explain how neurological, psychological and social factors may account for emotional difficulties in people with neurological conditions
7. explain the potential impact of emotional problems on a patient's rehabilitation outcomes and quality of life.

Introduction

Many neurological conditions in which the brain is affected are associated with changes in emotion, mood and motivation (Cappa 2001). For many patients and their families, the emotional 'fallout' of a neurological condition may be one of the most difficult problems they have to cope with. Health professionals working with patients who experience emotional distress may also find this to be challenging.

Despite the prominent place that emotion occupies in the lives of most of us, the scientific study of 'emotion' was neglected for a considerable period of time. The main barriers were that it was problematic to define 'emotion' in the first place, while traditional methods used to study the topic (e.g. introspection) were criticised for being 'unscientific'. Instead, the realm of emotion was considered to belong to artists, who – with prose and poetry, on canvas and through music – were considered to be much more capable of conveying emotion and its impact than any scientist. As a result, the scientific exploration of 'emotion' lay dormant until relatively recently, when neuro imaging technology emerged. An exciting era lay ahead; for the first time, scientists and clinicians were able to explore the neural correlates of emotion and mental illness such as depression and schizophrenia. As a result, scientific activity in this topic area has soared. However, 'emotion' is often neglected in textbooks of cognitive psychology. Given the prevalence and impact of emotional difficulties in people with neurological conditions, it is important that health-care professionals have a good understanding of this topic.

The aim of this chapter is to explore what is meant by 'emotion' and whether this is a purely personal experience that defies generalisation. Given its common occurrence in the general population, as well as in people with neurological conditions, we will then move on to discuss depression, its possible causes and treatment options in more detail. This will be followed by an introduction to some of the most frequently reported difficulties with emotion and motivation in people with stroke, traumatic brain injury (TBI), Parkinson's disease (PD) and Alzheimer's disease (AD). We will discuss various explanations for problems with emotion and motivation, beginning with a biomedical perspective – by investigating neurological consequences of the various conditions and identifying those brain areas and physiological processes that play a key role in emotion and motivation. We will then move on to a more psychosocial perspective by exploring how neurological conditions may affect the lives, experiences and aspirations of those affected – and the impact of coping strategies and social support. Finally, we will refer back to the previous chapter on executive function and explore how an intricate integration between executive function and emotion is required for rational behaviour that serves the survival of the individual.

Our intention is that this information will enable you to have a better understanding of, and empathy for, the patients and the families with whom you will be working.

Emotion: an overview

Emotion: can it be defined?

What is emotion? Try for a moment to remember an emotionally rich event in your life. Graduations are a useful example, where people typically feel intensely proud, experience a rush of pleasure and excitement, believe that the world is full of promise, and throw their mortar boards in the air, out of sheer joy. It is difficult to unpick this complex experience, but basically it comprises the following responses:

- Physiological (i.e. involving the endocrine, nervous and musculoskeletal systems)
- Psychological (i.e. thoughts, beliefs, expectations)
- Behavioural (i.e. expressed through voice, posture and movement).

A physiological response to an emotionally intense life event at the other end of the spectrum could be a frightening situation, such as a house fire. This situation would involve the release of stress hormones (e.g. cortisol), activation of the sympathetic nervous system and a preparation of the musculoskeletal system for a fright, flight or fight reaction. A psychological response in such a scenario could be your belief that you're in imminent danger, which in turn motivates you to flee, while a typical behavioural reaction would be to scream for help, adopt a defensive posture and run for safety.

Some psychologists have made attempts to define emotion. Here is an example by Smith (1993):

> 'An emotion may be defined as an innate and acquired predisposition to respond cognitively, physiologically and behaviorally to certain internal and external events that relate to important goals and motives'.

Although this is a very inclusive description, one could argue that its broadness jeopardises its specificity. It is probably more useful to have an understanding of different types of emotion, than to worry about comprehensively capturing this complex concept.

When we think of an emotion, we may be inclined to think that this is unique to each of us – specific to our own individual world of experience only. Although it is attractive to indulge in the notion of a strictly private world, ground-breaking work by Darwin in the 1850s confirmed that there are around six basic facial expressions, each conveying a distinct emotion, which are understood the world over

(Darwin 1865, cited in Berthoz 2003). These universal facial expressions communicate:

- sadness
- anger
- disgust
- surprise
- happiness
- fear.

Pioneering work by anthropologist Ekman in Papua New Guinea, where until that time no Westerner had set foot, confirmed these basic emotions; when told an emotionally charged story and asked to express what this felt like, local inhabitants showed facial expressions that could readily be understood by people from Western civilisations (Ekman 1984).

This universality in basic emotions makes sense from the perspective of survival: before the arrival of the communication technologies we use today, facial expressions were our primary means of communicating to our immediate social network how we felt. If there is danger, communicating fear is essential to warn others around us. Disgust may signal food that is inedible, while an angry face conveys a warning. This universality suggests that some of our emotional expressions are 'hardwired' in the brain – a topic we will come to later.

We will now turn to the topic of depression, one of the most common mental health problems in both the general population, and in people with long-term neurological conditions.

Depression

The group of conditions known as the affective disorders involve a disturbance of mood (with associated cognitive and emotional symptoms) associated with changes in behaviour, energy, appetite and sleep (the biological symptoms). Changes in our mood are regular occurrences and it is the highs and lows that we experience that give depth to our emotional existence. If we have had a bad day at work or university, then we will enjoy a relaxing and fun time with our friends all the more. So, ups and downs in our mood are not a bad thing, however if our mood strays to the pathological extremes of the normal continuum then that can result in significant problems. These pathological extremes can be manifest as either extreme excitement and elation (mania) or severe depression, or a swing between both. The affective disorders can be classified into two types:

unipolar (mania or depression) and bipolar (manic depression). As depression is the more common phenomenon to manifest itself after an injury or illness then we shall focus on that for the purpose of this chapter. Among the more common features of depression are:

- a persistent sad or 'empty' mood
- feelings of hopelessness
- feelings of guilt
- a loss of interest in what were previously pleasurable activities
- alterations in sleeping and eating patterns
- low levels of energy.

Classification of depression

Depression comes in different forms. It used to be thought that depression could be simply classified in two ways – reactive and endogenous. With reactive depression there is usually a very specific, clear psychological cause (e.g. a bereavement, the loss of a job, the break-up of a long-term relationship). This type of reactive change may occur following, for example, a stroke where the patient has had a significant loss of function and is no longer able to engage in certain activities and life roles that they were able to do pre-stroke. Unlike reactive depression, there appeared to be no clear cause for endogenous depression (hence the name). Patients suffering from endogenous depressions often express more severe symptoms (e.g. suicidal thoughts). It is important to correctly diagnose which form of depression an individual has, as evidence suggests that endogenous depression responds better to drug therapy (see later in this chapter).

An alternative way to consider depression is to classify the level of disability produced as being either a major depression or a dysthymia. A *major depression* will interfere quite markedly with the individual's ability to work, study, sleep, eat or enjoy pleasurable activities. Such a level of dysfunction may only occur once, but it is quite common for such a disturbance to occur on multiple occasions throughout life. Chronic major depression of this nature may require an extensive period of appropriate treatment. Dysthymic disorder, or *dysthymia*, produces symptoms of a less severe nature; however, they can still be chronic and long-lasting. Dysthymia does not necessarily seriously disable the individual, but it can keep them from feeling and functioning well. It is also possible that a person with dysthymia may also experience a major depressive episode at some point in their life.

Causes of depression

The actual cause of depression is still unknown. In some families it can be apparent that depression occurs from generation to generation, however, it can also occur in a person with no family history of depressive illness. It is also widely accepted that depression is a combination of genetic, psychological, social and environmental factors.

Current biomedical views on the cause of depression centre round the monoamine hypothesis, which was first proposed in 1965 by Schildkraut. This hypothesis puts forward the idea that depression occurs as a consequence of abnormalities in the levels of the monoamine neurotransmitters (noradrenaline [NA], serotonin [5-HT]) in the limbic system. As mentioned in Chapter 2, the limbic system is the 'emotional part' of the brain and this system will be described more in detail below. Research points to particular evidence that reduced serotonergic neurotransmission is involved. It is hypothesised that depression is caused, in part, by a number of biochemical/pharmacological changes within the limbic system.

These changes include a lower level of monoamine transmitters (NA, 5-HT) and/or an upregulation of presynaptic autoreceptors (located on the presynaptic terminal) and somatodendritic autoreceptors (located on the dendrites of the presynaptic cell) that control monoamine release. This increase in the presynaptic receptors and those found on the dendrites result in an enhancement of the normal negative feedback mechanism, thereby causing a subsequent greater reduction in further monoamine release. Over time this mechanism would result in a significantly lower release of the transmitters.

There are a number of key pieces of evidence that both support and refute the monoamine theory.

Evidence for the monoamine theory

It can be shown that drugs that deplete monoamine levels are depressant (e.g. the anti-hypertensive drug reserpine which inhibits the storage of NA and 5-HT). In addition, drugs that increase availability of monoamines (e.g. tricyclic antidepressants, monoamine oxidase inhibitors) improve mood in depressed patients and we shall discuss some of these drugs later in the chapter. When samples of cerebrospinal fluid are taken from depressed patients it can be shown that both the concentration of the monoamines, NA and 5-HT, and their corresponding metabolites are down. However, care should be taken when interpreting this type of information as secondary factors, such as diet and transport between the CSF and the blood, can impact on these levels.

Evidence against the monoamine theory

Despite the considerable evidence in support of the theory, there are some equally compelling arguments against the theory. There is a wide range of compounds that increase the availability of the monoamine transmitters (e.g. amphetamine, cocaine) but these agents have no ability to elevate the mood of depressed patients. It has also been noted that some of the atypical antidepressants work without affecting monoamine systems (e.g. trazodone or mirtazapine). The third, and final, piece of evidence that appears to suggest that there is more involved than the simple manipulation of the monoamine transmitters is the fact that there may be a 'therapeutic delay' of 2–3 weeks between the full neurochemical effects appearing and the start of the actual therapeutic effect.

As a consequence of the evidence that appears to refute the monoamine theory, it is possible to reach the conclusion that it is unlikely that monoamine systems alone are responsible for the symptoms of depression. A number of other systems that may be involved include GABA (γ-aminobutyric acid), neuropeptides (vasopressin, endogenous opiates) and various second messenger systems.

Having stated that other systems may be involved in the neuropharmacology of depression, it cannot be denied that some of the main, active antidepressant drugs do indeed exert their therapeutic effect through the manipulation of monoamine systems. Some examples of drugs that work via monoamine systems are discussed below, although for a full list of all of the mechanistic approaches you should refer to one of the pharmacology texts suggested at the end of Chapter 4.

Treatment of depression

The mechanisms of action of the antidepressants covered next can be seen in Figure 13.1. This diagram

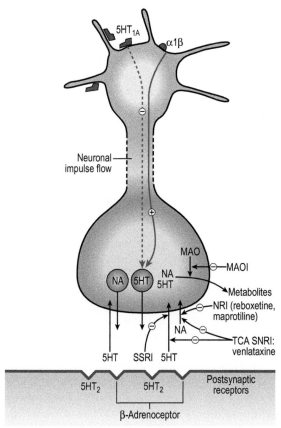

Fig. 13.1 • The mechanism of action of some antidepressants. (Based on Waller et al 2001, with permission)

shows a single synapse containing both NA and 5-HT, although in reality there would be either a noradrenergic synapse or a serotonergic synapse.

Tricyclic antidepressants

Examples of this class include amitryptyline, imipramine and nortryptyline. The tricyclic antidepressants (TCAs) inhibit the reuptake of both NA and 5-HT by competitively inhibiting the ATPase in the membrane pump used to take these transmitters back up into the presynaptic terminal. Different drugs within the class have more selectivity for one transmitter over another:

- Amitriptyline (Triptafen®) and imipramine (Tofranil®) have a greater impact on 5-HT uptake than NA uptake.
- Nortriptyline (Allegron®) and lofepramine (Gamanil®) have a greater impact on NA uptake than 5-HT uptake.

Selective serotonin reuptake inhibitors

Examples of this class include some of the most widely recognised antidepressant drugs including citalopram (Cipramil®), fluoxetine (Prozac®), paroxetine (Seroxat®) and sertraline (Lustral®). The selective serotonin reuptake inhibitors (SSRIs) reduce the neuronal reuptake of 5-HT, with little or no effect on NA reuptake. There are a number of unwanted effects with these drugs including sedation, weight gain, nausea, abdominal pain, diarrhoea, insomnia, agitation and anxiety, anorexia and a decreased libido. However, as they have no effect on NA, which could alter sympathetic activity on the heart, there is no evidence of any cardiotoxicity.

Serotonin and noradrenaline reuptake inhibitors

The serotonin and noradrenaline reuptake inhibitors (SNRIs) work in a similar way to the aforementioned TCAs in so far as they inhibit the neuronal reuptake of both 5-HT and NA, with a greater effect on 5-HT uptake at lower doses. One of the best known examples of an SNRI is venlafaxine (Efexor®). As with all of the antidepressant drugs, there are a number of unwanted side effects including drowsiness, dry mouth, nausea, constipation, dizziness and confusion.

Selective noradrenaline reuptake inhibitors

The noradrenaline reuptake inhibitors (NRIs) (e.g. reboxitine (Edronax®)) inhibit the neuronal reuptake of NA leading to increased noradrenergic activity at the somato-dendritic α1-adrenoceptors, which enhances serotonergic neurotransmission. So it can be seen that these drugs have an effect on the NA system, which in turn leads to a boost in the levels of 5-HT. Although the mechanism of action is slightly different, the drugs still possess a number of unwanted side effects including insomnia, sweating, dizziness, paraesthesia and postural hypotension.

Classical (non-selective) monoamine oxidase inhibitors

Examples of the monoamine oxidase inhibitors (MAOIs) include phenelzine (Nardil®) and tranylcypramine (Parnate®). These drugs work by inhibiting the enzyme responsible for the breakdown of the monoamine neurotransmitters, monoamine oxidase-A (MAO-A). Consequently, the inhibition of this enzyme leads to the elevation of the monoamine levels back to what they should be. It is not without cost though as can be seen with the unwanted side effects of dose-related hypotension, irritability and insomnia.

Non-pharmacological management of depression

It is important to note that drugs are only part of the answer to depression and it may be appropriate to use one or more alternative, or additional, management strategies.

One non-pharmacological approach to the management of depression is **cognitive behavioural therapy (CBT).** CBT is a collaborative, structured and time-limited intervention that is designed to assist patients in altering the behavioural patterns and/or negative thoughts that are associated with their condition (Donaghy et al 2008). For example, people with depression are characterised by their negative views about themselves, the world around them and the future (e.g. 'my family would be better off without me'). In CBT, patients are encouraged to explore and challenge these views, which are often automatic, and discover alternative ways of thinking and acting. There is a considerable body of evidence on the effects of CBT on depression and a range of other conditions (e.g. fatigue, chronic pain) since it was introduced over 30 years ago. A meta-analysis comparing CBT with antidepressants in people with depression found that CBT was equally effective, however CBT seemed to be slightly more effective at 12 months follow-up, while the chance of relapse was reduced (NICE 2009).

Current UK recommendations for the treatment for depression in adults can be found in the National Institute for Health and Clinical Excellence Clinical Guideline 90 (NICE 2009). This comprises a stepped care model with a range of treatment approaches, ranging from education and active monitoring to psychological and psychosocial interventions, medication, electroconvulsive treatment and inpatient care for different levels of depression.

Another type of non-pharmacological intervention for depression is **physical activity**, defined as 'any bodily movement produced by skeletal muscle that requires energy expenditure above that used at rest'(USDHHS 2008). A specific type of physical activity is exercise, defined as physical activity that is planned, structured, repetitive and purposive in the sense that it aims to improve or maintain one or more components of physical fitness (cf. Caspersen et al 1985). Research on the effects of physical activity on depression in the general population has been ongoing for several decades (see Biddle and Mutrie 2008). A Cochrane systematic review examining the effects of exercise on depression found that, compared to a control intervention, exercise had a large clinical effect at the end of the intervention, which diminished to a moderate effect at follow-up (Mead et al 2009). Interestingly, when exercise was compared with cognitive therapies (e.g. CBT) and antidepressants, exercise was equally effective. Although many factors remain uncertain (e.g. there is insufficient evidence to recommend any specific type or intensity of exercise), current guidance recommends exercise for people with mild to moderate depression, preferably a form of exercise that they enjoy (Mead et al 2009, NICE 2009).

Explanations for the effects of exercise on mood include physiological factors (e.g. the release of endorphins that result in the experience of pleasure, and neurotransmitters such as monoamines that improve mood; a reduction of stress hormones such as cortisol), psychological factors (e.g. distraction from negative thoughts; the acquisition of new skills and goal attainment that yield a sense of mastery, as well as improved body image that enhances self-esteem), in addition to social factors (e.g. peer support).

Research on the effects of exercise specifically in people with neurological conditions is less well developed, however. In stroke, a number of small-scale qualitative studies indicate that physical activity can improve mood (e.g. Carin-Levy et al 2009, Reed et al 2010, Sharma et al 2011). However, a recent Cochrane systematic review on exercise and physical fitness training after stroke reported that effects on mood were inconsistent between trials, and that no conclusions could be drawn (Brazzelli et al 2011). In PD, a meta-analysis of the effects of exercise on mood only included four studies, none of which reported a significant improvement of depression following exercise (Goodwin et al 2008). In MS, an RCT comparing endurance training with a control intervention did not find any significant improvements in depression (Dettmers et al 2009).

However, based on evidence from the general population, it would be reasonable to speculate that physical activity has the potential to improve depression in people with long-term neurological conditions, but further robust clinical trials need to be undertaken to put this hypothesis to the test.

Emotional difficulties in people with common long-term neurological conditions: an overview

In this section, we will provide an overview of frequently reported difficulties with emotion and motivation in people with the most common conditions of the central nervous system, i.e. stroke, AD, PD and TBI.

Stroke

The most common emotional difficulties after stroke comprise depression and anxiety, while emotionalism, so-called 'catastrophic' reactions, anosognosic excitement, indifference reactions and disinhibition can also be seen.

Depression is reported in 20–40% of patients in the first 2 weeks, in 19–55% at 1 year and in 9–41% at 3 years after stroke (Staub and Carota 2005). There is overlap between the symptoms of depression and those of anxiety, which makes it difficult to distinguish between these two problems. **Generalised anxiety disorder (GAD)** involves excessive worry about everyday events, with a range of autonomic symptoms such as dizziness, increased heart rate and shortness of breath. In a 3-year follow-up study in Sweden, 28% of stroke patients in the acute stage were classified as having GAD, of which half also had major depressive symptoms (Åström, 1996). At 1 year, 24% of stroke survivors had GAD, of which again more than half had concurrent major depression; and at 3 years, these figures were virtually unchanged.

Estimates of mood disorders after stroke vary widely between studies because of differences in definitions and assessment tools, as well as difficulties in assessing mood in a population where fatigue, cognitive and communication problems are also common (Hackett et al 2005). Despite these variations, there is no doubt that anxiety and depression are common and important problems after stroke. In a needs survey in the UK (McKevitt et al 2010), mood disorders were reported by stroke survivors as some of the most important 'unmet needs'. This is because the impact of post-stroke anxiety and depression can be extensive and affect rehabilitation outcomes such as independence in activities of daily living (ADL) and morbidity and mortality in the longer-term, as

well as family relations (Platz 2010). It can be difficult to identify from the literature which is 'chicken' and which is 'egg'; depression may lead to functional impairment, and conversely functional impairment may cause depression (Staub and Carota 2005). People who are depressed may lack the motivation for rehabilitation and see little point in engaging in this process, resulting in poorer outcomes. Conversely, poor physical function may make people feel helpless and hopeless, which are hallmarks of depression. Early diagnosis and treatment of post-stroke mood disorders is, therefore, of utmost importance.

A Cochrane systematic review of interventions for depression after stroke (Hackett et al 2008) found that antidepressants could lead to a complete remission and symptom improvement. However, there was also an increase in adverse events (e.g. gastrointestinal problems and confusion). There was no evidence that psychological interventions (including counselling, motivational interviewing, cognitive-behavioural therapy) were effective, although very few studies were included in the review.

Emotionalism (also known as pathological laughing and crying, or emotional liability), is described as 'the habit of weakly yielding to emotion' (House et al 1989). It affects around 20–25% of patients in the first 6 months after stroke and, although some recover, about half continue to experience this problem in the longer term (Hackett et al 2010). Patients with emotionalism typically react more quickly and/or more strongly to situations that would not normally evoke an emotional reaction such as crying or laughing. Patients – and their families – often find emotionalism upsetting, and in some people it may lead to social withdrawal to avoid embarrassment. There is tentative evidence that antidepressants may be effective in reducing emotionalism after stroke (Hackett et al 2010).

So-called **'catastrophic' reactions**, e.g. a patient showing increasing feelings of upset, sometimes followed by an outburst of crying, may be seen in stroke survivors with severe sensory and motor impairments of the right side of the body accompanied by Broca's dysphasia (Gainotti 2003). In these patients, problems with expressive communication (yet with often largely intact comprehension, see Chapter 11) compound an already difficult situation. Imagine yourself in a situation where you have had a stroke, are unable to explain how you feel or ask questions, and yet you are acutely aware that others are struggling to understand you – and you can probably begin to understand some of the background to 'catastrophic' reactions.

'**Anosognosic excitement**' may be observed in patients with mild sensori-motor disability and Wernicke's dysphasia. As the chapter on communication will explain, patients with this type of dysphasia may produce speech that sounds fluent, but may not make much sense. The person affected, however, is often unaware of this as their key problem is speech comprehension, including understanding their own speech. The animation sometimes seen in such patients is, therefore, known as 'anosognosic excitement' (Gainotti 2003); in other words, it is excitement in a person who does not seem to be fully aware of their situation.

Indifference reactions may be observed in patients with unilateral neglect, particularly following right parietal or frontal lobe lesions (see Chapters 9 and 12). The apparent lack of concern for one's situation may be related to a lack of attention to, and awareness of, the affected side of the body (Gainotti 2003). In the chapter on executive dysfunction, we have seen that frontal lobe lesions may be associated with an apparent lack of concern, or apathy.

In contrast to indifference reactions, '**disinhibition**' refers to a situation where a person has difficulty controlling their emotions (e.g. frustration), or adjusting their verbal and non-verbal communication to a situation. Disinhibition is more common in people with traumatic brain injury, as will be explained below.

Parkinson's disease

Emotional problems encountered most frequently in people with PD include depression, anxiety and psychosis. **Depression** is the most common emotional disorder in this population and has been reported in 40% of cases (Stocchi and Brusa 2000). Patients diagnosed with this neurodegenerative condition may have low mood, feel pessimistic, sad and irritable, have suicidal thoughts (although relatively few suicidal actions), but may lack the feelings of guilt that can be found in endogenous depression. Patients who experience the 'on-off' phenomenon (i.e. a reduction in symptoms when medication is active, compared with when its impact ceases) apparently have a higher chance of experiencing depression. Depression also places a considerable burden on the patient's carer and wider family.

The causes of depression in PD are complex and poorly understood; underlying mechanisms include the role of neurotransmitters, existing susceptibility

to depression, side effects of medication, while psychosocial factors such as the response to the illness and relationship difficulties may also play a role.

Diagnosing depression in PD is not straightforward, as the signs and symptoms of depression overlap to some extent with the motor symptoms of PD (e.g. fatigue, slowed physical function). Therapists may erroneously label patients with PD as 'uninterested' or 'lacking in motivation', therefore it is essential to understand that signs such as a lack of facial expression and spontaneous behaviour, dysprosody (i.e. the lack of emotional expression in speech) or low mood may well be physiological manifestations of the disease itself, and/or depression. Health professionals need to look out for possible signs of depression in people with PD and refer appropriately.

At present, there is insufficient evidence to recommend any specific form of antidepressant therapy in PD, while some antidepressant medications that are effective in the general population may worsen the motor symptoms of PD. It is clear that more research is required in this area to improve treatment for this debilitating condition (National Collaborating Centre for Chronic Conditions 2006).

Psychosis is a mental health condition in which the person has lost their connection with reality. Examples are hallucinations, in which the person perceives stimuli that aren't there (e.g. believing there to be someone in the room with them), and delusions, in which the person has a belief that is unfounded (e.g. that the country is staging a party to celebrate their discharge from hospital). Around 40% of people with PD may have hallucinations (Fenelon et al 2000), although some patients may not report their symptoms, out of fear of being judged insane.

The causes of psychosis in PD are not well understood but may be related to polypharmacy (i.e. the ingestion of multiple pharmacological agents for a range of co-morbidities and symptoms), concurrent illness (e.g. infection) or dementia, which is commonly associated with PD (Aarsland et al 2003). In any case, health-care professionals should carefully explain to patients and carers the organic basis of their psychosis, to alleviate any anxieties about patients 'losing their mind'.

Alzheimer's disease

The hallmark of AD, a specific form of dementia, is cognitive decline. However, a range of **behavioural and psychological symptoms of dementia (BPSD)** associated with AD are now recognised as a major component of the dementia syndrome. These symptoms, which occur in up to 90% of cases (Robert et al 2005), have a major impact on the quality of life of the patient and their family, and determine to a large extent the type of care that is required.

The most commonly found emotional disorders in AD are apathy, anxiety and depression (Robert et al 2005). Depression and anxiety are estimated to occur in around 40% of people in the early stage of the disease (Gainotti 2003). This is thought to arise from patients' awareness of the condition and its prognosis, which is often still intact at that time. As the illness progresses and self-awareness diminishes, the prevalence of depression is likely to decrease. Common behavioural symptoms in AD include irritability, aberrant motor behaviour, agitation, aggression and disinhibition.

The causes underlying BPSD in AD are complex and likely to reflect an interaction between biological factors associated with the disease process, and psychological as well as social factors. It terms of biological factors, apathy has been associated with reduced perfusion in the anterior cingulate and subcortical structures in the frontal lobe. Depression in AD is associated with reduced cerebral blood flow in frontal, temporal and parietal lobes, while in patients demonstrating agitation, cholinergic deficits and a higher number of neurofibrillary tangles in the orbitofrontal cortex and anterior cingulate region have been found (Robert et al 2005). In terms of psychological factors, aggression can be a defensive reaction in response to fear in an individual who feels disoriented in time and place. Some relatively simple methods (e.g. colour coding) may be effective in helping people remember important locations such as the bathroom. The nature of social interaction can also have a considerable influence on the behaviour of the person with AD and education can assist family and carers in managing challenging behaviour.

Given the complexity of BPSD, management strategies for people with AD are recommended that adopt a comprehensive biopsychosocial approach, including pharmacological interventions, counselling, patient and family education, carer support, respite care as well as legal advice (NICE–SCIE 2007, Haberstroh et al 2010).

Traumatic brain injury

Following the acute stage of traumatic brain injury (TBI), common behavioural and emotional disorders are emotional outbursts, apathy, depression and anxiety (Gainotti 2003).

Some of these problems are a direct result of the injury, e.g. during a closed head injury, the acceleration and deceleration forces primarily affect the orbitofrontal region, damaging pathways between the frontal lobes and the limbic system. The frontal lobes are involved in governing behaviour, while the limbic system is involved in emotion, and the pathway between them plays an essential role in governing emotion and motivation. As we have seen in Chapter 12, a common consequence of TBI is **executive dysfunction**, characterised by difficulties setting goals, sticking to plan, initiating action, solving problems and governing one's behaviour and emotions. Especially since TBI affects predominantly young adult males (Bruns and Hauser 2003) who are often at a stage in their lives where they are establishing independence, these problems can have a major impact on relationships, leisure opportunities and employment prospects. Social isolation is common in the later stages after TBI, which can lead to further depression (Morton and Wehman 1995). Some people with TBI may need to return to their parental home following discharge for the required supervision and care, while others need longer term support in behavioural units.

Emotional outbursts may be explained as being the direct neurological consequences of damage to pathways and centres that govern emotion, often in combination with a reaction to the situation, which may be a prospect of permanent disability, limited self-expression and reduced autonomy. A combination of frustration and sense of helplessness can contribute to such emotional outbursts.

One of the difficulties with challenging behaviour in TBI is the lack of insight (**anosognosia**) that affects a considerable proportion of patients. This can make interaction with the person affected particularly difficult, as patients may not be aware of their disruptive behaviour or how this affects others. Patients may be seen as 'insensitive', placing further strain on relationships with family, friends and health-care professionals. Spouses may indicate that the person 'is not the one they married' and many relationships are affected by these behavioural changes. Interventions for emotional problems in TBI are manifold, as we discussed in the case of stroke or AD, ranging from pharmacological interventions to behavioural strategies and counselling in individual, family as well as group settings (Gainotti 2003).

Explanations for emotional difficulties in people with neurological conditions

From the previous sections, we hope that it has become clear how complex a phenomenon 'emotion' really is. Unsurprisingly, there is no simple explanation for disorders of emotion in people with neurological conditions. Broadly speaking, explanations can be formulated from two different perspectives:

- A biomedical perspective, i.e. at the levels of the nervous system as an organ, its constituting parts comprising neural pathways, centres, individual neurones, neurotransmitters and other molecules
- A psychosocial perspective, i.e. at the levels of psychological functions and social circumstances of the individual in their context.

A biomedical perspective on emotion: emotion and the brain

A biomedical perspective tries to explain emotional disorders (e.g. depression) on the basis of specific lesions in brain areas, neural pathways and neurotransmitter systems, with a view to design interventions that target these structures and functions.

The search for a brain area responsible for emotion in the first half of the 20th century was dubbed by LeDoux (1998) as a quest for the 'holy grail' (p. 73). Having identified specific cortical areas responsible for speech and vision (Chapter 5), scientists set out to discover the centre dedicated to emotion. Early attempts in 1930 led to a circuit proposed by Papez. In 1949, MacLean proposed the limbic system theory (also known as rhinencephalon or 'smell brain'). The term 'limbus' (which is Greek for 'rim') alludes to the shape of the system that includes the amygdala, hippocampus and thalamus (see Fig. 13.2). MacLean proposed his 'Triune Brain' theory in 1970, which purports that the brain consists of three different layers, each of which developed through evolution of the species. The most primitive part is the reptilian brain, which is concerned with survival and emotion. The next layer up is the paleomammalian brain, which governs social behaviour. Finally, homo sapiens has a top layer, i.e. the neomammalian brain, which is in charge of sophisticated behaviour such as language and reasoning. You will have noticed that

'emotion' in this model is assigned to the bottom layer, consistent with the idea that emotions prevail if this most 'primitive' part of the brain dominates the more developed parts. MacLean's limbic system theory was ground-breaking, as it provided an innovative synthesis of evolution theory, psychology and biology. It captured the public imagination to such an extent that references to the 'limbic system' can still be found in popular books on the topic. However, a number of weaknesses eventually led to the demise of this theory, including the fact that the anatomical description of the 'limbic system' is inconsistent (depending on which textbook you consult, you may come across different component parts). Furthermore, it is now known that some parts of the limbic system are not dedicated to emotion but to other functions (e.g. the hippocampus is mainly involved in memory). Importantly, the theory is overly simplistic; one only has to compare the serious attacks that can be committed by humans, with the intricate collaborative behaviour of ants, to question the assumption of the function of the 'neomammalian brain'.

In this section, we have only given an overview in a nutshell of the search for the brain centre of emotion and readers are referred to LeDoux (1998) for a more in-depth discussion. We conclude this fascinating story here by saying that the quest for the holy grail ran out of steam. When you think about the logic underpinning this endeavour, this is perhaps not surprising: consider the complexity of our emotional lives and the diversity of body systems involved in emotion, and it is clear that 'emotion' is not a single entity. A 1–1 correspondence between 'emotion' and 'the brain' is thus implausible, and the quest for a single centre responsible for emotion was therefore misguided.

A more contemporaneous interpretation is that the scientific investigation of emotion should distinguish between different types of emotions (e.g. fear, sadness, disgust). Each emotion has a different function and is supported by a dedicated, integrated neural network (Greenfield 2000). As you can see, this interpretation of the neural basis of emotion fits in with the more contemporary view of 'functional localisation' of the brain, discussed earlier (Chapter 5).

Pathways mediating emotion

The circuitry linking the various brain areas involved in processing emotional information utilises a number of chemical neurotransmitters. The neurotransmitters implicated in processing the ascending information are the monoamines serotonin (5-hydroxytryptamine; 5-HT), noradrenaline (NA) and dopamine (DA). Details of these neuronal pathways can be seen in Figures 13.2–13.4.

The main point of origin for the serotonergic neurones is the raphe nucleus (see Fig. 13.2), with one of the key destinations being the limbic system (the hypothalamus, the hippocampus and the amygdala). The noradrenergic pathways, on the other hand, primarily originate in the locus coeruleus. However, it is those noradrenergic pathways that have their cell bodies in the lateral tegmental nuclei (see Fig. 13.3) that project up to the limbic system. Finally, there are a number of dopaminergic pathways in the brain (see Fig. 13.4), but it is the mesolimbic projections that are involved in emotion. It is these ascending pathways travelling to the limbic areas that have a key role to play in emotional behaviour.

In MacLean's model of the triune brain, emotion was seen as a primitive force, which had to be firmly kept in check by reason. In a way, 'emotion' was judged to be inferior to reason; a potent source of bias that could cloud and confound our thinking and decision making. Should we attempt to ban emotions from our reasoning altogether? Intuitively, we might think this is a good idea; decisions should be rational and not biased by our subjective feelings. However, in a thought-provoking book, Damasio (1994) elegantly argues that it is precisely the *absence* of

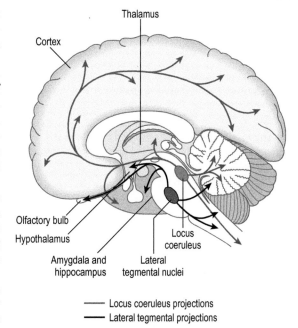

Fig. 13.3 • Noradrenergic pathways in the brain. From Brody, with permission

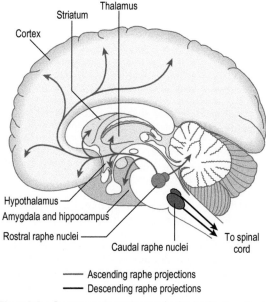

Fig. 13.2 • Serotonergic pathways in the brain. From Brody, with permission

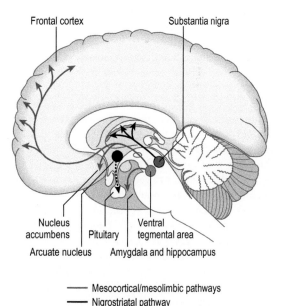

Fig. 13.4 • Dopaminergic pathways in the brain. From Brody, with permission

emotion in decision making that can lead to disastrous errors. He uses detailed case studies of people with executive dysfunction to support his theory. As we have seen in Chapter 12, people with executive dysfunction typically have a reduced ability to make decisions and a limited awareness of their situation. Interestingly, when asked to imagine fictitious scenarios (e.g. being fired by their employer, or rejected by their loved one), they also tend to demonstrate diminished emotional reactions compared to healthy controls.

Normal people tend to experience emotions when considering such scenarios. Damasio labelled these 'secondary emotions', as they are associated with the consideration of imaginary outcomes, i.e. the feelings associated with a prediction of what might happen. Consider choosing between the following two options: 'I will/will not get out of bed and arrive at work on time to see my first patient'. Without much difficulty, most of us would choose the former, probably because we experience a pang of fear and shame, associated with imagining the second option! Damasio argues that people routinely use such secondary emotions, which act as 'somatic markers', to make decisions. These emotions are called 'somatic' because of their physical quality, and Damasio's theory is known as the **'somatic marker hypothesis'**. Options associated with a strong negative somatic marker (as in our example) are quickly ruled out, which reduces the number of options, which in turn simplifies the decision-making process.

So, how does the lack of secondary emotions in people with executive dysfunction affect their decision making? The diminished ability to conjure up secondary emotions renders the emotional landscape 'flat' as it were; with no particular option standing out either way. Therefore, people with executive dysfunction may easily choose the wrong option, and arrive late for their first patient. You only need to do this a few times and you lose your job. So on the face of it, the decision not to get out of bed is clearly irrational, as it jeopardises one's social survival, but its origin can be found in a lack of emotional guidance, the absence of an emotional 'gut feeling' (or somatic marker) that steers one's decisions.

Although we have only discussed the tip of the iceberg of Damasio's somatic marker hypothesis here, you can probably see the importance of a sound partnership between emotion and reason, or feeling and executive function, in making decisions in the interest of survival.

Interestingly, from a neuroscience perspective, neural networks mediating emotion and executive functions also partially overlap, including the prefrontal cortex and limbic system, and pathways connecting these areas. Thus, any type of brain lesion affecting part of this system may lead to problems with reasoning and decision making, as well as difficulty governing one's emotions.

A psychosocial perspective on emotion

We need to be cautious against an overly simplistic interpretation of emotion as a purely biomedical phenomenon, however. Interestingly, the degree of emotional difficulty experienced by a disabled person is often not correlated with the degree of disability itself (Gainotti 2003). Consider the clinical Case study 13.1. on the next page.

As the comparison of these two patients shows, the key question is: what does the disability *mean* to the individual? How does it impact on their lives? Try and imagine the impact of a neurological condition on one's state of mind. A traumatic brain injury or stroke is an acute event, which inflicts a crisis on the life of the individual and family.

Robert McCrum (2008) published his own moving personal account of the impact of stroke on his life:

'The conundrum of stroke recovery is that while one's conscious efforts are devoted to recovering one's lost self, the cruel fact is that this former self is irretrievably shattered into a thousand pieces, and try as one may to glue those bits together again, the reconstituted version of the old self will never be better than a cracked, imperfect assembly, a constant mockery of one's former, successful individuality' (p. 148).

It is only months later that the full impact of what happened fully emerged:

'I realised, as I got better, that I was wanting to say goodbye to a person who had, in a sense, died nine months before, and I had to say goodbye to his life as well. I came to believe that just as a part of my brain was now irretrievably dead, so a part of my former activity and lifestyle was defunct, too.' (p. 205)

So while in the early stage after his stroke, McCrum attempted to re-habilitate (i.e. restore his previous self), eventually he realised that in his case this was unrealistic, and that he needed to accept that life would never be the same again. From then

Case study 13.1

Different emotional responses to cognitive impairment following traumatic brain injury

Two young adults with traumatic brain injury, independently of each other, attend a regional neurological rehabilitation centre for a routine check-up of their orthotics.

The patients come from completely different backgrounds but are comparable in terms of level of disability, lesion type and level of cognitive impairment, characterised by distractibility, poor memory and high levels of fatigue when engaged in activities such as reading and problem solving.

However, where they differ considerably is in terms of their emotional reaction to their cognitive impairment. The first patient experiences very high levels of anxiety; she worries constantly, feels 'useless' and has problems getting to sleep. In contrast, the second patient appears at peace with his situation, despite his considerable cognitive difficulties.

A key factor explaining the difference in anxiety between these two patients is the personal significance of the cognitive impairment and the impact this has on their individual lives; the first patient came to the UK from a developing country with the aim to undertake a PhD – a prestigious project for the student's extended family, which required considerable financial investment. The patient indicates she feels under tremendous pressure to be successful in the eyes of her family who have expressed their hope that she will lift them out of poverty following the completion of her PhD.

In contrast, the second patient works in the family business; a role has been created especially for him that allows him to have a meaningful occupation within his now limited abilities. His role has been adapted to such an extent that he is unable to identify any issues with his work and appears unaware of his actual level of cognitive impairment.

on, he focused his efforts more on 'habilitation'; developing new activities and a new lifestyle.

In conditions where some recovery may be possible, there is the important element of hope. In neurodegenerative conditions such as PD and AD, however, hope may eventually be extinguished, potentially rendering the emotional landscape of the patient and their family particularly bleak.

In conclusion, emotional difficulties, including depression and anxiety, loss and grief reactions, are common in people with long-term neurological conditions – whether as a biological consequence of the condition, a reaction to the situation as a whole, or a mixture of the two. Important psychological factors related to the emotional experience associated with (neuro)disability are the personal significance to the individual, their ability to cope, and their awareness of the situation (Gainotti 2003). Family and significant others can play a crucial role in coping with what may be a life-changing condition.

Summary and implications for rehabilitation

This chapter has given an overview of the most frequently reported emotional problems in people with stroke, PD, AD and TBI. These problems, which include depression and anxiety, apathy and emotional outbursts, are common – however they are often under-reported, under-diagnosed and under-treated. Despite our limited understanding of the complex causes underlying these disorders, they can have a major impact on rehabilitation outcomes, autonomy, employment, relationships and quality of life in general. They are often amongst the most difficult problems for the patient and their families to cope with. In addition, they are challenging for the health professionals involved, who need a sound understanding of the aetiology of these problems in order to understand and support patients and their family, and in order to refer for assessment and treatment as required.

Given the multifactorial nature of emotional disorders associated with long-term neurological conditions, no single approach is likely to be sufficient. As we have seen, a comprehensive, patient-centred, biopsychosocial approach is often required, integrating pharmacological, behavioural and psychosocial interventions for the patient and their family.

It is clear that much more research is urgently required into the causes of these debilitating problems, in order to inform the design of more effective treatment strategies.

SELF-ASSESSMENT QUESTIONS

1. Explain the difficulties associated with defining the concept of 'emotion'.
2. Describe the most common emotional disorders in people with stroke, TBI, PD and AD, and their potential impact on rehabilitation outcomes and life in general.
3. Explain these emotional disorders in terms of their neurological, psychological and social factors.
4. Outline the basic principles of our current understanding of the biological relationship between the brain and emotion, in particular in the case of depression.
5. Discuss the strengths and limitations of the main theories related to depression.
6. Explain the mechanism of action of the major classes of antidepressant medication.
7. Discuss the importance of understanding emotional difficulties in people with long-term neurological conditions from a comprehensive biopsychosocial perspective.

Further reading

Beauby, J.D., 1998. The Diving Bell and the Butterfly. Fourth Estate, London.

Pritchard, P., 1999. The Totem Pole and a Whole New Adventure. Constable, London.

Redfield-Jamison, K., 1995. An Unquiet Mind. A memoir of mood and madness, Picador, London.

References

Aarsland, D., Andersen, K., Larsen, J.P., et al., 2003. Prevalence and characteristics of dementia in Parkinson Disease: an 8-year prospective study. Arch. Neurol. 60, 387–392.

Åström, M., 1996. Generalized anxiety disorder in stroke patients. A 3-year longitudinal study. Stroke 27, 270–275.

Berthoz, A., 2003. Emotion and Reason. The cognitive neuroscience of decision making. Oxford University Press, Oxford.

Biddle, S.J.H., Mutrie, N., 2008. Psychology of Physical Activity: Determinants, well-being and interventions, second ed. Routledge, Oxon.

Brazzelli, M., Saunders, D.H., Greig, C.A., et al., 2011. Physical fitness training for stroke patients. Cochrane Database Syst. Rev 11, CD003316. doi:10.1002/14651858.

Bruns, Jr., J., Hauser, W.A., 2003. The epidemiology of traumatic brain injury: a review. Epilepsia 44 (S10), 2–10.

Cappa, C.F., 2001. Cognitive Neurology. An introduction. Imperial College Press, London.

Carin-Levy, G., Kendall, M., Young, A., et al., 2009. The psychosocial effects of exercise and relaxation classes for persons surviving a stroke. Can. J. Occup. Ther. 76, 73–76.

Caspersen, C.J., Powell, K.E., Christenson, G.M., 1985. Physical activity, exercise, and physical fitness: definitions and distinctions for health-related research. Public Health Rep. 100, 126–131.

Damasio, A., 1994. Descartes' Error. Emotion, reason and the human brain. Penguin Books, New York.

Darwin, C., 1865. The Expression of Emotion in Man and Animals. Vol. 23 of the Works of Charles Darwin.

Dettmers, C., Sulzmann, M., Ruchay-Plössl, A., et al., 2009. Endurance exercise improves walking distance in MS patients with fatigue. Acta Neurol. Scand. 120, 251–257.

Donaghy, M., Nicol, M., Davidson, K., 2008. Cognitive-behavioural Interventions in Physiotherapy and Occupational Therapy. Butterworth Heinemann Elsevier, Edinburgh.

Ekman, P., 1984. Expression and the nature of emotion. In: Sherer, K., Ekman, P. (Eds.), Approaches to Emotion. LEA, Hillsdale, NJ.

Fenelon, G., Mahieux, F., Huon, R., et al., 2000. Hallucinations in Parkinson's disease: prevalence, phenomenology and risk factors. Brain 123, 733–745.

Gainotti, G., 2003. Assessment and treatment of emotional disorders. In: Halligan, P.W., Kischka, U., Marshall, J.C. (Eds.), Handbook of Clinical Neuropsychology. Oxford University Press, Oxford, pp. 368–386.

Goodwin, V.A., Richards, S.H., Taylor, R.S., et al., 2008. The effectiveness of exercise interventions for people with Parkinson's disease: a systematic review and meta-analysis. Mov. Disord. 23, 631–640.

Greenfield, S.A., 2000. The Private Life of the Brain. Allen Lane, The Penguin Press, London.

Haberstroh, J., Hampel, H., Pantel, J., 2010. Optimal management of Alzheimer's disease patients: Clinical guidelines and family advice. Neuropsychiatr. Dis. Treat. 6, 243–253.

Hackett, M.L., Yapa, C., Parag, V., et al., 2005. Frequency of depression after stroke: a systematic review of observational studies. Stroke 36, 1330–1340.

Hackett, M.L., Anderson, C.S., House, A., et al., 2008. Interventions for treating depression after stroke. Cochrane Database Syst. Rev. 4, CD003437. doi:10.1002/14651858.

Hackett, M.L., Yang, M., Anderson, C.S., et al., 2010. Pharmaceutical interventions for emotionalism after stroke. Cochrane Database Syst. Rev. 2, CD003690. doi:10.1002/14651858.

House, A., Dennis, M., Molyneux, A., et al., 1989. Emotionalism after stroke. Br. Med. J. 298 (6679), 991–994.

LeDoux, J., 1998. The Emotional Brain. Simon & Schuster, New York.

McCrum, R., 2008. My Year Off. Rediscovering life after a stroke. Picador, London.

McKevitt, C., Fudge, N., Redfern, J., et al., 2010. The Stroke Association UK Stroke Survivor Needs Survey. The Stroke Association, London.

Mead, G.E., Morley, W., Campbell, P., et al., 2009. Exercise for depression. Cochrane Database Syst. Rev 3, CD004366. doi:10.1002/14651858.

Morton, M.V., Wehman, T., 1995. Psychosocial and emotional sequelae of individuals with traumatic brain injury: a literature review and recommendations. Brain Inj. 9, 81–92.

National Collaborating Centre for Chronic Conditions, 2006. Parkinson's Disease: National clinical guideline for diagnosis and management in primary and secondary care. Royal College of Physicians, London.

National Institute for Health and Clinical Excellence (NICE), Social Care Institute for Excellence (SCIE), 2007. Dementia: A NICE–SCIE Guideline on supporting people with dementia and their carers in health and social care. Available online from: http://www.nice.org.uk/nicemedia/

pdf/CG42Dementiafinal.pdf (accessed 20.011.2011).

National Institute of Health and Clinical Excellence, 2009. Clinical guidance 90: The treatment and Management of depression in Adults (update). Available online: http://publications. nice.org.uk/depression-cg90 (accessed 08.01.2012).

Platz, T., 2010. Depression and its effects after stroke. In: Nudo, R.J., Cramer, S.C. (Eds.), Brain Repair after Stroke. Cambridge University Press, Cambridge, pp. 145–162.

Reed, M., Harrington, R., Duggan, A., et al., 2010. Meeting stroke survivors' perceived needs: a qualitative study of a community-based exercise and education scheme. Clin. Rehabil. 24, 16–25.

Robert, P.H., Verhey, F.R.J., Byrne, E.J., et al., 2005. Grouping for behavioral and psychological symptoms in dementia: clinical and biological aspects. Consensus paper of the European Alzheimer disease consortium. Eur. Psychiatry 20, 490–496.

Schildkraut, J.J., 1965. The catecholamine hypothesis of affective disorders: a review of supporting evidence. Am. J. Psychiatry 122, 609–622.

Sharma, H., Bulley, C., van Wijck, F., 2011. Experiences of an exercise referral scheme from the perspective of people with chronic stroke: a qualitative study. Physiotherapy doi:org/10.1016/j. physio.2011.05.004.

Smith, R.E., 1993. Psychology. West Publishing Co, Minneapolis/Saint Paul.

Staub, F., Carota, A., 2005. Depression and fatigue after stroke. In: Barnes, M., Dobkin, B., Bougousslavsky, J. (Eds.), Recovery after Stroke. Cambridge University Press, Cambridge, pp. 556–579.

Stocchi, F., Brusa, L., 2000. Cognition and emotion in different stages and subtypes of Parkinson's disease. J. Neurol 247 (Suppl. 2) II/114–II/121.

U.S. Department of Health and Human Services (USDHHS), 2008. Physical Activity Guidelines for Americans. Chapter 1: Introducing the 2008 Physical Activity Guidelines for Americans. Available online at: http://www.health.gov/paguidelines/ guidelines/chapter1.aspx (accessed 04.11.2011).

Waller, D.G., Renwick, A.G., Hillier, K., 2001. Medical Pharmacology and Therapeutics, second ed. W.B. Saunders, Philadelphia.

Other disorders associated with neurological conditions: fatigue, sleep disorders, incontinence and sexual dysfunction

14

CHAPTER CONTENTS

LEARNING OUTCOMES

At the end of this chapter, you should be able to:

1. demonstrate an understanding of the prevalence and impact of a range of problems on the lives of people with neurological conditions, i.e. sleep disorders, fatigue, dysphagia, incontinence and sexual dysfunction

2. describe typical alterations in patterns of sleep and fatigue in people with neurological conditions compared to healthy people, and discuss the impact fatigue may have on quality of life

3. explain the physiological processes underlying normal continence function, and discuss which treatments may be available for incontinence in people with neurological conditions

4. explain the physiological processes underlying normal sexual function, and describe some common forms of sexual dysfunction that may result from a neurological condition

5. discuss the potential impact that sexual dysfunction may have on relationships and discuss which treatments may be available for people with a neurological condition.

Introduction

The previous chapters of this book have discussed a range of common problems that can be encountered in people with different neurological conditions, including perceptuo-motor impairments, cognitive and communication impairments, executive disorders and problems with emotion and motivation. This chapter is slightly different in that it is intended to provide you with an overview of a range of different types of problems, some of which may be under-reported, but which nevertheless may be distressing and have a considerable impact on people's lives.

We will begin by introducing you to problems with sleep and fatigue, which are very common across different neurological conditions, and which can have a detrimental effect on rehabilitation outcomes and quality of life. We will then discuss problems with swallowing, which have important safety implications. We will finish this chapter with a discussion on problems with continence and sexual function. These problems may be 'hidden' in some cases, as for many patients it can be difficult to disclose that they are experiencing difficulties in these areas, while some therapists may be too embarrassed to ask – or are unaware of possible treatments. However, it is important to acknowledge problems in these domains, as they can have a tremendous impact on relationships and quality of life, while solutions may be available. For each of these problems, we will explain the possible causes, explore the possible impact on people's lives, and look what solutions may be available.

Sleep and fatigue

Sleep is important. We would also consider that it is relatively easy to define: it is surely quite simple; — when we are not awake, we are asleep. Without sleep we can become irritable and less able to concentrate. Being awake, however, is not even that simple a concept. There can be some days where we feel really alert, vibrant and ready to take on any challenge; while there can be other days when we feel sluggish, disinterested and lacking in concentration. These different levels of consciousness are set by neural systems that influence the cerebral cortex, the activity of which can be modified by various neurological disorders – but more on that later.

Unlike sleep, fatigue is much more difficult to define as it is very subjective. There is a real grey area where it can be difficult to differentiate between tiredness and fatigue. Under normal circumstances fatigue is caused by a relative level of overexertion and can, therefore, be reversed by an adequate period of rest. Another problem with reaching a definition is that the fact that, under certain circumstances, fatigue can be enjoyable, e.g. the stimulation of the reward pathway that must be taking place as the athlete wins his/her Olympic marathon [I'll have to assume that this is correct as the only running I have ever done was a bath]. Since it is difficult to define fatigue in general terms it is, of course, difficult to define it from the clinical perspective as well. To put it as simply as possible, fatigue can be defined as a problem with starting and/or maintaining some level of activity. Our level of fatigue is dependent on a number of complex interactions between various systems within our body (voluntary effort and central motor systems, homeostatic mechanisms, the autonomic nervous system, the motivational and emotional centres of our brain), as well as on external factors, such as temperature of the environment.

Sleeping and waking

It would be helpful to start by identifying the changes that are going on in the brain that lead us from wakefulness into sleep. The feeling of drowsiness that we experience as we approach sleep occurs as the cells of the cerebral cortex become synchronous. This synchrony is brought about by a regular sequence of pulses travelling up to the cortex from non-specific nuclei. As a consequence of this pulsing, neuronal signals arriving in the cerebral cortex from the peripheral sensory receptors are no longer received properly, making us unaware of them. This ' thalamic pulsing' of the cortex does not take place when we are awake. During our waking hours the thalamus is under an excitatory control from the **reticular formation** of the brain stem, which switches off the pulsing. It is the way that the aforementioned brain areas interact with each other that is responsible for the control of our regular **sleep/wake cycle**, including aspects of sleep such as depth and periods of dreaming. There are a number of neurotransmitters thought to be involved in the control of our sleep/wake cycle, but those with a major role include serotonin (5-HT), noradrenaline and acetylcholine.

The sleep/wake cycle

As mentioned above it is a part of the brainstem known as the reticular formation that plays a key role in controlling our sleep/wake cycle. More specifically, it is the neuronal clusters found in the raphe nuclei (RN) and nucleus locus coeruleus (NLC), which are under the control of impulses arriving from the hypothalamus. The activity of both the RN and NLC increases and decreases daily, under the influence of our ' biological clock' in the hypothalamus. The activity of these pathways can also be affected by external stimuli, which enter our system via the sensory receptors, and which can either keep us awake or arouse us from sleep.

The 'biological clock'

The circadian rhythm set by our ' biological clock' of approximately 16 hours awake/8 hours asleep is controlled, specifically by the suprachiasmatic nucleus of the **hypothalamus.** The pattern of 16/8 varies from person to person and will also change as we go through life from birth to old age. If an individual was allowed to go to sleep in an environment with no cues as to the time of day, they would develop a regular sleep/wake cycle of approximately 25 hours' duration. It is the various external factors that we employ (use of an alarm, daylight entering the bedroom, social habits and activities) that result in the 'training' of the cycle to 24 hours.

Arousal

The cortex of our brain is constantly bombarded by information coming in through all of our senses (visual, auditory, touch, taste, smell, proprioception) and as this information passes up through the brain via the various pathways, collaterals branch off and send impulses to the reticular formation. The more sensory input there is, the greater the excitation of the reticular formation will be. If there is sufficient stimulation of the reticular formation, it will fire impulses up to the thalamus, switching off the thalamic pulsing to the cortex – and we waken. This process helps to explain why we can sometimes find it difficult to get to sleep, even if we want to, if there is a high level of sensory stimulation. Conversely, it also helps to explain why we can drop off to sleep at inappropriate moments, e.g. a warm lecture theatre with the lights dimmed, the quiet monotonous voice of the lecturer (not us obviously!). In this situation

there will be less reticular formation stimulation, leading to a reduced firing to the thalamus and a subsequent return of thalamic pulsing to the cortex.

Patterns of sleep

Once we have fallen asleep, if we sleep for long enough, our level of consciousness varies and we alternate between two distinct types of sleep: REM (rapid eye movement) sleep and non-REM sleep (see Fig. 14.1). The two types of sleep pattern are easily distinguishable, one from the other, by their distinct patterns of mental activity, cardiorespiratory patterns, muscle activity and, particularly, electroencephalogram (EEG) activity (see Chapter 1).

Non-REM sleep

Four separate stages (I–IV) of non-REM sleep have been identified using EEG recordings. Stage IV is often referred to as deep sleep, or slow wave sleep due to the characteristic EEG trace observed, and it is during this level of sleep that we are most difficult to rouse. It is also during stage IV that sleepwalking, talking, tooth-grinding and nightmares occur in some individuals (particularly the young). The time spent in stage IV does start to reduce as we grow older, so we can say that there may be some advantages to being older!

There is a rapid progression through the first four stages of sleep, followed by a short time spent at level IV and then a return back up through the stages. This occurs in a cyclical fashion throughout the period of sleep, with each cycle lasting about 90–100 minutes, although the depth lessens as the night progresses.

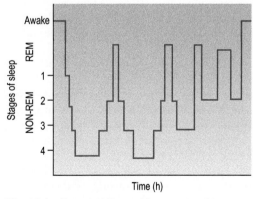

Fig. 14.1 • Stages of sleep with respect to time. From Waller et al. 2001, with permission

REM sleep

As well as the four stages of non-REM sleep, a distinctly different form occurs at regular intervals throughout the period, namely REM sleep. There are four key features associated with REM sleep:

- Rapid eye movements (REM)
- Dreaming
- Marked muscle relaxation
- Increases in blood pressure, heart rate and respiratory rate.

As we move from non-REM to REM sleep there is a notable change in EEG pattern, i.e. it starts to resemble the EEG pattern observed in an awake individual. However, as the individual is still very much in a deep sleep, this has resulted in REM sleep also being labelled '**paradoxical sleep**'. As noted above, dreaming occurs during the REM phase and the term REM sleep is derived from the fact that the eyeballs are moving as the mind of the individual is following the events unfolding in their dream. It is also during REM sleep that, even though our motor activity is significantly reduced, occasional twitches can occur. As well as the increases in the cardiorespiratory parameters noted above, there is also a greater variability in these values compared to non-REM sleep. During periods of both REM and non-REM sleep there is a general level of muscle relaxation; however, it is during the transition from REM to non-REM that we would change our body position.

Alteration in levels of fatigue and sleep in neurological disorders

Post-stroke fatigue

Fatigue is common after stroke, its prevalence ranging from 16% (Glader et al. 2002) to 70% (Carllson et al. 2003), depending on the definition of fatigue and the population studied.

There is often an increase in the level of fatigue felt by an individual after a stroke, particularly if the level of ischaemia has occurred subcortically, in the brainstem or in the thalamus. In fact, in certain cases, fatigue can be the only major disability and is often accepted as a common part of the disease process. Since, as we stated earlier, the definition of fatigue is so vague, it can be difficult to identify what actually causes it after a stroke. Consequently, it often goes undiagnosed – and thus untreated. In order to mediate this problem, a case definition and interview protocol was developed by Lynch

et al. (2007), with one version for inpatients and one for people living in the community. The **definition of post-stroke fatigue** for inpatients is as follows (p. 543):

> '*Since their stroke, the patient has experienced fatigue, a lack of energy, or an increased need to rest every day or nearly every day. This fatigue has led to difficulty taking part in everyday activities (for inpatients this may include therapy and may include the need to terminate an activity early because of fatigue).*'

Despite the fact that post-stroke fatigue is commonplace, very little is known on the actual extent of the problem or, in fact, what impact it has on the recovery of the individual affected. It does beg the question of how much impact an undetermined level of fatigue could be having on the return to 'pre-stroke' levels of activity. There is some evidence that post-stroke fatigue may be slightly more commonplace in females (Glader et al. 2002). However, there are also many studies which find that there is no demographic link with the level of occurrence. There is further contradictory evidence when looking at the severity of the fatigue being experienced. Several studies have linked the severity of fatigue to poor general health, pain, anxiety and depression post stroke. However, other studies report no link between fatigue levels and depression post stroke (Naess et al. 2005, van der Werf et al. 2001). There also appears to be no link between the level of fatigue experienced and either the time since the stroke or the level of disability associated with the stroke (van der Werf et al. 2001).

It therefore appears that, although post-stroke fatigue is a very real issue, there is much we do not know about the factors affecting the occurrence and severity of the fatigue experienced by a patient post stroke. In terms of interventions, a Cochrane systematic review only identified three studies, the results of which were inconclusive (McGeough et al. 2009). Exercise can be effective in reducing fatigue; however a Cochrane systematic review on exercise and fitness training after stroke reported insufficient evidence on this issue (Brazzelli et al. 2011). The unknown aspects of post-stroke fatigue could make the role of the therapist involved in post-stroke rehabilitation particularly difficult. It is clear that a considerable amount of further research is required in this important area.

Fatigue in multiple sclerosis

A **definition** of multiple sclerosis (MS) fatigue is 'a subjective lack of physical and/or mental energy that is perceived by the individual or caregiver to interfere with usual and desired activities' (Multiple Sclerosis Council 1998).

Fatigue in patients suffering from MS is very commonplace; in an audit of people with MS living in Oxfordshire, nearly half of the respondents reported fatigue (Wade and Green 2001). One particular problem mentioned is the fact that fatigue can be experienced at rest and, if occurring following activity, is not helped by rest. Levels of fatigue may also vary within the individual. Another interesting aspect that has been uncovered in some studies is that the level of fatigue experienced appears to be worsened by stress as well as heat (e.g. due to a warm environment or exercise). The exact mechanism behind the occurrence of fatigue in MS patients is not really understood, despite the fact that significant levels of information have been gathered from patients. However, it is thought that fatigue in MS may be associated with depression, cognitive impairment and muscle weakness, as well as disability, and, therefore, a comprehensive biopsychosocial approach to the assessment and management of fatigue should be taken.

It is clear that fatigue can have a considerable impact on rehabilitation and life in general; the high and variable levels of fatigue mean that it is often difficult for individuals with MS to plan their activities. They may only be able to engage with rehabilitation to a limited extent, and therapists need to carefully balance the need to avoid over-exertion with the need for sufficient physical activity to maintain optimum function. Outside rehabilitation, together with cognitive impairment, fatigue is one of the most important factors affecting employment prospects of people with this condition.

Fatigue in Parkinson's disease

As is the case with both stroke and MS patients, fatigue is also widely observed in Parkinson's disease (PD), with prevalence ranging from 33 to 58% (Friedman et al. 2007), and about half of patients reporting fatigue as a major symptom (Friedman et al. 2007). Having said that, it is not always clearly defined as a symptom by the patient who may not actually use the word 'fatigue' spontaneously. The problems with defining fatigue, mentioned in the context of stroke and MS, also apply to PD and there is currently no consensus on the best tool for assessing fatigue in people with PD (Friedman et al. 2007). Therapists, therefore, need to listen carefully for expressions such as 'tiredness', 'exhaustion' or 'lack of energy' (Brown et al. 2005).

Both depression and cognitive impairment are often linked to fatigue, but this is not necessarily the case in PD patients. Chronic fatigue has been observed in some PD patients, lasting as long as 9 years since diagnosis in some cases, while there is evidence to indicate that fatigue increases with time since diagnosis (Friedman et al. 2007).

In conclusion, fatigue is a real issue for PD patients, with a number of the people affected having to deal with a level that is both all-encompassing and persistent.

Post-stroke sleep disorders

There are three separate sleep disorders which can appear in patients who have suffered a stroke: **sleep disordered breathing (SDB); sleep–wake disorders (SWD);** and **insomnia**.

One of the most common forms of SDB is obstructive sleep apnoea (see later). Approximately 65% of stroke survivors will show symptoms associated with SDB, in which the patient usually experiences abnormalities in their respiratory pattern resulting in significant interruptions in their sleep patterns. The knock-on effects of this disrupted sleeping pattern are a marked level of fatigue during the day coupled with a difficulty in focusing their attention on any particular task. One aspect of SDB that has been identified was the fact that those suffering from it exhibited a worrying increase in both blood pressure and clotting factors (Golbin et al. 2008, Robinson et al. 2004). In addition to this, other studies suggest that abnormalities in breathing during sleep may increase the risk of vascular disease. However, it has to be pointed out that there is a lot of debate around this controversial area. A number of clinical studies have been carried out which suggest that habitual snoring actually increases the risk of developing high blood pressure and stroke (Lees et al. 2008, Neau et al. 2002). Interestingly, however, such findings have not been backed up in further work when other risk factors such as age, body mass index (BMI) and smoking were controlled for.

Around 30% of those individuals surviving a stroke will display symptoms of SWD, which affects the normal circadian rhythms (mentioned earlier), so that the usual pattern is no longer governed by day/night changes. The consequences of the sleep disturbances observed in SWD can be a high level of fatigue, some level of depression and a degree of attention/memory problems. The sleep fragmentation that can derive from SDB can result in a form of SWD.

Sleep disorders in Parkinson's disease

Various studies have shown that somewhere between 60 and 88% of PD patients will show some level of night-time sleep disturbance, coupled with a marked increase in the level of daytime sleepiness (Kales et al. 1971, Larsen 2003, Lees et al. 1988, Tandberg et al. 1998). A number of these patients report a range of marked night-time problems, including broken sleep and regular waking, which do not appear to be helped with use of sleep medications (hypnotics such as Zolpidem®) (Dauvilliers 2007, Gjerstad et al. 2007, Oerlemans and de Weerd 2002, Tandberg et al. 1998). Any form of sleep fragmentation appears to be more commonplace during the lighter stages I and II, with the patients noting that if they waken they find it exceptionally difficult to fall back asleep.

Sleep apnoea is most commonly found in individuals with a high BMI, a factor not frequently found in PD patients. Despite this, the occurrence of sleep apnoea is much higher than predicted in PD patients. It has been observed in a group of patients with a BMI within the normal range (approximately 19–25 kg/m^2) that almost 50% have a significant level of sleep apnoea. Around one-quarter to one-half of PD patients exhibit symptoms of **REM sleep behaviour disorder (RBD)** where there is an increased level of muscle activity during REM sleep. One key piece of research by Iranzo et al. (2006) showed that RBD may even precede the onset of the clinical symptoms of PD. Further research is required to see if RBD could be an early marker for PD. Another common complaint in about 15% of PD patients is **excessive daytime sleepiness (EDS)** which results in sleep 'attacks' and a danger of, for example, car accidents.

It can be seen that sleep disturbance and fatigue is a common feature of a number of neurological conditions, but it still remains an area that is not greatly understood.

Fatigue and sleep disorders: summary

This section has shown that sleep disorders and fatigue are very common in people with diverse neurological conditions, often under-reported by patients, under-diagnosed by health professionals and under-treated. For many patients, the experience of fatigue is intense and distressing, and affects everyday activities, social participation, relationships, employment and mood. Fatigue is a complex phenomenon, comprising both physiological and psychological components, that is poorly defined, difficult to assess and poorly understood in the context of neurological conditions. It is clear that much more research is needed into the causes of fatigue and optimal ways to treat this – often debilitating – symptom.

Eating, drinking and swallowing problems

Introduction

As adults we may take the ability to eat and drink safely for granted but it is actually a very complex skill that we develop from the first time we drink milk as a newborn to eating a sirloin steak in adulthood. Can you imagine how you would feel if you were told that you were no longer able to eat or drink normally, but could only eat food that was pureed and drinks that were thickened to the texture of a smoothie? Or even more severe measures such as not being able to eat or drink at all but having to be fed through a tube down your nose (**naso-gastric tube – NG tube**) or through your stomach (**percutaneous endoscopic gastrostomy – PEG tube**). Do you think that you would look forward to mealtimes? How would you feel about going out to a restaurant for a family meal? While our very lives depend on our ability to take in adequate nutrition and hydration for the healthy functioning of our bodies as well as for growth and repair, eating and drinking is also a central socialising activity which we often use for building and maintaining relationships.

The intricacies of how we manage different types of food and drink can be influenced by the strength and coordination of our musculature such as lips and tongue, closing off our nasal passage as we swallow, coordinating our breathing as we eat and drink and getting the food to go into our stomach rather than into our airway. It is also influenced by how alert we are, our posture (have you ever tried drinking whilst lying down?) and the amount and texture of the food and drink we put into our mouths. Eating, drinking and swallowing problems (**dysphagia**) can be experienced by people with acquired neurological diseases, and depending on the particular type of neuropathology, dysphagia can be transient (for example as a result of a transient ischaemic attack), persistent (for example, in stroke) or deteriorating (e.g. motor neurone disease (MND)).

Due to the different ways that dysphagia is reported, it is difficult to ascertain the exact incidence and prevalence of the problem. However, some studies have given insight into the extent of people experiencing dysphagia – 64–90% of people in the acute phase of stroke (SIGN 2010); 68% of people with dementia in residential homes (Steele et al. 1997); more than 90% of those with MND; 41% of patients with PD, and 33% of patients with MS (Hartelius and Svensson 1994). While problems eating and drinking can cause poor quality of life it can also cause choking or risk of aspiration (where food or liquid spills into the airway rather than stomach) which in turn can lead to chest infections and pneumonia, malnutrition and dehydration. Patients who are undernourished and dehydrated take longer to recover from illness, and aspiration pneumonia can in some cases lead to death.

Anatomy and physiology of swallowing

In order to understand the difficulties patients with dysphagia are experiencing, it is useful to know the anatomy and physiology of the eating, drinking and swallowing process. There are various anatomical structures that are involved in the swallowing process (see Figs 14.2 and 14.3) and damage to any of the motor or sensory nerves innervating these structures or affecting their coordination can cause an unsafe

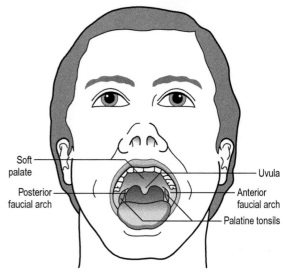

Fig. 14.2 • A frontal view. Anatomical structures involved in the swallowing process. Adapted from Hardy and Morton Robinson (1999), with permission from Pro-ed, Austin, Texas, USA.

swallow. There are different stages involved in eating and drinking and problems can arise in any one.

Oral phases

The first phase prepares the food so that it is in a suitable format for swallowing and involves the various structures in your oral cavity. Have a look inside your mouth using a mirror. You can see many of the

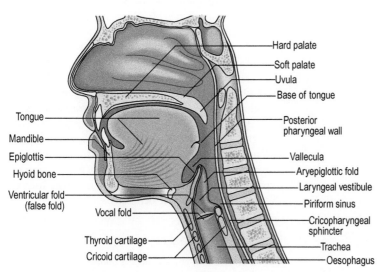

Fig. 14.3 • A sagittal view. Anatomical structures involved in the swallowing process. Adapted from Hardy and Morton Robinson (1999), with permission from Pro-ed, Austin, Texas, USA.

structures which include the lips, teeth and tongue, and looking towards the back of your mouth you can see the soft palate (velum), uvula (dangling soft tissue) and faucial arches (see Fig. 14.2). The tongue is an amazing structure which is composed almost entirely of many muscle fibres. It is composed of six regions – the tip, blade, front, centre, back and the base. The first five regions are largely under voluntary cortical control and are involved in the oral phases of the swallow. The sixth region, the base of the tongue, is employed during the pharyngeal phase of the swallow (see below) and is largely under involuntary neural control coordinated in the brainstem. It is also important to note the oral crevices (spaces) between your upper and lower lips and gums and between your cheeks and gums where food can lodge if not cleared by our tongue.

During the first preparatory phase, food is placed on the tongue and is then mixed with saliva. This saliva is created by three large salivary glands (parotid glands, sub-mandibular glands and sublingual glands) as well as lots of smaller glands positioned in the mucous membrane of the tongue, lips, cheeks and roof of the mouth. Solid food requires mastication where we chew and grind the food down with our teeth, use side to side and rotary movements of our tongue and jaw, and mix it with saliva in order to make it into a form that we can easily swallow. During this process the muscle tension in our lips and cheeks prevents the food from spilling out of our mouth as well as from lodging in our oral crevices. The velum is pulled forward to touch the back of the tongue preventing food or drink from prematurely spilling into the pharynx before the swallow is triggered (Fig. 14.4). There are two methods by which we can safely hold the bolus in our oral cavity before the swallow is triggered. Around 80% of the population holds the bolus between the tongue and frontal portion of the hard palate (known as a tipper pattern). However, in the remaining 20% it is held on the floor of the mouth in front of the tongue (known as a dipper pattern). So are you a dipper or a tipper? Next time you're eating why not find out! So now the food is ready for the second oral phase where the food travels back along the tongue in a very controlled manner to the back of your oral cavity. When the food reaches the area between the faucial arches, a complex sequence of actions occurs in the pharynx (cavity between mouth and larynx) and larynx (at your Adam's apple) which ends the oral phase of the swallow (takes approximately 1–1.5 seconds).

Oral phase swallowing difficulties

As we get older we experience subtle changes in our eating and drinking physiology, but this does not cause us significant difficulties. However, for patients with neurological impairments a wide range of problems in the oral phases can result in less efficient and unsafe swallowing. Normal muscle tone is essential for food to be controlled and manipulated in the mouth so if a patient's condition results in them having problems at this stage then food or liquid may spill from their mouths, go up their nose or spill into their pharynx before the food is ready to be swallowed. Apart from being unpleasant and embarrassing this can be very dangerous causing the patient to choke or **aspirate** (food going into the lungs rather than the stomach). In addition, in order to manipulate the food/drink to prepare it for swallowing, you need to be able to sense where it is in your mouth (this is why dentists advise us not to eat or drink for some time after an anaesthetic!). Patients who experience reduced sensation may find that food builds up in their mouth. Patients with dementia, for example, frequently hold food in their mouth without swallowing it, due to reduced awareness. Lack of awareness or poor muscle tone can also cause a premature spillage of food into the pharynx before the swallow is triggered, putting the patient in danger of aspiration. Poor muscle control and reduced sensation are often experienced by people with stroke, head injury, PD and MND amongst others.

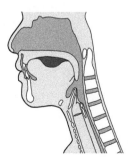

Fig. 14.4 • Oral phase of swallowing. Adapted from Logemann (1998). Evaluation and treatment of swallowing disorders, with permission from Pro-ed, Austin, Texas, USA.

Pharyngeal phase

The next phase of the swallow is called the pharyngeal phase and involves structures that are not readily visible without instrumental tools (see Fig. 14.3) – the base of your tongue, epiglottis, pharyngeal wall, aryepiglottic folds and the cricopharyngeal sphincter (which is the valve that opens to allow the food into your oesophagus). As with your oral cavity, there are crevices (called the valleculae and pyriform sinuses) where food can potentially build up if someone has dysphagia. It is not known exactly what causes the actual swallow to trigger, however it is thought that stimulation of the oral structures (e.g. tongue and faucial arches) sends sensory information to the reticular formation (the swallow centre) in the brainstem which sends motor commands back to the pharynx and larynx to initiate the muscular movements of this stage of the swallow. During this stage there are various actions which serve to prevent food/drink entering your nasal cavity or your airway. These movements also create pressure which helps propel the bolus through the pharynx (Fig. 14.5) into your oesophagus. As this is happening the cricopharyngeal sphincter relaxes and opens to allow the food to pass into the oesophagus, which brings the food to your stomach (Fig. 14.6). This very complex stage of the swallow takes only approximately 1 second to complete.

Pharyngeal phase swallowing difficulties

As with the oral phases, our physiology changes as we age, for example resulting in us taking longer to trigger our swallow, but again this doesn't cause us

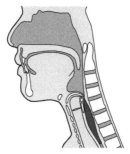

Fig. 14.6 • Cricopharyngeal sphincter relaxes and opens for bolus to pass into the oesophagus. Adapted from Logemann (1998). Evaluation and treatment of swallowing disorders, with permission from Pro-ed, Austin, Texas, USA.

significant problems. However, for patients with neurological impairment, a delay in triggering the swallow (which can be totally absent in severe cases) may cause food or liquid spilling into an unprotected airway and can result in aspiration. This is thought to be the most commonly occurring swallowing problem experienced by patients with stroke or head injury. Some patients with paresis or paralysis of the tongue base may have difficulties building up enough pressure to propel the bolus safely to the oesophagus and other issues can include leakage of food or liquid into the nasal passage. In addition, if the food/liquid isn't fully transferred to the oesophagus it may cause a build-up of residue in the crevices and can potentially spill over into an unprotected airway.

Once the bolus has passed into the oesophagus and travels into the stomach, the cricopharyngeal sphincter stops it from re-entering the pharynx. However, it is important to be aware that some patients who have digestive tract problems may find that it interferes with the swallowing process.

Assessment

There are perhaps some obvious signs that someone is having problems eating and/or drinking, including spillage from their lips (due to poor lip seal), taking a long time to finish their meal, regurgitation of food (oral or nasal), if they are showing weight loss or coughing and choking. Other symptoms which are perhaps less obvious include dehydration, malnutrition or frequent chest infections (suggestive of aspiration). Due to the large number of patients with post-stroke dysphagia, Scottish Intercollegiate Guideline Network (SIGN) guidelines recommend that all patients are screened for dysphagia before being given food or drink. The speech and language

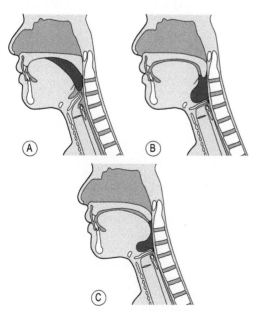

Fig. 14.5 • Pharyngeal phase of swallowing. Adapted from Logemann (1998). Evaluation and treatment of swallowing disorders, with permission from Pro-ed, Austin, Texas, USA.

therapist (SLT) is considered an expert in the assessment, diagnosis and treatment of dysphagia and works closely with a multidisciplinary team. The composition of the team will vary depending upon the setting; however, it is likely to include a dietitian, occupational therapist, physiotherapist, consultant, nursing staff and radiographer. The dietitian will assess the patient's level of nutrition and hydration, dietary preferences and current feeding pattern, and so works closely with the SLT to establish the safest and most nutritious diet for the patient.

A screening process (usually carried out by a trained nurse) is used to identify those patients who should be referred to an SLT for full clinical assessment. A preliminary risk assessment will be carried out and include observations of the patient's level of consciousness, degree of postural control and ability to control their own saliva. The SLT takes a detailed case history and carries out an oro-motor examination to evaluate the strength and coordination of the patient's oral musculature. If safe to do so a water swallow test is often used to identify the risk of aspiration. This assessment involves the patient being given teaspoons of water and the initiation of their swallow is observed. If there are no adverse signs then the patient is given a larger quantity to drink from a glass. This is considered a useful and reasonably sensitive screening test which has a reported sensitivity of >70% and a specificity of 22–66% for the prediction of aspiration (SIGN 2010). We've all experienced times when food or drink goes 'down the wrong way' which resulted in us coughing in order to clear our airway of the food or liquid. However, it is important to note that while coughing is a sign of material penetrating the airway, the absence of a cough does not indicate a safe swallow – up to 68% of patients who were seen to aspirate during a videofluoroscopy (dynamic swallow X-ray) assessment failed to cough (Perry and Love 2001). Throughout the assessment the SLT will make clinical judgements as to whether the patient can be assessed on solid food and other liquid, and will determine the safety of the patient eating, drinking and swallowing. Depending on the presentation of the patient and the difficulties they experience this may involve assessing their ability to swallow a variety of bolus size, pacing of their feeding and the temperature, texture and viscosity of the food and drink. Think about the different skills you need for eating a dry crumbly biscuit compared to some custard, or drinking a thick creamy hot chocolate versus a glass of extra cold fizzy juice. In order to

observe the pharyngeal phase, patients may also be assessed using instrumental procedures such as a **videofluoroscopic evaluation of swallowing (VFES)** and/or **fibre-optic endoscopic evaluation of swallowing (FEES)**. These allow the SLT to gain a dynamic view of the swallow structures and function, and assess the presence and cause of aspiration. Evidence suggests that for some individuals their swallow function may continue to improve over time and others with progressive diseases may worsen, therefore regular assessment and reassessment is appropriate as required.

Treatment

Following assessment the SLT will inform the patient, multidisciplinary team and carers of the nature of the swallowing problems and the recommended intervention. There are many interventions common in clinical practice but the evidence for them is limited. Some of these include diet modification (e.g. pureed solids and thickened fluids) or teaching the patient compensatory strategies such as postural changes and manoeuvres in order to improve swallow function and reduce or eliminate symptoms of dysphagia. Therapy targeting maintenance and/or improvement of oro-motor function may include the patient engaging in a range of motion, chewing and swallowing exercises, and thermal and tactile stimulation. The SLT is also involved in the education and assessment of carers and staff involved in feeding patients with dysphagia, and will provide advice on how to support the patient when they are eating and drinking, including bolus size and temperature, texture, pacing, positioning, utensils and the environment.

Eating and drinking problems: summary

The process of eating, drinking and swallowing involves a complex integration and coordination of many muscles and nerves which can be greatly impacted due to acquired neurogenic diseases. In-depth specialist assessment is required by an SLT who then makes recommendations for treatment that could involve exercises or modifying textures of food and drink to improve the efficiency and safety of the swallow. For people with unsafe swallows it may mean short-term or long-term alternative non-oral feeding such as NG or PEG tube feeding. The SLT works closely with the multidisciplinary team to determine the best method of ensuring that patients receive their required nutrition and hydration in a manner that reduces the risk of aspiration.

Continence

Introduction

Achieving continence is one of the milestones of child development, often accompanied by considerable praise and delight and then forgotten about. In adult life continence is rarely given a thought until it goes wrong, when the occurrence of incontinence can be accompanied by feelings of embarrassment, distress, shock and fear. Individuals may become housebound – not because of mobility problems, but due to fear of 'accidents', i.e. incontinence of bowel or bladder. Due to the embarrassing nature of this symptom, individuals may not mention it and it has been termed the unvoiced symptom. In a study of 115 patients with spinal cord injury, bowel dysfunction was considered to be one of the most distressing disabilities (Glickman and Kamm 1996).

Prevalence

Estimates of urinary incontinence vary because of differing definitions, but a study of people over 30 years living in their own homes revealed that 14% of women and 6.6% of men had experienced urinary incontinence. Half of those who answered positively had sought help from their GP (Brocklehurst 1993). Continence problems increase with advancing age, often secondary to conditions such as benign prostatic hypertrophy in men, incompetence of the urethral sphincter in women and post-menopausal hormonal changes. Age-related bladder instability is another cause, along with other morbidities such as diabetes mellitus and a variety of medications. More than one-fifth of people over 85 years may be affected by urinary incontinence.

Bowel incontinence is less common, but may be even more distressing for individuals and their families, and may be the trigger for moving from the community into residential or nursing care. One study reported a prevalence of 2.2% anal incontinence in the general population, with risk factors including female sex, advancing age, poor general health and physical limitation. The prevalence is higher amongst those in institutions with an estimate of 11–15% (Macmillan et al. 2004).

Neurological disease may affect bladder and bowel function directly or secondarily because of its impact on mobility, upper limb function and cognition. Amongst people with MS, approximately 75% may have lower urinary tract symptoms (Marrie et al. 2007) and 68% may have bowel dysfunction (Hinds et al. 1990). In a study of people with stroke, the prevalence of urinary incontinence varied with time from stroke, with 36% prevalence on admission and 8% at 6 months post stroke in one study (Nakayama et al. 1997). Similarly, approximately 30% of patients have problems with bowel dysfunction in the early phase and 11% at 12 months post stroke (Harari et al. 2003).

Urinary continence

Physiology

The bladder has two functions: storage and voiding. Control of the bladder depends upon intact neural connections between the sacral spinal cord and the pontine micturition centre, which in turn is influenced by input from the cortex – especially the medial aspect of the frontal lobes. The smooth muscle of the bladder, the detrusor muscle, is innervated by the sacral parasympathetic nerves from S2,3,4. Sympathetic nerves originating from the thoraco-lumbar cord have an inhibitory effect on the detrusor, but stimulate the bladder neck. The somatic pudendal nerves innervate the striated external sphincter and pelvic floor. These muscles are under voluntary control.

Storage

The unique structure of the bladder wall, with its high compliance, allows filling and expansion of the bladder to occur with minimal pressure rise. Bladder pressure is normally measured in terms of cm water and during normal filling to around 300 ml, pressure rise does not exceed 10 cm water. During bladder filling there is inhibition of parasympathetic activity (see Fig. 14.7). At approximately 300 ml there is the first sensation of a desire to void. This feeling can be suppressed via supraspinal and spinal pathways, which suppress the parasympathetic activity and maintain a closed urethra until an appropriate time and place for voiding is identified.

Disorders of storage may arise where detrusor contractions cannot be suppressed by supraspinal pathways. The individual will complain of *urgency, frequency* and *urge incontinence*. Urodynamic studies will reveal unstable contractions of the detrusor

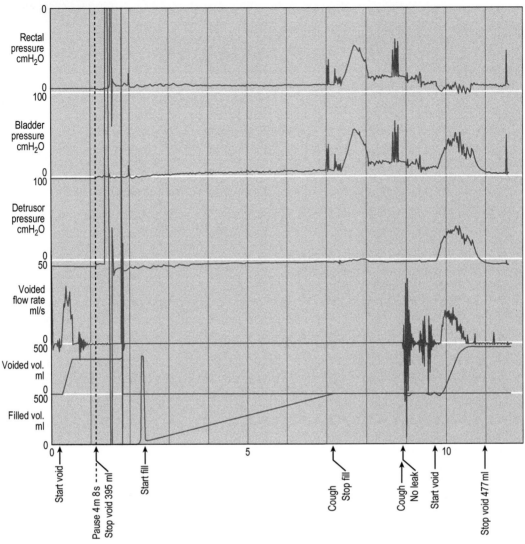

Fig. 14.7 • Cystometrogram (CMG) showing normal filling and voiding phases. To obtain the CMG the bladder is slowly filled via a catheter whilst pressure measurements are recorded. Detrusor pressure is derived by subtracting abdominal pressure, measured through a rectal probe, from bladder pressure measured via a bladder probe. In this normal CMG, when intra-abdominal pressure is increased by coughing there is no increase in bladder pressure or leakage. When voiding is initiated there is a pressure rise of < 40 cm water and a maximum flow rate of 20 ml/second. From: Chandler, B.J. Continence and stroke. In: Barnes, M., Dobkin, B., Bogousslavsky, J. (eds.). Recovery after stroke (2005). Cambridge, Cambridge University press, with permission. Cystometrograms kindly provided by Mr. R. Pickard, Consultant Urologist, The Newcastle upon Tyne Hospitals NHS Foundation Trust, Newcastle, UK.

which may generate high pressures within the bladder (see Fig. 14.8). This is seen in spinal cord pathology secondary to trauma, or disease such as MS. Supra-pontine pathology may also affect storage and the basal ganglia appear to have an inhibitory effect on the micturition reflex. Some of this inhibition is lost with the cell loss of the substantia nigra in PD (see Chapter 6), resulting in detrusor hyper-reflexia. In severe frontal lobe disease (e.g. in dementia),

there may be a loss of the modulating effect of higher centres, so that the bladder adopts an infantile pattern of function in which filling and voiding occur without voluntary control.

Voiding

Emptying the bladder involves a coordinated relaxation of the external sphincter and contraction of the detrusor muscle. This coordinated event is dependent upon intact connections between the sacral spinal cord and the pontine micturition centre. Patients with problems of voiding may complain of *difficulty emptying, interrupted stream, hesitancy* and *incomplete emptying*. However, this problem may pass unnoticed by the individual and more than 50% of people with neurological causes of voiding disorder may be unaware that they are failing to empty completely. In some cases, the complaint may be of increased frequency because the bladder is permanently holding more than 300 ml and any further increase in volume causes a desire to void.

In patients with spinal cord injury, the consequence of voiding disorder can be extremely serious and meticulous management of bladder function is essential. Lack of coordinated sphincter relaxation and detrusor contraction can result in high pressures being generated within the bladder as contraction occurs against a closed sphincter. This can lead to hypertrophy of the smooth muscle of the bladder wall and reflux of urine into the ureters and intrarenal reflux of urine that may often be infected. Obstruction to ureteric drainage can lead to ureteric dilatation and hydronephrosis. The risk of reflux is greatest in the first couple of years post injury. Prior to the outstanding work of the spinal injury centres in the mid-20th century, **renal damage** was a common cause of morbidity and death in spinal patients. Careful monitoring of renal and bladder function in spinal patients has transformed this situation.

Other causes of spinal pathology such as MS are not associated with such a risk of upper tract damage and so monitoring of the upper tracts is not a requirement for these patients. Nevertheless, active management of their lower urinary tract symptoms is essential. **Urinary tract infection** is a common problem and can lead to an exacerbation of symptoms and overwhelming **sepsis** if not actively managed. Due to the progressive nature of MS, the approach to management of bladder symptoms must keep pace with the changing level of disability. Very helpful guidelines in the management of the bladder in MS have been developed to guide clinical teams (Fowler et al. 2009).

Investigation and treatment of neurological urinary incontinence

Following a history and examination (including a prostate examination in men and an obstetric history and vaginal assessment in women), the key investigations are to test the urine for abnormalities such as

---

Box 14.1

Factors influencing continence

- Bladder function
- Bowel function
- Mobility
- Upper limb function
- Sensory neglect
- Visuo-spatial problems
- Communication difficulties
- Cognitive difficulties
- Type of clothing
- Presence of a carer
- Location of toilet
- Ease of access to toilet
- Time available in care plan for toileting

---

infection, glucose or protein; to ask the patient to keep a fluid balance chart which documents intake and the pattern and volume of output; and to assess post-void residual urine to check for incomplete bladder emptying. Other factors of importance include level of independence, cognitive capacity, etc. (see Box 14.1). Where there may be concern about the upper urinary tracts, further imaging of kidneys and ureters is required. If more detailed information is required about the activity of the bladder in storage and voiding phase, specialist urodynamic assessment is extremely helpful from a urology unit.

Detrusor instability (Fig. 14.8) may be improved with an anti-cholinergic drug. It is essential to monitor progress by repeating a post-void residual measurement to ensure that the bladder is continuing to empty fully. A more recent option in managing troublesome detrusor instability is intra-vesical Botulinum toxin (Duthie et al. 2011, and see Chapter 6).

If the problem is one of incomplete emptying, then assisted emptying using a bladder stimulator may be helpful in patients who are ambulant and have abdominal sensation. If this is not successful the next option would be intermittent catheterisation. Patients with degenerative disease such as MS often move through different options in treatment as the disease progresses and often a long-term catheter is eventually required. Ideally, this should be a suprapubic catheter as this causes less damage to the urethra and is often more comfortable. For a small proportion of people with persistent problems, urinary diversion is a further option.

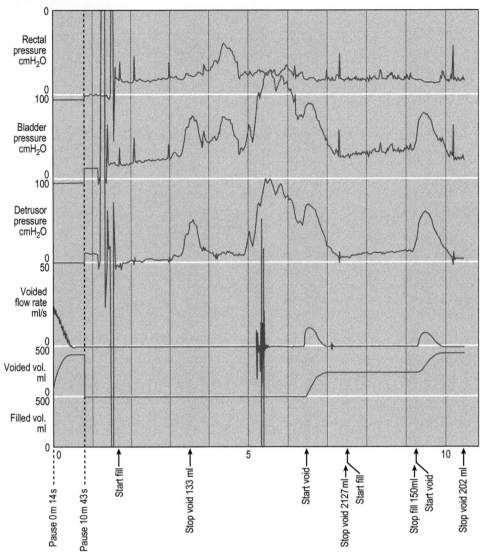

Fig. 14.8 • CMG showing detrusor instability, as might occur in a patient with a neurological condition. High detrusor pressures are generated both by the involuntary and voluntary contractions. The filling phase was curtailed because of the involuntary contractions leading to voiding. From: Chandler, B.J. Continence and stroke. In: Barnes, M., Dobkin, B., Bogousslavsky, J. (eds.). Recovery after stroke (2005). Cambridge, Cambridge University press, with permission. Cystometrograms kindly provided by Mr. R. Pickard, Consultant Urologist, The Newcastle upon Tyne Hospitals NHS Foundation Trust, Newcastle, UK.

Bowel function

Physiology

As with the bladder, the gastro-intestinal tract is under neurological control. It is supplied by the parasympathetic system via the vagus nerve as far as the splenic flexure of the colon and beyond this point by the sacral parasympathetic nerves (Fig. 14.9). The internal anal sphincter has input from the sympathetic nerves and maintains a high resting tone. The external sphincter is under voluntary control via the pudendal nerves. Sensation from the rectum, which gives awareness of rectal filling, passes via the inferior rectal branch of the pudendal nerve. Unlike the bladder, there is also a complex intrinsic nervous system which is influenced by the autonomic nervous system, but allows the gut to function even when it is separated from spinal and supraspinal control.

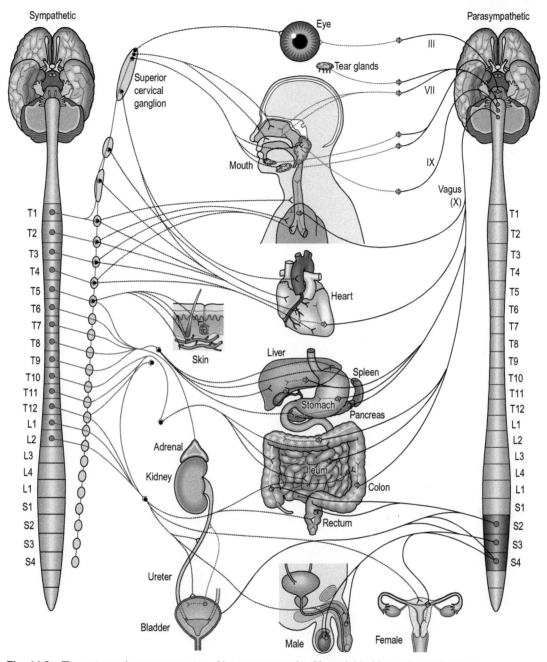

Fig. 14.9 • The autonomic nervous system. Note nerve supply of bowel, bladder and sexual organs.

The function of the colon and anorectum is to mix and dehydrate faecal materials, to provide for growth of symbiotic bacteria and to store faecal waste prior to elimination when socially appropriate. Material moves through the gut as a result of propulsive muscle activity in the gut wall. An increase in colonic activity occurs approximately 40 minutes after a meal, the gastro-colic reflex, which can be used in bowel training programmes to help establish a pattern of emptying. The 'storage organ' of the bowel is the sigmoid colon. Material moves from this area into the rectum prior to defecation. The rectum should be empty other than at this time. A common finding in patients with faecal impaction is a loaded rectum which indicates a lack of normal functioning. The resting pressure of the anal canal provides a passive barrier to leakage of stool.

Distension of the rectum with faeces results in relaxation of the internal sphincter, the recto-anal inhibitory reflex. Voluntary contraction of the external sphincter via supra-spinal and spinal tracts can delay emptying of the bowel until convenient. When defecation is appropriate, the external sphincter relaxes and passage of faeces occurs often helped by a Valsalva manoeuvre.

Treating bowel disorders

The principles of management of bowel disorders are similar to those of managing urinary problems, and for patients with neurological problems these will be most appropriately managed with advice from a specialist continence service. Nurse-led continence teams can assess, advise and give patients the time and security they need to deal with these problems, which are often felt to be so embarrassing and distressing. A detailed history of the bowel problem is required as well as an examination, (see Box 14.2); if there has been a recent change in bowel habit, weight loss or passage of blood this will require more detailed investigation in a gastrointestinal unit.

The commonest problem amongst people with neurological disorders is **constipation** with or without associated episodes of incontinence. The aim of management is to establish a regular bowel habit and this may involve a combination of adjustment to diet, use of laxatives, increasing fluid intake and giving more time for toileting. Problems are often multi-factorial.

Generally people prefer to struggle with constipation rather than risk episodes of incontinence. It may take some time to establish a regular bowel pattern that fits in with lifestyle. Laxatives can be taken orally to stimulate movement through the gut. If there is weakness of abdominal musculature, it may also be necessary to use additional stimulation to achieve evacuation with either suppositories or enema. Some spinal cord injury patients find digitally stimulating the bowel can induce the recto-anal inhibitory reflex, triggering evacuation. For patients with complex problems, referral to a specialist centre for more detailed investigation (see Box 14.3) and advice on treatment options is helpful. A detailed review of more invasive therapeutic options such as colostomy, anterograde continence enema, percutaneous endoscopic caecostomy, and electrical stimulation is beyond the scope of this

Box 14.3

Specialist investigations of bowel dysfunction

Colonic transit time is an objective measure of large bowel function and allows estimation of segmental and total colonic transit times

Defecography is a dynamic study of defecation and is helpful in patients with difficulty in expulsion of stool. Puborectalis relaxation, pelvic floor descent and completeness of evacuation as well as anatomic abnormalities like intussusception and rectocele can be assessed with this technique

Colonometrograms study the colonic pressure – volume relationships

Neurophysiological techniques study the striated pelvic floor and pudendal nerve function

Flexible sigmoidoscopy, colonoscopy and barium enema can assess the presence of structural abnormalities

Box 14.2

Factors to be considered in assessing bowel dysfunction in patients with neurological problems

- Colonic transit time
- Sensation of arrival of the stool in the rectum
- Ability to allow the rectum to serve as a temporary compliant reservoir
- Ability to effectively contract external sphincter and puborectalis muscles
- Stool volume and consistency
- Cognition:
  - Interpretation of sensory feedback
  - Motivation to make the appropriate responses
  - Awareness of social norms
- Communication
- Neurological integrity

- Fluid intake
- Diet
- Exercise
- Medications
- Mobility
- Dependency on help to move
- Upper limb function
- Muscle weakness/spasticity
- Bladder management
- Past history of obstetric injury to the external sphincter/pelvic surgery
- History of physical or sexual abuse
- Activity level, lifestyle and return to work issues

chapter. However, the key message for patients with bowel problems is that there are treatment options and having identified the difficulty, an appropriate referral to a continence service can be made and from there referral to more specialist units is possible.

Incontinence: summary

Bladder and bowel control are frequently affected in neurological conditions. This causes immense distress and can impede effective rehabilitation as well as life after discharge. The aetiology of problems is often multi-factorial and management involves a holistic approach which is offered though a nurse-led continence service. The first stage in helping people is acknowledging that the problem exists.

Sexual dysfunction

Introduction

Sexuality is a fundamental part of human life, influencing how individuals perceive themselves and how they interact with those around them. It encompasses many concepts (see Box 14.4) and behaviours. Research into sexuality has moved from studies of mating behaviour in animals to the use of complex imaging techniques such as measurement of regional cerebral blood flow (cRBF), positron emission tomography (PET scans) and functional magnetic resonance imaging (fMRI). These techniques, some of which were explained in Chapter 1, offer increased understanding of the neurophysiological basis of love, desire and sexual fulfilment.

Bancroft identifies three strands of **sexual development:** sexual differentiation and the acquisition of gender identity; sexual responsiveness; and the capacity for intimate relationships. These strands

develop at varying rates throughout childhood and adolescence, becoming more inter-connected as adulthood is reached. As described in Chapter 3, sexual development begins in utero with the genetic make-up of the foetus, influenced by the hormonal environment and responsiveness of the cells. With increasing maturity, the impact of cognitive and emotional responses further influences the physiological development. At its most basic level, sexuality is about finding a partner for reproduction and the passing on of genetic material, but for humans it is of course so much more than that. Sexual attraction can lead to the formation of an intimate relationship in which life experience is shared – and for some this is the context in which major stresses such as the acquisition of long-term illness will be experienced (see Box 14.5).

Neurophysiology of sexual function

The nervous system is central to the experience and expression of sexuality, and includes both excitatory and inhibitory pathways. Much of the understanding of the neural pathways involved in humans has come from studying people with various disorders of neurological functioning. More recently it has been possible to further this understanding through the use of functional imaging techniques. Bancroft refers to a psychosomatic circle to encompass how awareness of sexual response impacts on the experience of sexual arousal and expression (Bancroft 2009). There are links between cognitive processes and emotional responses that influence arousal and its peripheral manifestation. Apart from in fantasy or masturbation, sexual expression also involves a relationship. The influence of that relationship on the sexual

Box 14.5

Intimate relationships

Relationships may form on the basis of:
- Physical attraction
- Shared interests
- Sense of humour
- Shared upbringing and values
- Similar or contrasting approach to problem solving
- Sexual attraction
- Sexual experience
- Views of the future
- Love
- Commitment
- Trust

Box 14.4

Concepts within sexuality

- Sexual development
- Sexual awareness
- Sexual responsiveness, desire and arousal
- Self-image
- Self-esteem
- Gender
- Intimate relationships
- Roles
- Communication

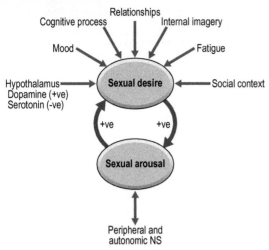

Fig. 14.10 • Factors influencing sexual desire and arousal. The interplay of neurotransmitters is complex and only two are shown in this simplified diagram. There is a positive feedback loop between desire and arousal that can be broken by any of the factors that may act in a negative manner. Adapted from: Chandler, B.J. Sex and relationships following stroke. In: Barnes, M., Dobkin, B., Bogousslavsky, J. (eds.). Recovery after stroke (2005). Cambridge, Cambridge University press, with permission.

experience is significant and is also affected by external factors such as social circumstances, past experience, fears and expectations. Understanding human sexuality is, therefore, not simply about a physiological system, but a complex interplay of biological, social, emotional and relationship factors.

There are both inhibitory and excitatory pathways of sexual arousal and a positive feedback between desire and arousal (see Fig. 14.10). Some of the neurotransmitters involved have been identified and alteration in the levels of these transmitters has an important role to play in some sexual disorders.

In the 1960s Masters and Johnson (1966) began research into the physiology of sex and produced a model of sexual response involving four stages: excitement, plateau, orgasm and resolution. They identified that changes for males and females were very similar. Their model also allowed classification of sexual disorders linked to these phases of response. Kaplan (1974) subsequently proposed a modified version with three phases: desire, excitement and orgasm. This model included the important phenomenon of sexual desire which is a common area of dysfunction and is included in the Diagnostic and Statistical Manual of Mental Disorders (DSM-IV, 1994) classification.

Imaging studies have shown that the cerebral response to sexual stimuli occurs in the anterior cingulate cortex (ACC) which has connections to the amygdala, an area of the brain with a crucial role to play in emotional response. The amygdala is active in response to visual sexual stimuli. The more caudal part of the ACC is involved with cognition and may have a modulating effect, processing potentially contradictory information to continue or cease sexual activity depending on circumstances. The putamen also appears active in relation to penile erection.

Love is a concept that cannot really be broken down into physiological component parts and yet studies have been undertaken to look at brain activity in response to viewing pictures of loved ones. Similarities and differences were identified in relation to maternal and romantic love, e.g. the dentate gyrus, and hypothalamus were more active in romantic love, possibly representing an overlap with sexual arousal.

The spinal cord is the neurological connection between the brain and the periphery. The genitalia are richly supplied with sensory nerve endings which travel in the pudendal nerve to sacral segments S2,3,4. Both parts of the autonomic nervous system (see Chapter 2) are involved in the sexual response. The parasympathetic supply is also from S2,3,4, and the sympathetic supply is from the thoracic and upper lumbar rami. The simplest explanation of sexual response is that the parasympathetic system is responsible for erection in men and vasocongestion in women and the sympathetic system for ejaculation. However, evidence from animal studies and patients with spinal cord injury suggests there is also a sympathetic pathway involved in erection. Erection may occur as a spinal reflex or in response to brain activity. The complexity of pathways and neurotransmitters involved in sexual function is immense.

The response of the genitalia to sexual arousal is a neuro-vascular phenomenon. The blood supply to the penis stems from paired pudendal arteries, terminal branches of the internal iliac arteries. Erection of the penis occurs as blood fills three longitudinal structures within the penis called corpora. These consist of blood-filled spaces or sinusoids connected by multiple anastomotic channels with the small arteries of the penis. The walls of the sinusoids contain smooth muscle and fibroelastic tissue, whereas the corpora are surrounded by a layer of fibrous tissue, the tunica albuginea. The venous drainage is via small veins within the corpora which coalesce to form emissary veins passing through the tunica albuginea. With no sexual arousal, the penis is in a flaccid state with the corporeal smooth muscle contracted and the blood flow restricted. Stimulation via the parasympathetic system causes cavernous smooth muscle relaxation and blood flow into the sinusoidal spaces. The resultant expansion compresses the veins impeding venous outflow and increasing the vasocongestion resulting in erection. In women this physiological response results in vasocongestion of the vagina and vulva. The uterus becomes engorged and rises in the pelvis pulling the cervix effectively 'out of the way' and the upper part of the vagina expands.

The relaxation of smooth muscle to allow vasocongestion, occurs in response to a decrease in intracellular calcium. Cyclic GMP, cAMP and nitrous oxide all play a second messenger type role in this (see Chapter 4). Phosphodiesterase enzyme in the genital tissues is responsible for breaking down cGMP and this has allowed drugs which inhibit phosphodiesterase (e.g. Sildenafil or Viagra®) to become a valuable treatment for erectile dysfunction. This final step in the pathway will occur in response to sexual arousal at a conscious level transmitted to the periphery via long tracts in the spinal cord; or a reflex response at the level of the sacral cord may also occur in response to a variety of stimuli, when the cord is isolated from cerebral control, as in spinal cord injury.

Relationships

The context of most sexual expression is within a relationship. It is also within this context that many people will experience the life-changing impact of chronic disease or acquired disability. For some couples, problems of adjustment to the changes can be significant and place a strain on the relationship, sometimes leading to separation. For others, the impact of such stress can enhance their closeness.

Each partner brings into a relationship a set of characteristics that are given expression through thoughts, behaviours and emotions. These are influenced by upbringing and belief systems, family and social context. Each partner has a set of needs, expectations, fears and past experience that influence their response to new situations. There will be differing needs for autonomy and intimacy within the relationship and different roles will be assumed as a relationship progresses. One of the commonest divisions of role within a long-term relationship is with the arrival of children when, in some cases, one partner assumes the 'bread-winner' role and the other home-maker. Each partner has an image of self and an image of

the partner they have chosen and this includes an awareness of their physical and psychological health.

The onset of neurological disease and/or disability can present a great challenge to the stable state of a relationship. This may result in change of physical appearance and cognitive ability. The couple, having been partners in a familiar relationship, may find that now there is a carer and a partner who requires care. New roles may be taken on by one partner whilst roles must be relinquished by the other. The shared hopes and expectations for the future may alter. It is important to note that the greatest impact comes from disorders that alter cognitive and emotional responses – rather than just physical functioning. A not uncommon comment from wives of men with acquired brain injury is 'this is not the man I married'.

Sexual disorders and neurological disease

The complex nature of many neurological conditions that affect so many aspects of functioning leads almost inevitably to some impact on sex and relationships. For health professionals it is important to be aware that disorders of the peripheral, autonomic or central nervous system are likely to affect sexual function. How much of a problem this presents, depends on the nature of the dysfunction and the context of the individual. A number of studies using a simple scale of sexual dysfunction have found that, although 50% of respondents to separate surveys (including people with MS (Szasz et al. 1984) neurological disorders (Chandler and Brown 1998) or PD (Hand et al. 2010)) experienced a change in sexual function during the course of their disease, only 25% were actually concerned about the change. These findings indicate that, although many individuals and couples make adjustments to accommodate the changes within their intimate relationships, 25% of people with these conditions might want to seek help with their sexual difficulties.

Most often the problems are multi-factorial in origin, e.g. loss of sensation because of MS, which alters the sexual experience, together with fatigue causing a change in overall lifestyle; low mood as a response to loss; medication resulting in specific sexual dysfunction, such as delayed orgasm with the selective serotonin reuptake inhibitors (SSRI anti-depressants); social changes resulting from loss of income; or practical issues at home, such as no longer managing stairs and, therefore, sleeping in a separate room from the partner. Treating sex and relationship problems, therefore, demands a **holistic bio-psycho-social approach**.

Each specific neurological condition presents a set of challenges to the functioning of intimate relationships. Traumatic brain injury is well recognised as causing profound and often destructive effects upon the family and social networks (Lezac 1988). Increased depression and anxiety in the partner is common and can persist. Sexual problems are common post injury and in one study 50% of men identified dysfunction (O'Carroll et al. 1991). In a small proportion of patients, increased sexual drive and sexual disinhibition can be a problem and is more likely to occur with damage in the frontal lobes, in some cases as part of executive dysfunction (Chapter 12). Reduced sexual desire and reduced sexual interest are most common and result from the brain damage itself, the effect on the relationship, fatigue, depression, anxiety, low motivation and, in a small number of cases, low testosterone secondary to hypothalamic trauma.

On a more positive note, studies have shown that where more support can be given to families, in particular to ease the burden of caring, then the outlook is better (Ponsford et al. 2003); with flexibility in **coping** styles leading to a more positive outcome for partners (Katz et al. 2005).

Treatment

More often than not, the neurological disorder itself cannot be cured and, therefore, the treatment of the sexual and/or relationship problem is set within that context. The most important first step is to identify the problem. There is often a reticence on the part of the patient to present the difficulty, and reluctance on the part of the health professional to initiate discussion. A useful approach to management is to use the **P-LI-SS-IT model**, which will be detailed below. This is a hierarchical model which can be adopted by all health professionals.

Permission

Permission involves creating a trusting therapeutic relationship in which the individual can talk about issues without fear of ridicule or censure. The health professional should be aware of the unspoken issues and be alert to hints that may be dropped about concerns. Gentle questions or statements that indicate a

willingness to listen to problems will encourage the individual to talk. This alone may be of great benefit. If a problem is identified that may need more specific help, then it is really important to acknowledge this and offer to find an appropriate source of help for the individual.

Limited information

Often there is a lot of anxiety about resuming sexual activity and simple information about the nature of the condition can be of immense help. If spasticity or pain is a problem, then ideas about positioning and use of medication may help. As explained earlier in this chapter, fatigue is a major factor in many neurological conditions and advice about fatigue management can help with this area of life as well as others. Medication often has effects on sexual functioning, but is an essential part of disease management. Encouraging people to discuss their medication with their GP, specialist nurse or consultant may enable some changes to be made that will help. There is also good condition-specific literature available from many patient organisations and it can be helpful for patients to read through this and discuss any issues arising.

Specific suggestions

This may involve referring the person to their GP or to an organisation that can give psychosexual and relationship therapy, such as Relate (1997), or to a service within health psychology or rehabilitation. It is possible to assure people that, for example, there are specific treatments for erectile dysfunction with medication, such as the phosphodiesterase 5 inhibitors (e.g. Sildendafil) or non-drug treatments, such as the vacuum device. There are techniques to assist with resuming sexual activity, such as the Sensate Focus Programme (College of Sexual and Relationship Therapists 2010), which gives people a scheme to start exploring their sexual relationship with specific measures to reduce anxiety. Problems of loss of sensation can be approached using a technique of body mapping in which individuals or couples can identify those areas that can be sexually responsive. Most importantly a couple can be helped to communicate with each other.

Intensive therapy

Specialist intervention from a therapist trained in psychosexual or relationship therapy may be necessary, but only a small proportion of people will require this type of intervention. There are many useful resources about sexual and relationship problems in general, as well as resources associated with particular conditions. A few website examples are listed in the further reading list at the end of the chapter.

Sexual dysfunction: summary

Sexuality is part of our nature and forming and sustaining intimate relationships is central to life for many people. Supporting people as they adjust to changes and face difficulties associated with neurological conditions is as important in this area of functioning as in any other.

Summary

The aim of this chapter was to give you an overview of a range of problems that are very common in people with different neurological conditions, i.e. fatigue and sleep disorders, impaired swallowing, incontinence and sexual dysfunction. Despite the fact that these problems are common and often distressing – not only for the patient, but also for their family – they are often under-diagnosed and under-treated. The impact of the problems on

rehabilitation outcomes as well as quality of life after discharge can be considerable. The importance of health professionals being knowledgeable about relevant signs and symptoms, having the necessary skill and tact to enquire about potential problems in these areas, and being aware of potential solutions or referral routes, therefore cannot be overstated.

SELF-ASSESSMENT QUESTIONS

1. What is the prevalence of fatigue, dysphagia, incontinence and sexual dysfunction in people with different neurological conditions?
2. What impact may fatigue have on rehabilitation outcome and quality of life after discharge?
3. What are the physiological processes mediating normal bowel and bladder function, and which impairments may arise from neurological conditions? Which options are available to treat incontinence?
4. What are the possible psychosocial consequences of incontinence and how might these affect people?
5. What are the physiological processes underlying normal sexual function, and what are typical examples of sexual dysfunction that may result from a neurological condition?
6. What is the potential impact of sexual dysfunction on relationships? What treatment options could be explored for people with sexual dysfunction associated with a neurological disorder?

Further reading

Annon, J.S., 1976. The Behavioural Treatment of Sexual Problems: Brief therapy. Harper and Row, New York.

Arnold, E.P., 1999. Spinal Cord Injury. In: Fowler, C.J. (Ed.), Neurology of Bladder, Bowel and Sexual Dysfunction. Butterworth-Heinemann, Woburn, MA (Chapter 18).

Burridge, A.C., Williams, W.H., Yates, P., et al., 2007. Spousal relationship satisfaction following acquired brain injury: the role of insight and socio-emotional skill. Neuropsychol. Rehabil. 17, 95–105.

Chandler, B., 2009. About MS: sex and relationships. MS Matters 83, 14.

Comi, G., Leocani, L., Rossi, P., et al., 2001. Physiopathology and treatment

of fatigue in multiple sclerosis. J. Neurol. 16, 174–179.

Hardy, E., Morton Robinson, N., 1999a. Swallowing Disorders Treatment Manual, second ed. Pro-ed, Austin, Texas.

Kreuter, M., Sullivan, M., Siosteen, A., 1994. Sexual adjustment after spinal cord injury focussing on partner experiences. Paraplegia 32, 225–235.

Logemann, J.A., 1998. Evaluation and Treatment of Swallowing Disorders. Pro-ed, Austin, Texas.

Maria, B., Sophia, S., Michalis, M., 2003. Sleep breathing disorders in patients with idiopathic Parkinson's disease. Respir. Med. 97, 1151–1152.

Multiple Sclerosis Society, 2010. MS Essentials 12: Sex, intimacy and

relationships. Available online from: http://www.mssociety.org.uk/ms-resources/ms-essential-12-sex-intimacy-and-relationships (accessed 08.01.12).

Parkinson's, U.K., 1996. Sexual problems and Parkinson's. Available online from: http://www.parkinsons.org.uk/default.aspx?page=10808 (accessed 08.01.12).

Thomas, R., Chandler, B., 2007. Management of bowel dysfunction in neurological rehabilitation: a review. Critical Reviews in Physical and Rehabilitation Medicine 19, 251–274.

Wood, R.L.I., Liossi, C., Wood, L., 2005. The impact of head injury neurobehavioural sequelae on personal relationships: preliminary findings. Brain Inj. 19, 845–851.

References

Bancroft, J., 2009. Human Sexuality and its Problems, third ed. Churchill Livingstone Elsevier, Edinburgh.

Brazzelli, M., Saunders, D.H., Greig, C.A., et al., 2011. Physical fitness training for stroke patients. Cochrane Database Syst. Rev. 11, CD003316. doi:10.1002/14651858.

Brocklehurst, J.C., 1993. Urinary incontinence in the community: analysis of a MORI poll. Br. Med. J. 306, 832–834.

Brown, R.G., Dittner, A., Findley, L., et al., 2005. The Parkinson fatigue scale. Parkinsonism Relat. Disord. 11, 49–55.

Carllson, G.E., Mooler, A., Blomstrand, C., 2003. Consequences of mild stroke in persons < 75 years: a 1 year follow up. Cerebrovasc. Dis. (Basel, Switzerland) 16, 383–388.

Chandler, B.J., Brown, S., 1998. Sex and relationship dysfunction in neurological disability. J. Neurol. Neurosurg. Psychiatry 65, 877–880.

Chandler, B.J., 2005. Continence and stroke. In: Barnes, M., Dobkin, B., Bogousslavsky, J. (Eds.), Recovery after stroke. Cambridge University Press, Cambridge, pp. 415–435.

Chandler, B.J., 2005. Sex and relationships following stroke. In: Barnes, M., Dobkin, B., Bogousslavsky, J. (Eds.), Recovery after stroke. Cambridge University Press, Cambridge, pp. 436–455.

College of Sexual and Relationship Therapists, 2010. Available online from: http://www.cosrt.org.uk/ (accessed 08.01.12).

Dauvilliers, Y., 2007. Insomnia in patients with neurodegenerative conditions. Sleep Med. 8 (Suppl. 4), 27–34.

Diagnostic and Statistical Manual of Mental Disorders, DSM-IV, 1994. revised 2000. Available online from: http://psychiatryonline.org/ (accessed 28.12.11).

Duthie, J.B., Vincent, M., Herbison, G.P., et al., 2011. Botulinum toxin injections for adults with overactive bladder syndrome. Cochrane Database Syst. Rev 12, CD005493. doi:10.1002/14651858.

Fowler, C.J., Panicker, J.N., Drake, M., et al., 2009. A UK consensus on the management of the bladder in multiple sclerosis. J. Neurol. Neurosurg. Psychiatry 80, 470–477.

Friedman, J.H., Brown, R.G., Comella, C., et al., 2007. Fatigue in Parkinson's disease: a review. Mov. Dis. 22, 297–308.

Gjerstad, M.D., Wentzel-Larsen, T., Aarsland, T., et al., 2007. Insomnia in Parkinson's disease: frequency and progression over time. J. Neurol. Neurosurg. Psychiatry 78, 476–479.

Glader, E.L., Stegmayr, B., Asplund, K., 2002. Post-stroke fatigue: a 2 year follow-up study of stroke patients in Sweden. Stroke 33, 1327–1333.

Glickman, S., Kamm, M.A., 1996. Bowel dysfunction in spinal cord injury patients. Lancet 347, 1651–1653.

Golbin, J.M., Somers, V.K., Caples, S.M., 2008. Obstructive sleep apnea, cardiovascular disease and pulmonary hypertension. Proc. Am. Thorac. Soc. 5, 200–206.

Hand, A., Gray, W.K., Chandler, B., et al., 2010. Sexual and relationship dysfunction in people with Parkinson's disease. Parkinsonism Relat. Disord. 16, 172–176.

Harari, D.F., Coshall, C.M., Rudd, A.G., et al., 2003. New-onset fecal incontinence after stroke: prevalence, natural history, risk factors, and impact. Stroke 34, 144–150.

Hardy, E., Morton Robinson, N., 1999. Swallowing Disorders Treatment Manual, second ed. Pro-ed, Austin, Texas.

Hartelius, L., Svensson, P., 1994. Speech and swallowing symptoms associated with Parkinson's disease and multiple sclerosis: a survey. Folia Phoniatr. (Basel) 46, 9–17.

Hinds, J.P., Eidelman, B.H., Wald, A., 1990. Prevalence of bowel dysfunction in multiple sclerosis. Gastroenterology 98, 1538–1542.

Iranzo, A., Molinuevo, J.L., Santamaria, J., 2006. Rapid-eye-movement sleep behaviour disorder as an early marker for neurodegenerative disorder: a descriptive study. Lancet Neurol. 5, 572–577.

Kales, A., Ansel, R.D., Markham, C.H., et al., 1971. Sleep in patients with Parkinson's disease and normal subjects prior to and following levodopa administration. Clin. Pharmacol. Ther. 12, 397–406.

Kaplan, H.S., 1974. The New Sex Therapy. Ballière Tindall, London.

Katz, S., Kravetz, S., Grynbaum, F., 2005. Wives coping flexibility, time since husbands' injury and the perceived burden of wives of men with traumatic brain injury. Brain Inj. 19, 59–66.

Larsen, J.P., 2003. Sleep disorders in Parkinson's disease. Adv. Neurol. 91, 329–334.

Lees, A.J., Blackburn, N.A., Campbell, V.L., 1988. The nighttime problems of Parkinson's disease. Clin. Neuropharmacol. 11, 512–519.

Lezac, M., 1988. Brain damage is a family affair. J. Clin. Exp. Neuropschol. 10, 111–123.

Logemann, J.A., 1998. Evaluation and Treatment of Swallowing Disorders. Pro-ed, Austin, Texas.

Lynch, J., Mead, G., Greig, C., et al., 2007. Fatigue after stroke: the development and evaluation of a case definition. J. Psychosom. Res. 63, 539–544.

Macmillan, A.K., Merrie, A.E., Marshall, R.J., et al., 2004. The prevalence of fecal incontinence in community dwelling adults: a systematic review of the literature. Dis. Colon Rectum 47, 1341–1349.

Marrie, R.A., Cutter, G., Tyry, T., et al., 2007. Disparities in the management of multiple sclerosis related bladder symptoms. Neurology 68, 1971–1978.

Masters, W.H., Johnson, V.E., 1966. Human Sexual Response. Churchill, London.

McGeough, E., Pollock, A., Smith, L.N., et al., 2009. Interventions for post-stroke fatigue. Cochrane Database Syst. Rev 3, CD007030. doi:10.1002/14651858.

Multiple Sclerosis Council for Clinical Practice Guidelines. Fatigue and multiple sclerosis: evidence-based management strategies for fatigue in multiple sclerosis. Paralyzed Veterans of America. Available online from: http://www.mscare.org/cmsc/images/pdf/fatigue.pdf (accessed 08.01.12).

Naess, H., Nyland, H.I., Thomassen, L., et al., 2005. Fatigue at long term follow up in young adults with cerebral infarction. Cerebrovasc. Dis. 20, 245–250.

Nakayama, H., Jorgensen, H.S., Pedersen, P.M., 1997. Prevalence and risk factors of incontinence after stroke. Stroke 28, 58–62.

Neau, J-P., Paquereau, J., Meurice, J-C., Chavagnat, J-J., Gil, R., 2002. Stroke and sleep apnoea: cause or consequence? Sleep Med. Rev. 6, 457–469.

O'Carroll, R.E., Woodrow, J., Maouns, F., 1991. Psychosexual and psychosocial sequelae of closed head injury. Brain Inj. 5, 303–313.

Oerlemans, W.G., deWeerd, A.W., 2002. The prevalence of sleep disorders in patients with Parkinson's disease: a self-reported community-based survey. Sleep Med. 3, 147–149.

Perry, L., Love, C.P., 2001. Screening for dysphagia and aspiration in acute stroke: a systematic review. Dysphagia 16, 7–18.

Ponsford, J., Olver, J., Ponsford, M., et al., 2003. Long term adjustment of families following TBI where comprehensive rehabilitation has been provided. Brain Inj. 17, 453–468.

Relate, 1997. Available online from: http://www.relate.org.uk/home/index.html (accessed 28.04.11).

Robinson, G.V., Pepperell, J.C.T., Segal, H.C., et al., 2004. Circulatory cardiovascular risk factors in obstructive sleep apnoea: data from randomised controlled trials. Thorax 59, 777–782.

Scottish Intercollegiate Guidelines Network (SIGN), 2010. Guideline 119: Management of patients with stroke: identification and management of dysphagia. Available online at: Scottish Intercollegiate Guidelines Network (SIGN), Edinburgh. http://www.sign.ac.uk/guidelines/fulltext/119/index.html (accessed 08.01.12).

Steele, C.M., Greenwood, C., Ens, I., et al., 1997. Mealtime difficulties in a home for the aged: not just dysphagia. Dysphagia 12, 45–50.

Szasz, G., Paty, D.W., Lawton-Speert, S., et al., 1984. A sexual function scale in multiple sclerosis. Acta Neurol. Scand. 101, 37–43.

Tandberg, E., Larsen, J.P., Karlsen, K., 1998. A community-based study of sleep disorders in patients with Parkinson's disease. Mov. Disord. 13, 895–899.

van der Werf, S.P., van den Broek, H.L.P., Anten, H.W.M., et al., 2001. Experience of severe fatigue long after stroke and its relation to depressive symptoms and disease characteristics. Eur. Neurol. 45, 28–35.

Wade, D.T., Green, Q., 2001. A Study of Services for Multiple Sclerosis. Royal College of Physicians, London.

Waller, D.G., Renwick, A.G., Hillier, K., 2001. Medical pharmacology and therapeutics, second ed. W.B. Saunders, Philadelphia.

Synopsis and implications of neuroscience for neurological rehabilitation

15

CHAPTER CONTENTS

Introduction

The intention behind this book was to provide students from a range of health-care professions, especially allied health professions, with a foundation in neuroscience to inform their clinical practice. As we have seen, neuroscience is a complex, transdisciplinary area, comprising highly specialised lines of research. This cognate area has expanded tremendously over the last few decades, but despite the plethora of excellent textbooks and high-quality journals, this information is not always easily accessible to health professionals, while its relevance to practice is not always immediately apparent. Our key aim was to select, from the wealth of information available, a number of key topics that we felt would be useful for students in an allied health profession starting out in neurological rehabilitation. In addition, we hope that components of this text would be useful for students in related disciplines with an interest in neurological rehabilitation.

Synopsis

We started by laying the foundation of neuroscience. Following a brief synopsis of the fascinating history of neuroscience, we set out the basic structure and function of the nervous system, explored normal and abnormal changes in the nervous system across the life span, and examined the various ways in which drugs work. This was an area that could have had a whole textbook devoted to it and, indeed, there are many such books on the market. What we attempted to do was 'cherry-pick' the key areas that we thought would be of most interest and/or relevance.

Redundancy and plasticity

Having laid the foundation, we then moved on to explore how the brain works – or at least an exploration of our current, and still limited, understanding of how we think it works! This revealed the brain as the most complex structure in the universe; a complex, heterogeneous, integrated organ that exhibits both redundancy (i.e. spare capacity) and plasticity (i.e. the capability to change). Redundancy and plasticity are key phenomena in neuroscience and their relevance for rehabilitation cannot be underestimated. Redundancy implies that there is spare capacity that can be tapped into, and plasticity means that the brain responds to change – and thus to therapeutic input. Plasticity can go 'haywire', however, and the phenomenon of spasticity was used as an example of how disorganised movement may result from dysfunctional neural connections. The implications for health-care professionals are to provide timely therapeutic input of the right intensity and type, to drive neuroplastic changes that will ultimately enable long-term, functional improvement.

Interventions that involve intensive activity of a functional nature where possible, comprising an element of problem solving, currently seem to be the most likely candidates. Although there are promising lines of evidence in specific patient populations (e.g. constraint-induced movement therapy for people with some active hand movement after stroke), much more research is needed to establish a library of interventions that are effective, acceptable and meaningful to people with different levels of ability, wanting to achieve different rehabilitation goals.

Functional localisation

We saw how function is localised in the brain, which means that each specific function (e.g. colour perception), is mediated by a dedicated, complex, integrated neural network. An appreciation of the level of integration of brain function is essential; a function can only be executed successfully if the brain is able to receive the right information at the right time, process this using all necessary connections, relay the information to the areas involved in planning, sequencing and finally execution, and complete this on time. So there is much more to action than meets the eye! The role of the health professional is to unravel this complexity by carefully and systematically assessing the patient (often involving other members of the multidisciplinary team), and test various hypotheses as to the main causes of the patient's problems.

Having explored generic principles of the structure and function of the nervous system in general and the brain in particular, we then went on to examine a range of problems that are commonly found in people with neurological conditions.

Perceptuo-motor control and learning as a problem-solving activity

We started off with normal motor control and explored the role of different levels of the nervous system in the control of reflex, as well as voluntary movement. We looked at various expressions of disordered motor control, and compared and contrasted spasticity with rigidity and hypertonia, which highlighted the importance of differentiating between neural and biomechanical contributions to soft-tissue stiffness.

Next, we looked at more complex processes involved in perceptuo-motor control and introduced various theoretical models. We focused on an information processing approach, which describes successive stages of motor control from sensory input to planning, programming, execution and, finally, feedback. According to this approach, movement is coordinated by a generalised motor programme (GMP) that stores the equivalent of a 'blueprint' for each class of action. This template can be fine-tuned to the specific requirements of the task within the environment in which the action takes place. Although there is no consensus (yet) regarding the most convincing theoretical model of motor control, most movement scientists would agree that purposeful movement is a problem-solving activity. In the search for a solution to this problem, motor control operates at the interface between the individual with their particular characteristics, the specific task requirements, and the environmental conditions.

The implications for therapists are that they need to consider this interface in its entirety, as focusing on perfecting movement per se (e.g. gait) without training this in the environment in which the walking is to take place, and without exploring relevant task variations (e.g. sideward stepping to avoid obstacles, or holding a shopping bag while walking) is unlikely to carry over into a walking activity that is useful for the patient following discharge.

We then moved on to explore skill acquisition, i.e. processes involved in the learning of new skills or re-learning skills that were previously mastered. Based on the information processing approach discussed earlier, we identified a number of factors that can influence this process, including strategies for structuring practice and feedback. But first, we identified goal setting as an important prerequisite to tap into the patient's motivation for rehabilitation. It is only when we understand what the person really wants to achieve through their rehabilitation, and have agreed their goals with them, that we can begin to design an appropriate treatment plan that the patient wants to engage with. Next, strategies for practice and feedback were explored. Here we came across some research findings that appeared – at least initially – to be counter-intuitive. For example, the superiority of random over blocked practice seems to go against common sense (and this is exactly why we need to do research!). During random practice, participants performed considerably worse than their counterparts using blocked practice; but on delayed transfer tasks, it emerged they had learned far more. On more careful consideration, this finding makes sense: during blocked practice, the individual only learns something new at the start, but once the task is familiar, the exercise becomes merely repetitive. The participant can effectively 'switch off', and no further learning takes place. In contrast, those undertaking random practice have to problem solve each time – and so they continue to learn. However, it is important to remember that this evidence base was mainly established on the basis of healthy, young participants. When we try to generalise this to people with cognitive impairment, that is when it becomes problematic, as we have seen in work with people with Alzheimer's disease. It is clear that much more research is needed in the area of skill acquisition in people with different neurological conditions. Meanwhile, health professionals need to be cognisant of the literature, as well as to carefully consider individual patients' cognitive abilities.

Attention as a gatekeeper

The prevalence of impairments in attention and memory is high, across the spectrum of neurological conditions that affect the brain. This is not surprising, given the extent of neural networks involved in both of these functions. We spent some time exploring hemi-inattention, a particular problem that may be encountered in patients with stroke, a brain tumour or head injury. This difficulty in paying attention to, detecting and processing information, as well as responding to information from one side of the body and/or space, shows the complex integration between neural networks mediating attention, perception, cognition and action.

When exploring memory, we highlighted that memory is not a 'filing cabinet', where information is simply stored and 'replayed'. Instead, it is an active process of reconstruction, and it is vulnerable to processes such as interference and decay. Furthermore, 'memory' comprises different functions that are supported by different neural networks. This explains seemingly counter-intuitive phenomena such as the preservation of one type of memory together with

severe impairment of another type of memory in the same person. An example is a patient with Korsakoff's syndrome who shows evidence of motor learning (i.e. intact procedural memory), but does not remember having met the therapist before (i.e. impaired episodic memory).

Taking an information processing approach, 'attention' can be seen as the gatekeeper to learning while memory enables a person to build on information they have stored before. Impairments of attention and memory can have a considerable impact on rehabilitation outcomes. Problems with attention and memory are not directly observable and, therefore, need to be inferred, so health-care professionals need to look out for signs such as increased distractibility, inability to remain focused, disengagement from an activity and forgetfulness. Input from a clinical psychologist can be indispensible for diagnosing problems and formulating treatment plans.

Network processing in sensation and perception

The chapter on sensation and perception explained how sensation, in principle a bottom-up process, can be influenced by previous experience, expectation and knowledge. Such top-down influences enable us to make sense in scenarios where information is incomplete and/or corrupted, however it may also lead us to misconstrue information. We focused on the perception of pain, particularly in stroke, to demonstrate the intricate connectivity between bottom-up and top-down processes. Neurological conditions may affect sensation and perception in a myriad of different ways and since these processes are not directly observable, we often – at least initially – infer sensory or perceptual impairments through problems with movement or action. For example, a child with cerebral palsy may fall over objects when walking, not primarily due to a motor impairment, but due to the fact that his eye movements are too slow to pick up relevant information at the right time for the nervous system to act upon. This is where multidisciplinary team work is essential to establish the nature, severity and impact of the deficit(s), and formulate treatment plans.

Communication

Communication – verbal and non-verbal – is *the* vehicle for interaction between patients, family and health-care professionals. We explained the various processes involved in communication, highlighting the complexity of this myriad of different functions. We were careful to avoid the impression that communication impairment can be divided into simple categories, such as 'expressive' or 'receptive' aphasia. Given the diversity of communication, it is not surprising that different neural networks have been identified that support different communicative functions. This redundancy can be exploited by therapists and patients in search for alternative communication routes. Input from a speech and language therapist is invaluable in identifying the nature of the communication problems, and advising patients, family and staff regarding optimum communication support for an individual.

Executive function

Executive function is a broad term for a collection of functions, which together enable us to prioritise goals, make plans to achieve our goals, initiate action and monitor progress to check that we keep on track. Meanwhile, it also monitors our conduct to ensure it is appropriate under the circumstances. We have seen, especially (but not exclusively) in individuals with frontal lobe involvement, that executive function is often compromised. Executive dysfunction may have severe consequences for rehabilitation outcomes and for life after discharge in general. Although the term 'executive' conjures up images of a rational, goal-orientated function, we have learned that emotional dysregulation is part and parcel of this syndrome. This tight integration between executive function and emotion, based on contemporary neuroscience and clinical research, questions traditional Cartesian thinking that has separated cognition and emotion, mind and body, for centuries and calls for a comprehensive biopsychosocial approach to neurological rehabilitation.

Emotion

Emotional difficulties associated with neurological conditions may be among the most difficult problems that patients and families have to face. Depression and anxiety are particularly common, while apathy and emotional outbursts may also be seen. Emotional problems may be caused directly by the brain lesion itself, due to impact on neural networks and

neurotransmitter systems, or associated with the psychosocial impact of the situation on the person and their family. We have seen that the level of emotional difficulty may not match the severity of the disability, and important factors are the personal significance of the disability to the person, and their ability to cope with the situation. Social support can make a huge impact on the emotional landscape of the patient and this is where loved ones, family and friends enter the picture. One of the privileges (and sometimes challenges) of working in neurological rehabilitation is the interaction with the patient and their family, making the rehabilitation process a genuine team effort.

Other problems

We covered a range of other problems, including sleep disorders and fatigue, incontinence and sexual problems. These problems can have an enormous impact on patients' ability to engage in rehabilitation and, following discharge, on their quality of life and opportunities to participate in social events, relationships and employment. However, the topics of continence and sexuality are often taboo in our society, and therefore under-reported and under-treated. Much research is still required to establish effective interventions strategies for many of these problems, however health professionals who look out for the relevant signs and symptoms and have an awareness of possible treatment options, may be in a position to make a considerable contribution to the quality of life of patients and their family.

Neuroscience and neurological rehabilitation: some reflection and challenges ahead

As we mentioned in the introduction to this chapter, our primary aim for this book was to select a number of key topics that we felt were important for health professionals in neurological rehabilitation. However, despite the awe-inspiring advances in neuroscience, its translation into routine rehabilitation practice is tentative in many areas, while in other areas (e.g. consciousness) there are still significant gaps in our knowledge and understanding. Given the state of the art in neuroscience and the complexity of neurological rehabilitation, this textbook is unable to offer answers to even some of the most elementary questions. For example, skill acquisition research is often based on healthy, young participants, and we need to be very cautious in extrapolating evidence from these studies to patients with neurological conditions. In cases where neurological populations have been involved in research, sample sizes are often small, there may be a number of confounding factors (e.g. the neurological condition may be heterogeneous while patients may have additional co-morbidities), and often there are difficulties standardising therapeutic input and measuring outcomes. This chapter is not the place to comprehensively appraise the rehabilitation literature, but it is clear that methodological limitations and flaws pose a challenge for health professionals wanting to apply evidence from neuroscience and neurological rehabilitation research to their routine clinical practice. Clinical reasoning needs to be informed by relevant evidence, but the evidence needs to be critically appraised in the context of the situation of the individual patient.

Despite these limitations, we hope that this textbook will enhance health professionals' awareness of the observable and, especially, of some of the more 'hidden' sequelae of neurological conditions. We hope that it will enhance their understanding of some of the most commonly found phenomena associated with perception, cognition and action, emotion and motivation, as well as other functions including communication, sleep and sexuality, that can impact on the process and outcomes of neurological rehabilitation. Ultimately, our hope is that the information in this book will enhance therapists' understanding of some of their patients' most commonly found difficulties, and enable them to make better informed decisions regarding interventions. There are certain challenges on the horizon for health professionals in neurological rehabilitation, as well as some unique opportunities.

A global recession forces governments to justify spending on health care, and any cuts are likely to affect neurological rehabilitation services as well. Health professionals need to think smartly and creatively about interventions that are relevant for patients, clinically effective as well as cost-effective. A patient-centred, long-term view needs to be taken to ensure that interventions – where possible – meet targets that patients feel are meaningful to them, and yield benefits after therapy input has ceased. Opportunities for face-to-face, individual treatment sessions are

diminishing and therapists need to find other ways to deliver interventions and enable patients to engage in self-management of their (often long-term) condition. It is, therefore, more important than ever to use evidence to inform practice.

What areas of neuroscience research are particularly needed to further inform, improve and innovate neurological rehabilitation? Here are just some examples. In terms of screening and assessment, more accurate biomarkers (e.g. specific neuroimaging data) are needed, together with better prediction models to improve estimates of recovery in different neurological conditions. Avoiding unnecessary delays involved in trying treatments that ultimately prove to be ineffective, early and accurate prediction will enable clinicians to make the most of the window of neuroplastic opportunity by selecting those treatments that are most likely to be effective. Based on predictions, options such as electrical stimulation, mental imagery, constraint-induced movement therapy, or robot-assisted therapy may be selected from a library of options, to assist the individual patient to achieve their goals.

In terms of interventions, it is clear that many more robust and sufficiently powered randomised controlled trials (RCTs) are required in almost all areas of allied health in neurological rehabilitation. However, despite the unquestionable strengths of RCTs in establishing the effectiveness of interventions, this type of study design cannot provide the answer to all types of questions. For example, some fascinating proof-of-concept single case studies have been carried out on brain-computer interfaces and there is now evidence that EEG can be used by individuals who have no action capability (e.g. due to a brain stem stroke) to steer a wheelchair through an environment. This very exciting line of evidence not only points towards novel interventions, but can also be used to shed light on processes (e.g. mental imagery) that were previously difficult to investigate. Furthermore, more rigorous qualitative studies are required to evaluate whether interventions are acceptable and meaningful to patients. To summarise, not only do we need more robust research to examine *whether* treatments are effective, we also need a sufficient body of research elucidating *how* treatments work and whether patients are likely to accept these.

Research is particularly urgent in interventions that can be delivered in groups, or remotely. There are interesting developments in the application of games technology (e.g. the Nintendo Wii or Microsoft Kinect) to home-based therapeutic activities.

Individual patients can be connected through virtual reality and play therapeutic games together, adding a social element to the mix. Therapists can employ telemedicine applications to check up on patients, motivate them, provide feedback and progress them through an intervention.

In terms of outcome assessment, information can be gathered through body-worn sensor systems including activity monitors and sensors in equipment itself (e.g. remote controls and robotic devices), on the performance and outcomes of therapeutic activities. This information can be used to provide feedback to individuals, as well as – provided that consent has been given – contribute to the evidence base of the intervention involved. Neuroimaging data, comparing before and after treatment, can provide further evidence of neuroplastic changes associated with behavioural outcomes.

With regards to developments in neuroscience, we are living in an unprecedented and exciting time. Health professionals have the challenging, yet privileged opportunity to be working with patients, in an area where science is really coming to life. Despite the gaps in the evidence base mentioned above, using state-of-the-art science to try and understand patients' problems, designing interventions to enable patients to achieve their rehabilitation goals, and seeing the outcomes from therapeutic interventions, can be a hugely exciting and rewarding journey. In addition to health professionals improving patients' lives, they also have an important voice in deciding the direction of neuroscience research in the future.

Index

Catheterisation, intermittent, 193
Caudal neuropore, 22
Cell(s)
  assembly, 117–119
  body, 16
  differentiation, 22–23
  drug targets, *28*
  enzymes, *28*, 29
  membrane, 29
  types, 27–28, *28*
Central nervous system, *12*
  injury, 42
  mechanisms, 42
  plasticity, 43, *44*
Cerebellum ('little brain'), 14, *35*,
  60–61, 121, 161
  voluntary movement, 54–55
Cerebral asymmetry, 45
Cerebral cortex, 11–12, *35*
  synchrony, 182
Cerebral hemispheres, 132
Cerebral palsy (CP), 61–63, *62*
Cerebrospinal fluid (CSF),
  15–16, 21
  Galen, 3
'Chaining', 6
Chest infections, 189–190
Chiasma, 130–131
Chlorolabe, 129–130
Cholinergic system, 161
Chromatolysis, 41, *41*
Chronic depression, neural correlates,
  37
Chunking information, 116
Ciliary neurotrophic factor (CNTF), 23
Circadian rhythms, 183, 185
Citalopram, 169
Cocaine, 29
Codeine, *138*, *138*
Cognitive behavioural therapy (CBT),
  170
  vs exercise, 170
Cognitive impairment, *177*
Cognitive level, analysis, 6–7
Colon, 194–196
Colonic transit time, *196*
Colonometrograms, *196*
Colonoscopy, *196*
Commissural fibres, 34–35, *36*
Communication
  non-verbal, 151, 152
  right hemisphere, 149–150
  speech and language processes,
    142–143, *142*

synopsis, 207–208
Communication disorders, 141–153
  motor speech, 150–151
  see also Aphasia
Comparator stage, motor control model,
  70
Compensatory strategies
  executive function, 162
  swallowing problems, 190
Complex systems, theory of self-
  organisation, 80
Comprehension, 142
  impairments, 152
  language, 147
Conduction aphasia, 144, *146*, 148
'Conduite d'approche', conduction
  aphasia, 148
Constant practice, 96, 97
Constipation, 196–197
Constraint induced movement therapy
  (CIMT), 43, *44*
Context-dependency, 116–117
Contextual information, 48
Contextual interference, 91, 97, 100
Continence, 191–197
  bowel *see* Bowel disorders
  overview, 191
  prevalence, 191
  urinary *see* Urinary continence
Contractures, joint, 57–58, 61
Control parameters, 80
Coordination, 66–69
  defined, 67–68, 79
  developmental coordination disorder
    (DCD), *75*
  Degrees of freedom
  gait, *90*
  Parkinson's disease (PD), *82*
  synergies, 80–81
  see also Movement
Corpora, 198–199
Corpus Hippocraticum, 2
Cortex
  arousal, 183
  functional organisation, 5, 36–40
  pain, 134
Cortical areas, 119, 121
  maps, 40
Cortical blindness, 39
Coughing, 189–190
Covert practice, 93–94, 95
Cranial nerves, 14, *14*
Cranioscopy, 4–5
Cricopharyngeal sphincter, 188–189

Critical fluctuations, 80
Critical slowing down, 80
Crying, pathological, 171
'Cueing' strategy, 74
  cues, to behaviour, 158
  Parkinson's disease (PD), *66*, 89, *90*
Cyanolabe, 129–130
Cycloheximide, 24
Cystometrogram (CMG), *192*
Cytoarchitectonic maps, 38, *38*, *38*

D

Dax–Broca theory (left hemisphere
  dominance), 143
Daytime sleepiness, 186
  excessive (EDS), 186
De humanis corporis fabrica (Vesalius),
  3
Declarative memory, 119, 121
Deep sleep (slow wave sleep), 183
Defecation, 194–196
Defecography, *196*
Degrees of freedom, 68–69, *68*
  problem, 67, 80–81
Dehydration, 189–190
Delusions, Parkinson's disease (PD), 172
Dementia, Parkinson's disease (PD),
  172
Dendrites, 16
Denervation supersensitivity, 42–43, *43*
Deoxyhaemoglobin (deoxy-Hb), 9
Depression, 2, 167–170, 208
  Alzheimer's disease (AD),
    172–173
  causes, 168
  classification, 167–168
  common features, 167
  fatigue and, 184
  management, non-pharmacological,
    170
  multiple sclerosis (MS), 185
  Parkinson's disease (PD), 172, 185
  sexual function, 200
  sleep-wake disorders (SWD), 185
  stroke, 171–172
  treatment, 168–170, *169*
Dermatomes, 6
Descartes' error (Damasio), 4
Descartes, René, 3–5
  see also Cartesian thinking
Detrusor contractions, 191–193, *192*,
  194

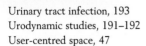

CPI Antony Rowe
Chippenham, UK
2017-08-17 15:37